Food Protein Induced Enterocolitis (FPIES)

Terri Faye Brown-Whitehorn
Antonella Cianferoni
Editors

Food Protein Induced Enterocolitis (FPIES)

Diagnosis and Management

Springer

Editors
Terri Faye Brown-Whitehorn
Division of Allergy and Immunology
University of Pennsylvania
Perelman School of Medicine
Children's Hospital of Philadelphia
Philadelphia, PA
USA

Antonella Cianferoni
Division of Allergy and Immunology
University of Pennsylvania
Perelman School of Medicine
Children's Hospital of Philadelphia
Philadelphia, PA,
USA

ISBN 978-3-030-21228-5 ISBN 978-3-030-21229-2 (eBook)
https://doi.org/10.1007/978-3-030-21229-2

This Springer imprint is published by the registered company Springer Nature Switzerland AG
The registered company address is: Gewerbestrasse 11, 6330 Cham, Switzerland

Preface

Food protein-induced enterocolitis syndrome (FPIES) is a severe condition causing acute vomiting and diarrhea that classically starts 2 hours after an ingestion of a specific food. In some cases, the symptoms can progress to dehydration and shock brought on by low blood pressure and poor blood circulation. The diagnosis of FPIES is a purely clinical one as there are no biomarkers to diagnose with certainty the food allergic reaction in the acute phase or food testing to predict the reactivity to foods. The fact that the diagnosis is clinical is one of the biggest frustrations of parents or caregivers of infants and toddlers.

FPIES symptoms are non-specific and are common manifestation of other common pediatric diseases, such as viral infections, sepsis, and pyloric stenosis. Therefore, if the clinician is not well versed and does not collect a focused history when a baby has a reaction, most often, he/she is diagnosed with "stomach flu." It is indeed not unusual that the parents make the diagnosis themselves after noticing that no one else gets sick, symptoms resolve, and all is well until the offending food is reintroduced. "Too much of a coincidence" remarked one family who searched the Internet and came across FPIES. In the adult world, where shellfish is often the cause, patients will self-diagnose themselves with "stomach flu" or food poisoning and if recurs will often avoid the food (without knowing its etiology). Then, the parent and adult patients have to find a provider who is knowledgeable about the disease.

To make things more complicated over the last few years, it has become clear that two distinct presentations of FPIES exist, acute and chronic. In the acute version, vomiting, lethargy, and, at times, diarrhea develop 2 hours after ingestion of a specific food(s). Twenty percent present in shock. Most often, these babies are otherwise growing well and thriving. In the chronic form, infants are often ill-appearing and not growing and present with vomiting and diarrhea. The removal of food leads to the improvement in symptoms, and the reintroduction leads to a more acute reaction.

We were happy to be coauthors (with many of our coauthors writing chapters in this book) of the first summary statements on FPIES published in 2017 after an international working group through the Adverse Reactions to Foods Committee of the American Academy of Allergy, Asthma, and Immunology (AAAAI) and the International FPIES Association advocacy group convened [1]. These guidelines were an important milestone to globally define FPIES and create a solid base for clinician education worldwide.

Although there is much to learn, there is a bit of an urgency to disseminate an accurate up-to-date information. This book was designed to introduce the clinicians (pediatricians, family practice clinicians, internists, nurse practitioners, physician assistants, emergency department specialists, intensivists, gastroenterologists, nutritionists, and allergists), the families, and the public to FPIES.

We are grateful to the Springer publishers for inviting us to initiate and edit this text and to Daniel Dominguez and Caitlin Primm of Springer publishers for their patience and guidance. We are also indebted to our coauthors, clinicians, researchers, and parents who have contributed chapters to this text. Each chapter builds on another and is written by experts in their respective fields.

We are grateful to our patients and families who entrusted their children to our care.

We are also thankful for our families, Matthew, Gregory, Michael, John, and Claire, for their support in both writing this book and their understanding of our commitment to them as well as our patients and families with FPIES.

Philadelphia, PA, USA — Terri Faye Brown-Whitehorn
Philadelphia, PA, USA — Antonella Cianferoni

Reference

1. Nowak-Wegrzyn A, Chehade M, Groetch ME, et al. International consensus guidelines for the diagnosis and management of food protein-induced enterocolitis syndrome: executive summary—workgroup report of the Adverse Reactions to Foods Committee, American Academy of Allergy, Asthma & Immunology. J Allergy Clin Immunol 2017;139:1111–26.

Contents

Contributors

Ozge Nur Aktas, MD Pediatrics, University of Illinois at Chicago, Chicago, IL, USA

Mary Grace Baker, MD Pediatrics, Division of Allergy and Immunology, Icahn School of Medicine at Mount Sinai, New York, NY, USA

M. Cecilia Berin, PhD Pediatrics, Icahn School of Medicine at Mount Sinai, New York, NY, USA

J. Andrew Bird, MD Pediatrics, Division of Allergy and Immunology, University of Texas Southwestern Medical Center, Dallas, TX, USA

Terri Faye Brown-Whitehorn, MD Division of Allergy and Immunology, University of Pennsylvania, Perelman School of Medicine, Children's Hospital of Philadelphia, Philadelphia, PA, USA

Jean-Christoph Caubet, MD Pediatric Allergy, University Hospitals of Geneva, Geneva, Switzerland

Antonella Cianferoni, MD, PhD Division of Allergy and Immunology, University of Pennsylvania, Perelman School of Medicine, Children's Hospital of Philadelphia, Philadelphia, PA, USA

Sherri Shubin Cohen, MD, MPH Gastroenterology, Hepatology, and Nutrition, Children's Hospital of Philadelphia, Philadelphia, PA, USA

Amy Dean, MPH, RD, LDN Department of Clinical Nutrition, Children's Hospital of Philadelphia, Philadelphia, PA, USA

Gayle Diamond, MD Gastroenterology, Hepatology, and Nutrition, Children's Hospital of Philadelphia, Philadelphia, PA, USA

Ashley A. Dyer, MPH Northwestern University Feinberg School of Medicine, Chicago, IL, USA

Alessandro Giovanni Fiocchi, MD Allergy Department, IRCCS Ospedale Pediatrico Bambino Gesù, Rome, Italy

Rebecca D. Ganetzky, MD Pediatrics, Division of Human Genetics, Children's Hospital of Philadelphia, Philadelphia, PA, USA

François Graham, MD, MSc, FRCPC Pediatric Allergy, University Hospitals of Geneva, Geneva, Switzerland

Ruchi S. Gupta, MD, MPH Northwestern University Feinberg School of Medicine, Chicago, IL, USA

Ann & Robert H. Lurie Children's Hospital of Chicago, Chicago, IL, USA

Jialing Jiang, BA Northwestern University Feinberg School of Medicine, Chicago, IL, USA

Shyam R. Joshi, MD Section of Allergy and Immunology, Oregon Health and Science University, Portland, OR, USA

Jacob D. Kattan, MD Pediatrics, Icahn School of Medicine at Mount Sinai, New York, NY, USA

Judith R. Kelsen, MD Division of Gastroenterology, Hepatology and Nutrition, Children's Hospital of Philadelphia, Philadelphia, PA, USA

Colleen Taylor Lukens, PhD Department of Child and Adolescent Psychiatry and Behavioral Sciences, Children's Hospital of Philadelphia, Philadelphia, PA, USA

Chaya Nautiyal Murali, MD Molecular and Human Genetics, Baylor College of Medicine, Houston, TX, USA

Rory E. Nicolaides, MD Pediatrics, Division of Allergy and Immunology, University of Texas Southwestern Medical Center, Dallas, TX, USA

Anna Nowak-Wegrzyn, MD, PhD Division of Allergy and Immunology, Department of Pediatrics, Elliot and Roslyn Jaffe Food Allergy Institute, Icahn School of Medicine at Mount Sinai, New York, NY, USA

Trusha Patel, MD Division of Gastroenterology, Hepatology and Nutrition, Children's Hospital of Philadelphia, Philadelphia, PA, USA

Valentina Pecora, MD, PhD Allergy Department, IRCCS Ospedale Pediatrico Bambino Gesù, Rome, Italy

Melanie A. Ruffner, MD, PhD Division of Allergy & Immunology, Children's Hospital of Philadelphia, Philadelphia, PA, USA

Department of Pediatrics, University of Pennsylvania Perelman School of Medicine, Philadelphia, PA, USA

Fallon Schultz Matney, MSW, LCSW, CAM International FPIES Association (IFPIES), Point Pleasant Beach, NJ, USA

Scott H. Sicherer, MD Pediatrics, Icahn School of Medicine at Mount Sinai, New York, NY, USA

Jonathan M. Spergel, MD, PhD Division of Allergy & Immunology, Children's Hospital of Philadelphia, Philadelphia, PA, USA

Department of Pediatrics, University of Pennsylvania Perelman School of Medicine, Philadelphia, PA, USA

Sophia Tsabouri, MD, PhD Department of Pediatrics/Paediatric Allergy, University Hospital of Ioannina, Ioannina, Greece

Kathleen Y. Wang, MD Allergy and Immunology, Children's Hospital of Philadelphia, Philadelphia, PA, USA

Christopher M. Warren, PhD(c) Northwestern University Feinberg School of Medicine, Chicago, IL, USA

Maria S. White, MSN, BA, RN, CCRN Wilmington, DE, USA

Historical Perspective

1

Jacob D. Kattan and Scott H. Sicherer

The first descriptions of what is now referred to as food protein-induced enterocolitis syndrome (FPIES) emerged in the 1960s and 1970s when features of this disease were described in case series of milk- and soy-"intolerant" infants that likely included those with a variety of disorders. These early reports began to elucidate the peculiar roughly 2 hour delayed onset of severe vomiting and/or diarrhea following ingestion of the trigger food, with additional systemic symptoms. These symptoms were found to reoccur when milk or soy was reintroduced to the diet after a period of elimination in an infant who had chronic gastrointestinal symptoms from prior chronic ingestion.

Early Descriptions and Characterization of Milk/Soy Enterocolitis

In 1967, Joyce D. Gryboski published a paper titled *Gastrointestinal milk allergy in infants* [1]. While she did not use the terms milk-induced enterocolitis of infancy or food protein-induced enterocolitis syndrome, she was likely the first to describe a cohort of patients with this disorder. She detailed 21 patients ranging in age from 2 days to 2 and ½ years who were admitted to Yale-New Haven Hospital in the previous 16 years with the diagnosis of gastrointestinal milk allergy. In this cohort, the predominant complaint was chronic diarrhea, and all of the patients had gross or occult blood in the stools at some point. The age of onset of the diarrhea was between 2 days and 4 and ½ months, though most children became symptomatic within the first 6 weeks of life. Vomiting occurred as the first symptom in four of the infants. Seven infants developed what was described as "cardiovascular collapse" after milk challenge, with two of them having gastrointestinal hemorrhage.

J. D. Kattan (✉) · S. H. Sicherer
Pediatrics, Icahn School of Medicine at Mount Sinai, New York, NY, USA
e-mail: Jacob.kattan@mssm.edu

T. F. Brown-Whitehorn, A. Cianferoni (eds.), *Food Protein Induced Enterocolitis (FPIES)*,
https://doi.org/10.1007/978-3-030-21229-2_1

Most of the infants became asymptomatic when placed on an extensively hydrolyzed formula or a soy-based formula, though 3 infants did not tolerate these products and only improved after being switched to a formula prepared from lamb. Half of the patients in this cohort became cow's milk tolerant by 1 year of age, and almost all of the subjects could ingest cow's milk by 3 years of age. Eight children underwent sigmoidoscopy and biopsy, which revealed changes consistent with colitis, which normalized after elimination of milk from the diet. In her summary, Gryboski wrote, "It is suggested that milk-induced colitis be considered a histologically documented and distinct entity."

In May of 1976, Powell published a report describing two cases of enterocolitis in low-birth-weight infants that was associated with milk and soy protein intolerance [2]. The two infants developed vomiting, abdominal distension, septic appearance, and bloody diarrhea after ingestion of cow's milk-based formula and, later, soy-based formula. She described that the purpose of the report was to describe two infants with a syndrome indistinguishable clinically from necrotizing enterocolitis and to provide carefully documented evidence of an association between their symptoms and intolerance to whole proteins from milk and soy in the neonatal period.

The first patient, Patient N.A., was a male born at 32 weeks gestation weighing 1600 g. He was on cow's milk-based formula until 15 days of age when he developed watery diarrhea. No pathogens were found in blood or stool cultures and the diarrhea resolved when he was given intravenous fluids and was started on soy-based formula. Nine days later, the infant was again placed on cow's milk-based formula, and within 8 hours he developed watery stools. He was placed back on soy-based formula, and again, his stools normalized. Three days after resuming the soy-based formula, however, he developed bloody diarrhea, lethargy, hypothermia, and marked abdominal distension with hypoactive bowel sounds. While a leukocytosis was noted, there were no pathogens in blood, urine, or stool cultures. He was diagnosed with necrotizing enterocolitis and IV fluids, blood, and antibiotics were administered with improvement in his symptoms. On day of life 43, he was again given a single 10 mL feeding of soy-based formula, resulting in vomiting and watery, guaiac-positive diarrhea for 3 days. On day of life 50, he was given Nutramigen, an extensively hydrolyzed formula, which he tolerated well. In preparation for discharge, he was given 30 mL of soy-based formula on day of life 61 and 40 mL of cow's milk-based formula on day of life 66, both of which led to watery, guaiac-positive diarrhea that began 2–6 hours after each challenge. Ultimately, he remained asymptomatic at home with a normal growth rate on Nutramigen.

The second patient, Patient B.W., was a male with a birth weight of 2000 g. He was started on cow's milk-based formula on day of life 2 and developed diarrhea on day of life 4. He was switched to soy-based formula and was placed on antibiotics, but the diarrhea continued, his dehydration worsened, and he began projectile vomiting. Blood, stool, and spinal fluid cultures were negative, and symptoms resolved with intravenous therapy. On day of life 14, soy protein-based formula was restarted, and he again began vomiting and had increasing diarrhea. A nasoduodenal tube was placed and a drip of cow's milk-based formula was started. He had watery stools that gradually increased in frequency, and on day of life 32 he became hypothermic and appeared septic. His abdomen became distended with a bluish discoloration; he had a positive blood culture and severe coagulation abnormalities; and he was diagnosed with necrotizing enterocolitis with sepsis and disseminated intravascular coagulation. He improved over the next 13 days, but developed bloody stools on day of life 46 when he was given a single 15 mL feeding with soy-based formula. He was ultimately switched to an extensively hydrolyzed formula with good weight gain and no diarrhea and was discharged home on day of life 68.

These patients continued to do well with stools that were normal in consistency and negative for pathogens and blood. They were both readmitted at 7–8 months of age. They had normal white blood counts and differentials. They both underwent oral food challenges with cow's milk based formula with similar responses, they both developed projectile vomiting 2 hours after the challenge, and watery diarrhea began 1 hour after that. Blood smears had large numbers of neutrophils, lymphocytes, eosinophils, and unidentifiable mononuclear cells. After 3 days of normal stools, the challenges were repeated with soy-based formula. Patient N.A. developed diarrhea 5 hours post-challenge, but not vomiting. Patient B.W. developed projectile vomiting and liquid stools within 3 hours post-challenge. Both infants again developed polymorphonuclear leukocytosis. They were sent home on the extensively hydrolyzed formula. Powell concluded that it seemed likely that the severe episode of distension, bloody diarrhea, and vomiting, similar in presentation to neonatal necrotizing enterocolitis, was due to intolerance of the whole proteins in milk- and soy-based formulas.

Two years after her initial report, in October of 1978, Powell characterized the syndrome in a paper she titled *Milk- and soy-induced enterocolitis of infancy* [3]. She described a cohort of 9 infants on a cow's milk-based formula who presented with severe, protracted vomiting and diarrhea, with symptoms that started between 4 and 27 days of life. The patients improved with substitution of a soy-based formula, but symptoms typically recurred 1–2 weeks later. At presentation, 7 of the 9 subjects were below birth weight and 8 subjects appeared acutely ill and underwent sepsis evaluations, all of which were negative. All of the infants had blood in their stool, low serum albumin, and elevated peripheral blood polymorphonuclear leukocyte counts. While in the hospital, the infants usually improved on intravenous fluids and then had a recurrence of severe symptoms with reintroduction of milk- or soy-based formula.

Each of the infants underwent follow-up oral food challenges with cow's milk- and soy-based formulas at a mean age of 5.5 months. Eight of the 9 patients reacted to milk and 6 of 9 reacted to soy. None of these patients had immediate symptoms of an IgE-mediated reaction such as urticaria, wheezing, or anaphylaxis. Ten of the 14 positive challenges resulted in vomiting, while all of the patients developed diarrhea with blood. All positive challenges were associated with a rise in peripheral blood polymorphonuclear cell counts 6 hours after ingestion, with a mean increase of 9900 cells/mm^3 (range 5500–16,800 cells/mm^3). The data collected in these reports led Powell to propose criteria for determining that a food challenge performed to diagnose food protein-induced enterocolitis of infancy was positive: patients would improve when not ingesting the causal protein, would have an oral food challenge that resulted in vomiting/diarrhea, evidence of gastrointestinal inflammation on stool studies, and a rise in the peripheral polymorphonuclear leukocyte count over 3500 cells/mL [4].

Examining the Pathophysiology

Interest in elucidating the pathophysiology emerged, and the understanding that findings from endoscopy and biopsy in these infants with enterocolitis were not specific, and that this was not an illness associated with IgE antibodies became evident. In this chapter, details about the pathophysiology of FPIES or laboratory findings in patients with this disorder will not be examined, as this will be reviewed in other chapters, but the early reports that helped lead to the current understanding will be discussed.

In a study from 1975, Fontaine et al. reported the findings of small intestinal biopsy from 31 infants with cow's milk protein intolerance, many of whom likely had FPIES [5]. These patients, ages 3–7 months except for one who was 20 months of age, were diagnosed with cow's milk protein intolerance based on having the onset of symptoms soon after the first cow's milk exposure, recovering clinically on a cow's milk-free diet, and having a return of symptoms with cow's milk challenge. They found mucosal damage, with partial villous atrophy being the most common finding. With a milk-free diet, recovery of normal mucosal appearance occurred between 3 and 13 months.

In 1977, Halpin et al. described 4 patients, ages 2 months to 4 months, with soy protein intolerance all of whom had vomiting, diarrhea, hematochezia, and weight loss of more than 10% [6]. These patients were fed soy formula because they were suspected of having cow's milk protein intolerance. This study detailed the existence of soy protein-induced colitis. Of 10 children seen at UCLA Center for the Health Sciences between 1973 and 1976 who were suspected of being intolerant to soy protein, 4 were followed prospectively to learn if the small bowel, colon, or both were affected. These patients underwent proctosigmoidoscopy and rectal biopsy within 24 hours of admission, and again after feeding was stopped, IV fluids corrected electrolyte deficits, diarrhea had ceased for 3 days, and the patients had achieved a 10% gain in weight. If the proctosigmoidoscopy and rectal biopsy was normal at that point, the patients underwent an oral food challenge with a soy formula. All four patients developed diarrhea, as early as 3 hours and as late as 5 days after systematic testing with soy protein. All four patients had both gross and microscopic evidence of an acute colitis on the initial proctosigmoidoscopy. These findings improved within 1 month of becoming asymptomatic. After being rechallenged with soy formula, all of the patients had evidence of an acute colitis with the presence of polymorphonuclear leukocytes within the lamina propria or in the walls of the rectal glands. The patients did not have any ulcerations of the mucosa, destruction of the crypts, or presence of granulomas before or after the challenge with soy formula. Two of the patients, both of whom had the presence of abnormal stool pH and increased amounts of reducing sugars after the soy challenge, had small bowel biopsy performed, which showed normal microscopic morphology.

These and other subsequent studies have demonstrated that the findings from endoscopy and biopsy in FPIES are nonspecific [1, 6–9]. Colonic biopsy specimens obtained from patients with symptoms reveal crypt abscesses and a diffuse inflammatory cell infiltrate with prominent plasma cells, while small bowel biopsy specimens demonstrate edema, acute inflammation, and mild villous atrophy.

FPIES has been described as a non-IgE-mediated disorder, and over the years it has been well documented that most children with FPIES do not demonstrate sensitivity to the causative food on skin prick testing or serum IgE testing [1, 10–13]. In her report in 1967, Gryboski discussed that gastrointestinal allergy is difficult to document by cutaneous testing as the patient's serum and tests for circulating antibodies are usually negative [1]. In that study, none of the 10 patients who had serum testing had circulating precipitins to cow's milk.

FPIES can involve antigen-specific T cells, antibodies, and cytokines as a cause of the inflammation found in the colon [12]. Heyman et al. demonstrated that tumor necrosis factor alpha (TNF-α) secreted by circulating milk protein-specific T cells increased intestinal permeability [14]. In reports from 1996 and 1999, Benlounes et al. reported that patients with FPIES showed significantly lower doses of intact cow's milk protein-stimulated TNF-α secretion from peripheral blood mononuclear cells than patients whose sensitivity resolved or those with skin manifestations of cow's milk hypersensitivity [15, 16]. Transforming growth factor β-1 (TGF-β1) is a cytokine that protections the epithelial barrier of the gut [17]. In 2002, Chung et al. reported that infants with FPIES demonstrated a depression of TGF-β1 expression and a decreased expression of the type 1 TGF-β1 receptor on immunohistochemical staining of duodenal biopsy specimens [18]. These early findings of T cell-related immune responses likely contributed to the decision to use corticosteroids during treatment.

Clinical Findings and the Label FPIES

In 1998, Sicherer et al. described a cohort with milk-, soy-, and solid food-induced enterocolitis and, in response to recognizing a number of characteristic features that warrant the designation "syndrome," coined the term food protein-induced enterocolitis syndrome (FPIES) [10]. Given that most patients become completely free of symptoms with the removal of the causal protein from the diet, making endoscopy and biopsy unnecessary, they did not perform biopsies to confirm inflammation in their cohort of patients. Setting forth a clinical criteria for the diagnosis of "typical" FPIES, subjects would receive this diagnosis if (1) they were younger than 9 months of age at initial diagnosis, (2) repeated exposure to the incriminated food elicited diarrhea and/or repetitive vomiting within 24 hours without any other cause of the symptoms, (3) there were no symptoms other than gastrointestinal symptoms elicited by the incriminated food, (4) removal of the offending protein from the diet resulted in resolution of the symptoms, and/or a standardized food challenge elicited diarrhea and/or vomiting within 24 hours after administration of the food. They also wrote that if monitored during a challenge, an increase in the absolute neutrophil count by over 3500/mm^3 at 5–8 hours after the challenge would add to the presumptive evidence of a positive challenge.

While most children do not have positive IgE testing to the causative food in FPIES, some patients have IgE to the trigger food and have been labeled as atypical [10–12, 20]. Sicherer et al. identified 16 patients with typical FPIES, as well as another 6 cases that were considered atypical. Of the patients with typical FPIES, 11 reacted to milk, 11 to soy, and 7 to both. The mean age at diagnosis was 7 weeks for milk reactivity and 8 weeks for soy reactivity. Another 2 patients had FPIES to rice and pea. FPIES to milk resolved in 6 of 10 patients and FPIES to soy resolved in 2 of 8 patients who were followed for a median period of 25 months. In the 6 subjects who were diagnosed with "atypical" FPIES, the subjects fulfilled the clinical criteria of FPIES, but were either older than 9 months of age at diagnosis or had IgE antibodies to the incriminated food. One subject experienced reactions to turkey and chicken at age 2 years. The other 5 subjects demonstrated positive IgE reactivity to the proteins that elicited typical FPIES. Interestingly, they reported that all of the patients who had specific IgE to the causal food remained sensitive, making this the first report that the presence of food-specific IgE is a poor prognostic sign for outgrowing FPIES, a finding supported by subsequent publications [11, 12, 19]. While it was hypothesized that atopy patch testing, designed to identify allergens that cause cell-mediated hypersensitivity, may be helpful in identifying patients with FPIES, studies have demonstrated that this modality is not helpful, largely due to a high rate of false-negative results [13, 20].

In 1993, Murray et al. reported the finding that some infants who were hospitalized for primary soy or cow's milk protein intolerance had transient methemoglobinemia [21]. In their cohort of 17 patients, 6 infants (35%) demonstrated this finding. Reexposure to the offending protein caused diarrhea, metabolic acidosis, and transient methemoglobinemia in all of the patients. The finding of transient methemoglobinemia was also reported by Sicherer et al. in one patient with FPIES who experienced dehydration [10]. The various case series added to the characterization that an FPIES reaction could be severe and include acidemia, methemoglobinemia, and hypotension/shock.

A Disorder Due to More than Just Milk and Soy

While once reported as a syndrome associated with milk and soy protein, in the early 1990s, case reports emerged describing "anaphylactoid" reactions consistent with FPIES due to solid foods. In 1992, Borchers et al. published a case report of an 8-month-old infant who presented with multiple hospital admissions for recurrent episodes of pallor, cyanosis, vomiting, diarrhea, hematochezia, dehydration, and lethargy, ultimately found to be due to ingestion of rice [22]. This patient initially presented at 5 weeks of age with 2 weeks of vomiting and 1 week of diarrhea after his formula was thickened with rice cereal for the treatment of gastroesophageal reflux. In 1994, Vandenplas et al. reported a case of a 9-month-old with an "anaphylactoid reaction," as well as colitis, after ingesting chicken [23]. This patient underwent a physician supervised oral food challenge after his mother noticed 4 episodes of vomiting and diarrhea 1–2 hours after the ingestion of chicken. Serum IgE testing to chicken was negative. Less than 2 hours after ingesting chicken in the food challenge, the patient developed biliary emesis, bloody diarrhea, and tachycardia, and he became pale. Colonoscopy, which had been previously normal when he was seen in the outpatient setting, showed a red, fragile, and hemorrhagic mucosa, with biopsies demonstrating a severe inflammation with an increased number of eosinophils. Serum IgE to chicken remained negative. This patient did also have an increased white blood cell count of 20,000/mm^3 with polynuclear cells increasing from 25 to 60%.

In 2003 Nowak-Wegrzyn et al. reported 14 infants with FPIES caused by solid food proteins [11]. The eliciting foods included grains (rice, oat, and barley), vegetables (sweet potato, squash, string beans, peas), and poultry (chicken and turkey). Nine (64%) of these patients also had cow's milk- and/or soy-FPIES, with 11 (78%) reacting to more than 1 food protein. The diagnosis of FPIES was delayed in these patients, coming after a median of two reactions (range, 2–5). More recent published case series have identified a plethora of FPIES triggers, including peanut [24], avocado [25, 26], fish [27–29], sesame [30], and egg yolk [31], in addition to published case reports of FPIES triggered by quail's egg (but not hen's egg) [32], short-neck clam and squid [33], oysters [34], corn [35], and mushrooms [36].

A review of 10 years of FPIES oral food challenges from one institution in New York included data on 160 subjects with FPIES and reported the most common foods to cause reactions were cow's milk (44%) and soy (41%), with rice (22.5%) and oat (16%) following as the next most common triggers [19]. In the largest cohort of patients with FPIES to date, with 462 cases seen at the Children's Hospital of Philadelphia, Ruffner et al. similarly reported the most common food triggers to be milk (67%), soy (41%), rice (19%), oat (16%), and egg (11%) [13].

A study from Australia found that neither milk nor soy were the most common trigger of FPIES in that country [37]. Mehr et al. used a survey through the Australian Paediatric Surveillance Unit, with monthly notification of new cases of acute FPIES in infants aged less than 24 months by 1400 pediatricians to identify 230 Australian infants with FPIES from 2012 to 2014. In that cohort, rice was actually the most common trigger (102), followed by cow's milk (75), egg (27), oat (21), chicken (19), fish (12), banana (9), sweet potato (7), pear (6), beef (6), avocado (5), potato (5), apple (4), pumpkin (4), and lamb (3). While rice and egg were the solid foods most frequently involved in FPIES in Australian children, Vila et al. reported that fish is the most common solid food trigger of FPIES in Spanish children [29]. The geographic variation in FPIES remains an interesting unsolved observation.

Still More to Learn

While the prevalence of FPIES is increasing [37, 38], reports on FPIES are still largely comprised of case reports, though publications on this topic are increasing in number. Entering the term "food protein-induced enterocolitis" into a search on PubMed currently provides 325 results [39], while the term "food protein-induced enterocolitis syndrome" yields only 208 results [40]. Reports on FPIES have been increasing in recent years, as more than half of the articles found in those PubMed searches were published in the past 5 years.

It was over 40 years ago that the initial reports on FPIES surfaced in the literature, yet many questions related to FPIES remain unanswered. There is no predictive test to confirm or rule out the diagnosis of FPIES prior to oral food challenge, there are no medications for home use to limit symptom development, the exact underlying mechanism of FPIES is not clearly understood, and it is difficult to predict whether a patient will have FPIES to one or multiple foods. Often the available data addressing these questions are contradictory. For example, there has been conflicting information as to whether patients with FPIES are likely to react to one food or multiple foods, with differing conclusions coming from a variety of geographic regions [13, 19, 37, 38, 41]. In an Australian cohort, Mehr et al. reported that 68% of infants with FPIES had one food trigger [37], similar to a report from New York by Caubet et al., where 65% reacted to only one food [19]. In a cohort of 66 Italian children with FPIES, Sopo et al. reported that 85% reacted to only one food [41]. In looking specifically at FPIES to milk and whether or not patients could tolerate soy, Sicherer et al. reported that among a New York cohort of 11 patients with cow's milk protein-induced FPIES, 64% had a coexisting allergy to soy [10]; in contrast, Katz et al. reported that in their Israeli cohort of 44 children with FPIES to milk, none of the patients had FPIES to any other foods [38]. Ruffner et al. specifically advised against introducing soy at home to a child with milk-triggered FPIES because 43.5% of their patients in Philadelphia with milk-triggered FPIES also reacted to soy [13]. Like the geographic variation in triggers, variation in rates of single versus multiple food FPIES remains an unresolved mystery likely to inform treatment and prevention strategies once understood.

Conclusions

Since the early observations described above, tremendous advances in understanding FPIES have been achieved. In 2017, an international workgroup convened through the Adverse Reactions to Foods Committee of the American Academy of Allergy, Asthma, & Immunology and the International FPIES Association advocacy group published the first international evidence-based guidelines to improve the diagnosis and management of patients with FPIES, representing a culmination in translating the literature to a guideline [12]. In the last 2 decades, the diagnostic definitions of FPIES have been refined, additional insights on pathophysiology noted, but much more research lies ahead toward better diagnosis, treatment, and prevention.

Key Points

- FPIES was first described in the 1960s and 1970s in case series that likely included infants with a variety of disorders. These early reports detailed a peculiar ~ 2 hour delayed onset of severe vomiting following ingestion of a trigger food.
- Increasing descriptions of the clinical features in the 1970s and 1980s further elucidated the defining characteristics that were used to propose initial diagnostic criteria.
- In 1998, in response to recognizing a number of characteristic features that warrant the designation "syndrome," the term food protein-induced enterocolitis syndrome was coined.
- While early reports focused on cow's milk and soy as triggers of FPIES, descriptions of a wide variety of solid food triggers have emerged since the 1990s.
- Over the past two decades, the diagnostic definitions of FPIES have been refined, additional insights on pathophysiology have been noted, but much more research lies ahead toward better diagnosis, treatment, and prevention.

References

1. Gryboski J. Gastrointestinal milk allergy in infancy. Pediatrics. 1967;40:354–62.
2. Powell GK. Enterocolitis in low-birth-weight infants associated with milk and soy protein intolerance. J Pediatr. 1976;88:840–4.
3. Powell GK. Milk- and soy-induced enterocolitis of infancy. J Pediatr. 1978;93:553–60.
4. Powell G. Food protein-induced enterocolitis of infancy: differential diagnosis and management. Comp Ther. 1986;12:28–37.
5. Fontaine JL, Navarro J. Small intestinal biopsy in cows milk protein allergy in infancy. Arch Dis Child. 1975;50(5):357–62.
6. Halpin TC, Byrne WJ, Ament ME. Colitis, persistent diarrhea, and soy protein intolerance. J Pediatr. 1977;91(3):404–7.
7. Jenkins H, Pincott J, Soothill J, Milla P, Harries J. Food allergy: the major cause of infantile colitis. Arch Dis Child. 1984;59:326–9.
8. Goldman H, Provjanksy R. Allergic proctitis and gastroenteritis in children. Am J Surg Pathol. 1986;10:75–86.
9. Coello-Ranurez P, Larrosa-Haro A. Gastrointestinal occult hemorrhage and gastroduodenitis in cow's milk protein intolerance. J Pediatr Gastroenterol Nutr. 1984;3:215–8.
10. Sicherer SH, Eigenmann PA, Sampson HA. Clinical features of food protein-induced enterocolitis syndrome. J Pediatr. 1998;133(2):214–9.
11. Nowak-Wegrzyn A, Sampson HA, Wood RA, Sicherer SH. Food protein-induced enterocolitis syndrome caused by solid food proteins. Pediatrics. 2003;111(4):829–35.
12. Nowak-Wegrzyn A, Chehade M, Groetch ME, et al. International consensus guidelines for the diagnosis and management of food protein-induced enterocolitis syndrome: executive summary-workgroup report of the Adverse Reactions to Food Committee, American Academy of Allergy, Asthma & Immunology. J Allergy Clin Immunol. 2017;139(4):1111–26.
13. Ruffner MA, Ruymann K, Barni S, Cianferoni A, Brown-Whitehorn T, Spergel JM. Food protein-induced enterocolitis syndrome: insights from review of a large referral population. J Allergy Clin Immunol Pract. 2013;1(4):343–9.

14. Heyman M, Darmon N, Dupont C, et al. Mononuclear cells from infants allergic to cow's milk secrete tumor necrosis factor alpha, altering intestinal function. Gasteroenterology. 1994;106(6):1514–23.
15. Benlounes N, Dupont C, Candalh C, et al. The threshold for immune cell reactivity to milk antigens decreases in cow's milk allergy with intestinal symptoms. J Allergy Clin Immunol. 1996;98(4):781–9.
16. Benlounes N, Candalh C, Matarazzo P, Dupont C, Heyman M. The time-course of milk antigen-induced TNF-alpha secretion differs according to the clinical symptoms in children with cow's milk allergy. J Allergy Clin Immunol. 1999;104(4 Pt1):863–9.
17. Planchon S, Martins C, Guerrant R, Roche JK. Regulation of intestinal epithelial barrier function by TGF-beta 1. Evidence for its role in abrogating the effect of a T cell cytokine. J Immunol. 1994;153(12):5730–9.
18. Chung HL, Hwang JB, Park JJ, Kim SG. Expression of transforming growth factor beta1, transforming growth factor type I and II receptors, and TNF-alpha in the mucosa of the small intestine in infants with food protein-induced enterocolitis syndrome. J Allergy Clin Immunol. 2002;109(1):150–4.
19. Caubet JC, Ford LS, Sickles L, et al. Clinical features and resolution of food protein-induced enterocolitis syndrome: 10-year experience. J Allergy Clin Immunol. 2014;134(2):382–9.
20. Jarvinen KM, Caubet JC, Sickles L, Ford LS, Sampson HA, Nowak-Wegrzyn A. Poor utility of atopy patch test in predicting tolerance development in food protein-induced enterocolitis syndrome. Ann Allergy Asthma Immunol. 2012;109(3):221–2.
21. Murray KF, Christie DL. Dietary protein intolerance in infants with transient methemoglobinemia and diarrhea. J Pediatr. 1993;122(1):90–2.
22. Borchers SD, Li BU, Friedman RA, McClung HJ. Rice-induced anaphylactoid reaction. J Pediatr Gastroenterol Nutr. 1992;15(3):321–4.
23. Vandenplas Y, Edelman R, Sacre L. Chicken-induced anaphylactoid reaction and colitis. J Pediatr Gastroenterol Nutr. 1994;19(2):240–1.
24. Robbins KA, Ackerman OR, Carter CA, Uygungil B, Sprunger A, Sharma HP. Food protein-induced enterocolitis syndrome to peanut with early introduction: a clinical dilemma. J Allergy Clin Immunol Pract. 2018;6(2):664–6.
25. Goodman M, Feuille E. Avocado: an emerging culprit in food protein-induced enterocolitis syndrome? Ann Allergy Asthma Immunol. 2018;122(2):218–20; Epub ahead of print.
26. Cherian S, Neupert K, Varshney P. Avocado as an emerging trigger for food protein-induced enterocolitis syndrome. Ann Allergy Asthma Immunol. 2018;121(3):369–71.
27. Infante S, Marco-Martin G, Sanchez-Dominguez M, et al. Food protein-induced enterocolitis syndrome by fish: not necessarily a restricted diet. Allergy. 2018;73(3):728–32.
28. Miceli Sopo S, Monaco S, Badina L, et al. Food protein-induced enterocolitis syndrome caused by fish and/or shellfish in Italy. Pediatr Allergy Immunol. 2015;26(8):731–6.
29. Vila L, Garcia V, Rial MJ, Novoa E, Cacharron T. Fish is a major trigger of solid food protein-induced enterocolitis syndrome in Spanish children. J Allergy Clin Immunol Pract. 2015;3(4):621–3.
30. Ovadia A, Nahum A, Tasher D, et al. Sesame: an unrecognized trigger of food protein-induced enterocolitis syndrome. J Allergy Clin Immunol Pract. 2018;7(1):305–6; Epub ahead of print.
31. Shimomura M, Tanaka H, Meguro T, Kimura M. Three cases of food protein-induced enterocolitis syndrome caused by egg yolk. Allergol Int. 2018;68(1):110–1; Epub ahead of print.
32. Sanlidag B, Babayigit Hocaoglu A, Bahceciler N. Quail's egg-induced severe enterocolitis in a child tolerant to hen's egg: first reported case. J Investig Allergol Clin Immunol. 2016;26(2):118–9.
33. Masumi H, Takemura Y, Inoue N, Takemura T. Food protein-induced enterocolitis syndrome in a 6-year-old girl after ingestion of short-neck clam and squid. Pediatr Int. 2018;60(4):380–1.
34. Sopo SM, D'Antuono A, Morganti A, Bianchi A. Food protein-induced enterocolitis syndrome due to oysters ingestion. Isr Med Assoc J. 2015;17(3):188–9.
35. Sopo SM, Filoni S, Giorgio V, Monaco S, Onesimo R. Food protein-induced enterocolitis syndrome (FPIES) to corn: a case report. J Investig Allergol Clin Immunol. 2012;22(5):391–2.

36. Serafini S, Bergmann MM, Nowak-Wegrzyn A, Eigenmann PA, Caubet JC. A case of food protein-induced enterocolitis syndrome to mushrooms challenging currently used diagnostic criteria. J Allergy Clin Immunol Pract. 2015;3(1):135–7.
37. Mehr S, Frith K, Barnes EH, Campbell DE, FPIES Study Group. Food protein-induced enterocolitis syndrome in Australia: a population-based study, 2012–2014. J Allergy Clin Immunol. 2017;140(5):1323–30.
38. Katz Y, Goldberg MR, Rajuan N, Cohen A, Leshno M. The prevalence and natural course of food protein-induced enterocolitis syndrome to cow's milk: a large-scale, prospective population-based study. J Allergy Clin Immunol. 2011;127(3):647–53.
39. National Center for Biotechnology Information. https://www.ncbi.nlm.nih.gov/pubmed/?term=food+protein+induced+enterocolitis. Accessed November 18, 2018.
40. National Center for Biotechnology Information. https://www.ncbi.nlm.nih.gov/pubmed/?term=food+protein+induced+enterocolitis+syndrome. Accessed November 18, 2018.
41. Sopo SM, Giorgio V, Dello Iacono I, Novembre E, Mori F, Onesimo R. A multicenter retrospective study of 66 Italian children with food protein-induced enterocolitis syndrome: different management for different phenotypes. Clin Exp Allergy. 2012;42(8):1257–65.

Epidemiology of Food Protein-Induced Enterocolitis Syndrome

2

Melanie A. Ruffner and Jonathan M. Spergel

Introduction

Food protein-induced enterocolitis (FPIES) has traditionally been thought to be a rare non-IgE-mediated food allergy syndrome. It was first described in 1967 in a case series of infants with prolonged diarrhea and vomiting following ingestion of cow's milk by Gryboski [1]. FPIES is distinct from infants with cow's milk proctocolitis in that the infants described presented with vomiting, diarrhea, bloody stool, and failure to thrive, yet symptoms resolved with removal of cow's milk. Almost 10 years later, Powell noted a similar condition following cow's milk formula introduction in a cohort of neonates and infants [2]. Patients presented with abdominal distension, hypothermia, peripheral blood neutrophilia, and elevated stool leukocytes. However, if milk was removed and reintroduced, reproducible symptoms of vomiting, diarrhea, hypotension, and neutrophilia developed 2–4 hours after ingestion. This initial chronic phase of the presentation of FPIES in young infants later came to be known as chronic FPIES due to the protracted symptoms of diarrhea, vomiting, and weight loss which can occur when the food antigen is a very frequent component of the infant diet [3].

The first medical reports of enterocolitis reactions to solid foods followed a similar timeline as those to milk. Ikola et al. published one of the earliest descriptions of an infant with acute rice and wheat enterocolitis [4]. However, this was not followed by additional reports of FPIES reaction to a solid food until approximately 20 years later when McDonald et al. described severe, delayed vomiting in three patients

M. A. Ruffner (✉) · J. M. Spergel
Division of Allergy & Immunology, Children's Hospital of Philadelphia, Philadelphia, PA, USA

Department of Pediatrics, University of Pennsylvania Perelman School of Medicine, Philadelphia, PA, USA
e-mail: ruffnerm@email.chop.edu

T. F. Brown-Whitehorn, A. Cianferoni (eds.), *Food Protein Induced Enterocolitis (FPIES)*, https://doi.org/10.1007/978-3-030-21229-2_2

upon first ingestion of hen's egg [5]. These studies highlighted that FPIES could present without chronic ingestion of a food and represent the earliest characterizations the acute FPIES phenotype presenting upon introduction of new foods in slightly older infants. This phenotype is characterized by delayed vomiting 1–4 hours after the ingestion of food antigen which can be accompanied by diarrhea, lethargy, pallor, hypotension, hypothermia, and leukocytosis with left shift. The phenotypic differences between acute and chronic FPIES are reviewed elsewhere in this text.

Limits and Advantages of Current Epidemiological Studies

In 1998 Sicherer et al. proposed diagnostic criteria describing the shared clinical and laboratory features of FPIES [6]. Despite these diagnostic criteria, many challenges remain to performing epidemiological studies of FPIES, and it remains inadequately studied. All of the current large studies on FPIES are from industrialized nations (Fig. 2.1); therefore, there is a paucity of data representing the presentation and natural history of this disorder in many regions, ethnicities, and cultures. The majority of studies are retrospective case series or case reports which have been derived from specialized referral centers. Therefore, this introduces reporting bias and may favor a representation of a more severe and complex FPIES phenotype within the published literature. Additional methodological limitations include the fact that there is a significant inter-study variation in the definition of FPIES used to include or exclude cases. An international classification of diseases (ICD-10) code for FPIES was introduced in 2015, which may permit more accurate identification of FPIES cases. Misdiagnosis of FPIES remains a significant clinical concern that results in patient morbidity and may also continue to result in underestimation of the

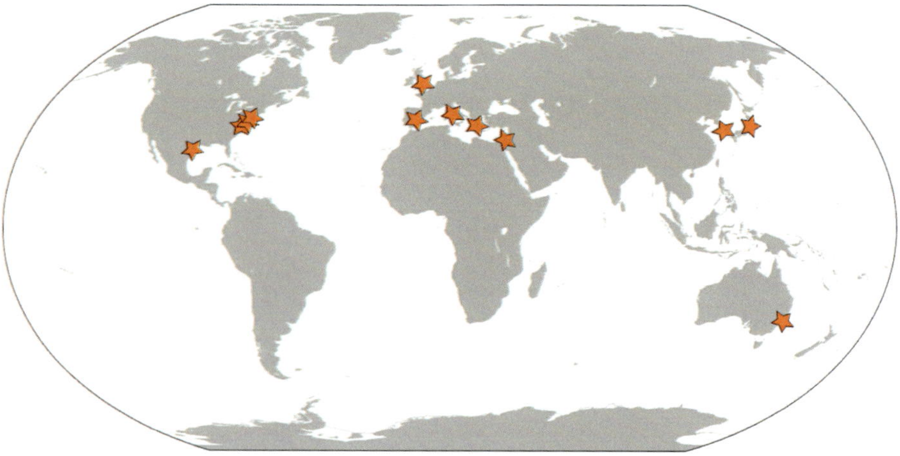

Fig. 2.1 Global distribution of food protein-induced enterocolitis syndrome case series, represented on the globe projection with orange stars

prevalence of FPIES as there are no biomarkers specific for FPIES [7]. International FPIES diagnostic criteria were published in 2017 to address the need for clinical and research consensus [3]; however, prior to that, the definitions used to classify FPIES in studies have varied. Therefore, the epidemiological study of FPIES has been challenging since its first description in the 1970s.

Nonetheless, the research conducted thus far has permitted identification of many important features of FPIES. Important commonalities have arisen from existing studies that have permitted the identification of factors that can assist with clinical management, such as age of presentation, common food antigen triggers, and potential risks of cross-reactivity.

Incidence and Prevalence

FPIES is thought to be a rare disease; however, as more peer-reviewed case series have been published over time, it has become clear that FPIES is not as rare as initially believed. Nonetheless, only a few prospective studies examining the true incidence of FPIES have been conducted. The first was conducted by Katz et al. and was a prospective birth cohort study conducted at a single Israeli hospital [8]. During the 2-year study interval, the cumulative incidence of cow's milk FPIES was 0.34%, whereas the incidence of IgE-mediated food allergy to cow's milk was 0.5% [8]. All of the infants with FPIES had onset of symptoms by 6 months of age, and 90% of the cohort had resolution of FPIES symptoms by 3 years of age. The cumulative incidence from this study by Katz et al. matches closely with a reported cross-sectional incidence of approximately 0.1% within a Japanese hospital system over retrospective review of records from 2003 to 2007 [9] and suggests that FPIES is not as rare as previously thought in relation to IgE-mediated cow's milk allergy.

Mehr et al. conducted the second prospective epidemiological study in Australia, a study of 1400 participating pediatric practices providing monthly reports into an existing national Australian Pediatric Surveillance Unit database. This was estimated to represent 50% of the pediatricians in Australia, and they provided pediatricians with a guideline for diagnosis that was consistent with the diagnosis of acute FPIES. This study determined the cumulative incidence of FPIES to be 15.4/100,000/year. Interestingly this was more common than the reported Australian rates of both Crohn disease and eosinophilic esophagitis in this age group [10, 11]. However, this estimate is considerably less than that observed in Katz et al. [8], which was from a single center. This may have been due to underreporting of less severe cases into the central databases in the Australian study by Mehr et al. or further epidemiological studies may yet demonstrate that there are bona fide variations in the geographic incidence of FPIES. However, these studies both help to establish that FPIES is more common than was initially appreciated based upon the first case series reports.

Indeed, the larger retrospective case series of FPIES patients indicate an estimated point prevalence of approximately 1% [12, 13]. One strength of these studies is that they provide information over several years' time. However, the cohorts likely reflect some referral bias and may fail to capture patients with mild symptoms. In several retrospective studies, the prevalence of FPIES appears to be increasing over time; however, without prospective population-based studies, this is difficult to confirm [12, 14, 15]. Recent evidence to suggest that a gap in clinician education remains regarding the diagnosis and management of FPIES, and therefore some of this increase may be due to increased provider awareness [16]. However, as the mode of inheritance and mechanism of FPIES remain largely unknown, it is unclear if there are unappreciated mechanistic factors that may be contributing to the current apparent increase in FPIES cases.

Risk Factors

Environmental Risk Factors Population-based studies have demonstrated some risk factors associated with the development of FPIES; however, the exact mechanism of FPIES remains unknown. In the birth cohort study conducted by Katz et al., development of FPIES was associated with Israeli Jewish ethnicity and birth by cesarean section [8]. Association of increased rates of cesarean births among patients with FPIES has been observed in other case series [17]. It is hypothesized that cesarean section may disrupt the microflora, predisposing to the development of food allergy, including FPIES. This is in keeping with other studies which have found risk of eosinophilic esophagitis, food allergy, and other atopic disorders with cesarean delivery and early neonatal antibiotic use [18–20]. Of note, the birth cohort study conducted by Katz at all did not observe any association between the development of FPIES and infant's gestational age, maternal age, birth order, age at cow's milk introduction, or maternal dairy consumption during pregnancy [8]. Additional case series have not examined the association of prenatal risk factors nor additional postnatal risk factors, including age of food introduction, with the development of FPIES.

Family History It is hypothesized that ingestion of food allergens in FPIES causes aberrant cellular and humoral immune system responses resulting in abnormal intestinal barrier function and inflammation. This occurs through a non-IgE-mediated immune reaction. However, a family history of atopy is frequent in FPIES patients. The reported rate of first-degree relatives with atopic conditions (including allergic rhinitis, asthma, IgE-mediated food allergy, and eczema) varies based on patient population (Table 2.1). The reported range varies between 21% and 80% depending on the study [15, 21].

FPIES has been reported to occur in siblings in a handful of studies. Mehr et al. reported an increased prevalence of FPIES in siblings, occurring in 7% of the siblings of FPIES patients in the study [10]. The chronic FPIES phenotype has been described to occur occasionally in identical and fraternal twins [22, 23], with both sets of twins reacting to the same food antigens. However, it does not appear that there is evidence that the association of FPIES in twins is particularly strong. This is significantly different than the pattern seen eosinophilic esophagitis which is also

Table 2.1 Summary of food protein-enterocolitis syndrome studies

	Year	Country	FPIES definition	No. of patients	Prevalent foods	Fam. Hx atopy	Multiple FPIES triggers	% male
Prospective								
Burks et al. [31]	1994	USA	–	43	Milk and soy FPIES studied	–	60% milk and soy	60%
Katz et al. [8]	2011	Israel	Sicherer et al.	44	Only cow's milk studied	–	–	52%
Hwang et al. [32]	2009	Korea	Powell et al.	23	Milk and soy FPIES studied	–	8.7% milk and soy	70%
Caubet et al. [28]	2014	USA	Powell et al.	160	Milk, soy, rice, and oat	77%	35% overall multifood	54%
Retrospective								
Gryboski [1]	1967	USA	–	21	Milk	66.6%	14% milk and soy	84%
Powell [2]	1976	USA	–	9	Milk and soy	–	–	–
Sicherer [6]	1998	USA	–	16	Milk, soy, and some solids	56%	43% milk and soy	50%
Levy and Danon [29]	2003	Israel	Sicherer et al.	6	Poultry, milk, soy, and *legumes*	–	83%	66%
Nowak-Wegrzyn et al. [21]	2003	USA	Sicherer et al.	44	Milk, soy, rice, and oat	71–80%	25%	59%
Fukuie et al. [9]	2008	Japan	Powell et al.	10	Milk and rice	–	30% milk and rice	–
Jarvinen-Seppo et al. [33]	2011	USA	–	76	Milk, soy, rice, wheat, and poultry	–	20%	–
Sopo et al. [15]	2012	Italy	Powell et al.	66	Milk, *fish*, egg, rice, soy, and corn	20%	15%	61%
Ruffner et al. [12]	2013	USA	Sicherer et al.	462	Milk, soy, grains, *egg*, and meat/fish	–	30% overall multifood	60.4
Ruiz-Garcia et al. [34]	2014	Spain	Sicherer et al.	16	Milk, *fish*, soy, rice, wheat, and chicken	–	6.3%	62.5%
Vasilopoulou [17]	2014	Greece	–	16	Fish FPIES only	44%	–	68%
Ludman et al. [7]	2014	UK	Powell et al.	70	Milk, *fish*, egg, soy, wheat, and chicken	–	30% overall multifood	59%
Other								
Mehr et al. [10]	2017	Australia	Sicherer et al.	230	Rice, milk, and egg	57%	33%	48%

a non-IgE-mediated food allergy syndrome but has a 57.9% concordance in monozygotic twins and 36.7% concordance in dizygotic twins [24]. A high rate of concurrent atopic disease has been reported in FPIES patients, ranging approximately 30–40% of patients in reported case series [10, 12, 21]; however, it is unknown if there are unique genetic risks distinct from other atopic disorders that are uniquely associated with FPIES.

Population Demographics

A majority of case series have noted a slight male predominance, ranging from 50% to 60% (see Table 2.1). The etiology of this is unknown. Interestingly, a male predominance has been noted in eosinophilic esophagitis, another non-IgE-mediated food allergy syndrome [25]. The majority of retrospective FPIES studies from western countries have included predominately patients with White racial backgrounds. From the retrospective design of these studies, it is difficult to discern if this reflects a true racial predilection in the presentation of FPIES or if referral or recruitment bias accounts for some of these findings.

In general, FPIES presents in infancy. It is uncommon for exclusively breast-fed infants to develop FPIES, and symptoms usually begin with the introduction of exogenous dietary protein via infant formula or weaning to solid food. The age of presentation of chronic of FPIES is different from that of acute FPIES and seems to be influenced by when food proteins are introduced into the diet (Fig. 2.2). As initially observed by Gryboski and Powell, chronic FPIES presents in newborns following the introduction of cow's milk or soy protein formulas. The median age of presentation was 1 week (observed range 4 days–3 weeks) and 4 weeks (observed range 3 days–4 months) in these studies [1, 2]. In these neonates, continued ingestion of the food antigen can lead to continuing emesis, diarrhea, and failure to thrive which can lead to dehydration and shock. However, elimination of the chronic FPIES food trigger resolves the symptoms. Subsequent feeding of the food antigen after this period of avoidance induces the characteristic acute FPIES reaction within 1 to 4 hours of antigen ingestion. This history is consistent with FPIES and distinguishes it from other diagnoses in the differential including celiac disease, eosinophilic gastrointestinal disorders, food protein-induced enteropathy, and very-early-onset inflammatory bowel disease.

Acute FPIES commonly occurs once cow's milk- or soy-based formula or solids alike are introduced into the infant's diet. As formula is often introduced earlier,

Fig. 2.2 Reported age of FPIES presentation. (**a**) Chronic FPIES to cow's milk or soy presents exclusively in the the first weeks of the neonatal period. (**b**) Acute FPIES to milk and soy presents at a younger age than FPIES to solid food like grain, egg, fish, and poultry. (Data are represented as mean ± 95% confidence interval from the case series indicated, unless denoted by §, indicating that data are displayed as mean ± range)

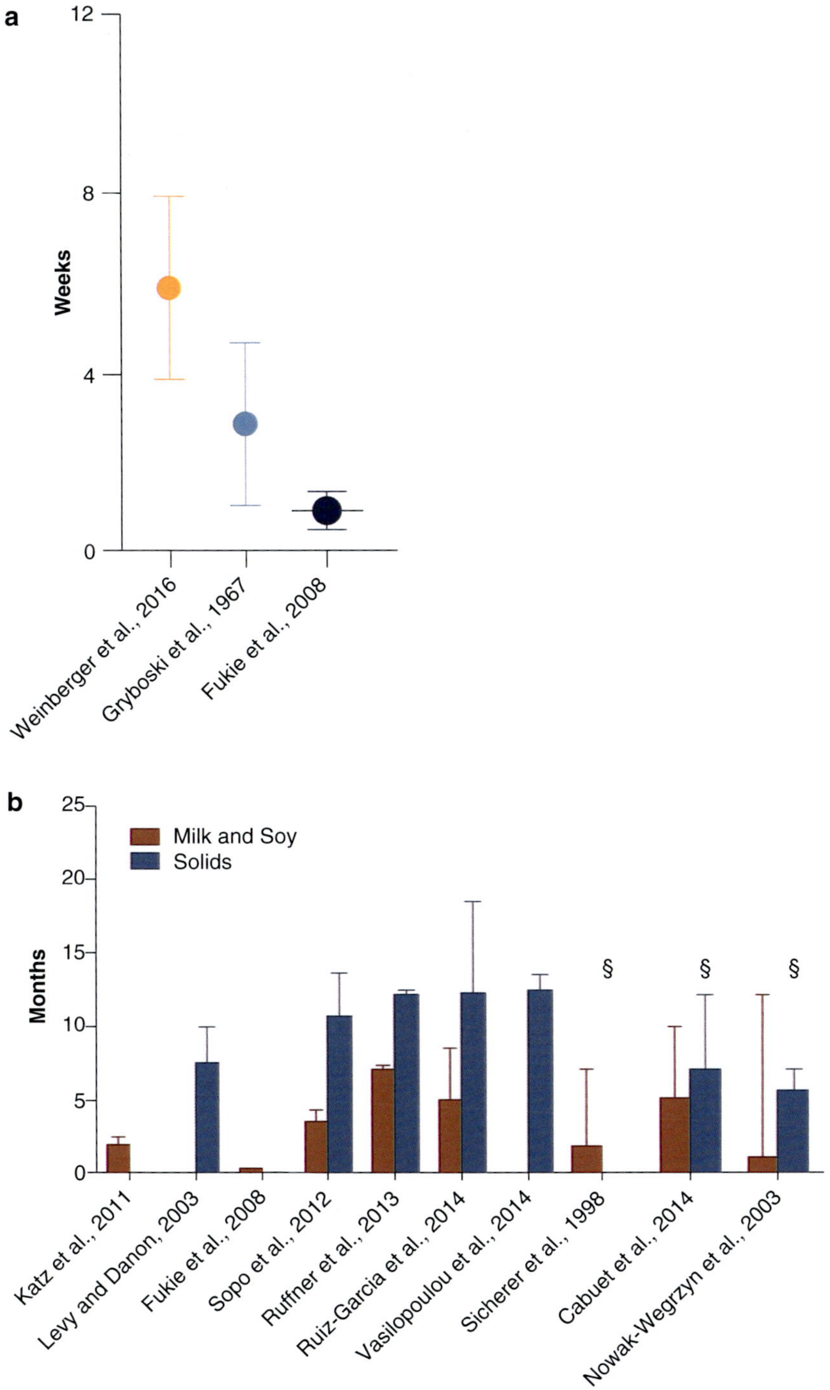
a
12
8
4
0
Weeks
Weinberger et al., 2016
Gryboski et al., 1967
Fukie et al., 2008
b
25
20
15
10
5
0
Months
Milk and Soy
Solids
§
§
§
Katz et al., 2011
Levy and Danon, 2003
Fukie et al., 2008
Sopo et al., 2012
Ruffner et al., 2013
Ruiz-Garcia et al., 2014
Vasilopoulou et al., 2014
Sicherer et al., 1998
Cabuet et al., 2014
Nowak-Wegrzyn et al., 2003

infants with cow's milk- and soy-induced FPIES will often present at a younger age (see Fig. 2.2b). In the majority of case series, most infants with grain-induced FPIES present between 5 and 7 months of age, whereas those with fish, egg, or poultry FPIES present slightly later.

Notably, there have been rare reports of FPIES developing in adults. These reactions were characterized by non-IgE-mediated vomiting beginning 1–4 hours after ingestion of the inciting allergens despite previous tolerance to the food. This is uncommon but has been reported to occur in adults ranging from 22 to 53 years of age [26, 27]. The most frequent food triggers reported in adults are with crustaceans, mollusks, fish, and egg.

Implicated Allergens

Regional Variance The most commonly reported allergens causing the acute FPIES phenotype are cow's milk, soy, grains (rice, oat, wheat), and egg; however, there is significant geographic variance in the overall frequency of implicated allergens. Cow's milk is the most frequent cause of FPIES in the United States and in European countries including Italy and Spain. Soy is a common FPIES trigger in the United States, where coincidence of soy FPIES has been commonly described in patients with FPIES to cow's milk [12, 21, 28]. Soy FPIES is significantly less common in Australia and Israel [8, 10]. For example, in Katz et al., 40 of 44 infants with cow's milk FPIES were challenged to soy; however, none of these patients reacted [8]. The mechanism of this difference is unclear but could relate to unknown combinations of genetic, atopic, and environmental risks or may be due to the early introduction of soy formulas in the United States.

Grains, including rice and wheat, are some of the most frequent solid food FPIES triggers. In Australia, rice is the most common FPIES trigger and, in several case series, appears to cause FPIES reactions more frequently than cow's milk [10, 14]. In several European countries including Italy, Spain, and the United Kingdom, FPIES reactions to fish have been commonly reported, although these are relatively uncommon in other regions of the world. Therefore, there may be underappreciated contributing factors beyond the age of food introduction that dictate which foods are common FPIES trigger allergens in a geographic region. The mechanisms behind these differences are perplexing. The reactions to fish in European countries have been postulated to relate to the more frequent use of fish as a weaning food in these regions. However, rice is a common weaning food in both the United States and Australia, and the frequency of FPIES reactions to different food types varies significantly between these two areas. Therefore, there may be underappreciated contributing factors beyond the age of food introduction that dictate which foods are common FPIES trigger allergens in a geographic region.

Multifood FPIES Reactions The majority of patients (65–80%) with FPIES will react to a single food. There are several well-described patterns of cross-reactivity among FPIES triggers. The mechanism underlying the co-occurrence of these multifood reactions in a subset of patients is unknown. The percentage of patients with cow's milk FPIES reacting to soy varies based on publication, with a rate of milk and soy co-allergy of approximately 30–40% across all studies [3]. This accounts for the majority of patients who have FPIES to more than one food in the majority of series [12, 28]. Approximately 16% of all patients with either milk or soy FPIES have had cocurrent solid food FPIES, whereas 25% of patients with solid food FPIES have had reactions to milk or soy [3]. Among solid foods, there is particularly high cross-reactivity among soy FPIES patients to other legumes, reaching 80% in some series [29]. Approximately half of all patients who have had a FPIES reaction to one type of grain in American studies will react to an additional grain [12, 21, 28]. Patients reacting to fish are typically able to tolerate poultry; however, approximately 40% of patients with FPIES caused by poultry (chicken, turkey) will have acute FPIES reaction if exposed to another form of poultry [3, 7, 30].

Conclusions

FPIES was first described in 1967, and studies regarding its epidemiology have made significant strides in describing the clinical scope of this disorder. The majority of large-scale studies have been retrospective case series, which have provided insights into the slight male predominance, occurrence mainly in infancy, atopic predilection, and common food allergen triggers which cause FPIES. These studies have helped to establish that FPIES is not rare; however, the exact incidence and prevalence in most regions of the world are still unknown. Further work involving population-based cohorts will likely provide additional epidemiological information regarding the frequency and clinical characteristics of FPIES.

Clinical Pearls
- Food protein-induced enterocolitis syndrome is rare; however, it occurs more frequently than thought when first studied after its discovery in 1967.
- Investigation into the epidemiology of FPIES has been limited to mainly industrialized countries, and therefore the effect of this disorder on populations around the world remains unknown.
- As physicians and providers become more educated regarding the presentation of FPIES, increases in the diagnosis rate of FPIES may be seen due to provider education.

References

1. Gryboski JD. Gastrointestinal milk allergy in infants. Pediatrics. 1967;40:354–62. https://doi.org/10.1111/j.1753-4887.1969.tb04937.x.
2. Powell GK. Enterocolitis in low-birth-weight infants associated with milk and soy protein intolerance. J Pediatr. 1976;88:840–4. https://doi.org/10.1016/S0022-3476(76)81128-6.

3. Nowak-Węgrzyn A, Chehade M, Groetch ME, et al. International consensus guidelines for the diagnosis and management of food protein–induced enterocolitis syndrome: executive summary—Workgroup Report of the Adverse Reactions to Foods Committee, American Academy of Allergy, Asthma & Immunology. J Allergy Clin Immunol. 2017;139:1111–1126.e4. https://doi.org/10.1016/j.jaci.2016.12.966.
4. Ikola RA. Severe intestinal reaction following ingestion of rice. Am J Dis Child. 1963;105:281–4. https://doi.org/10.1001/archpedi.1963.02080040283010.
5. McDonald PJ, Goldblum RM, Van Sickle GJ, Powell GK. Food protein-induced enterocolitis: altered antibody response to ingested antigen. Pediatr Res. 1984;18:751–5.
6. Sicherer SH, Eigenmann PA, Sampson HA. Clinical features of food protein-induced enterocolitis syndrome. J Pediatr. 1998;133:214–9. https://doi.org/10.1016/S0022-3476(98)70222-7.
7. Ludman S, Harmon M, Whiting D, Du Toit G. Clinical presentation and referral characteristics of food protein-induced enterocolitis syndrome in the United Kingdom. Ann Allergy Asthma Immunol. 2014;113:290–4. https://doi.org/10.1016/j.anai.2014.06.020.
8. Katz Y, Goldberg MR, Rajuan N, et al. The prevalence and natural course of food protein-induced enterocolitis syndrome to cow's milk: a large-scale, prospective population-based study. J Allergy Clin Immunol. 2011;127:647–53. https://doi.org/10.1016/j.jaci.2010.12.1105.
9. Fukuie T, Nomura I, Nakatani K, Gocho N, Saito A, Akashi M, Narita M, Akasawa A, Ohya Y, Arai K, Itou N. Food protein-induced enterocolitis syndrome in neonate: summary of 10 patients. In: JACI; 2008. p. S105.
10. Mehr S, Frith K, Barnes EH, Campbell DE. Food protein-induced enterocolitis syndrome in Australia: a population-based study, 2012-2014. J Allergy Clin Immunol. 2017;140:1323–30. https://doi.org/10.1016/j.jaci.2017.03.027.
11. Nowak-Wegrzyn A, Spergel JM. Food protein–induced enterocolitis syndrome: not so rare after all! J Allergy Clin Immunol. 2017;140:1275–6.
12. Ruffner MA, Ruymann K, Barni S, et al. Food protein-induced enterocolitis syndrome: insights from review of a large referral population. J Allergy Clin Immunol Pract. 2013;1:343–9. https://doi.org/10.1016/j.jaip.2013.05.011.
13. Miceli Sopo S, Monaco S, Badina L, et al. Food protein-induced enterocolitis syndrome caused by fish and/or shellfish in Italy. Pediatr Allergy Immunol. 2015;26:731–6. https://doi.org/10.1111/pai.12461.
14. Mehr S, Kakakios A, Frith K, Kemp AS. Food protein-induced enterocolitis syndrome: 16-year experience. Pediatrics. 2009;123 https://doi.org/10.1542/peds.2008-2029.
15. Sopo SM, Giorgio V, Dello Iacono I, et al. A multicentre retrospective study of 66 Italian children with food protein-induced enterocolitis syndrome: different management for different phenotypes. Clin Exp Allergy. 2012;42:1257–65. https://doi.org/10.1111/j.1365-2222.2012.04027.x.
16. Greenhawt M, Bird JA, Nowak-Węgrzyn AH. Trends in provider management of patients with food protein–induced enterocolitis syndrome. J Allergy Clin Immunol Pract. 2017;5:1319–1324.e12. https://doi.org/10.1016/j.jaip.2016.11.036.
17. Vasilopoulou I, Charitidou E, Trigka M. Food protein induced enterocolitis syndrome to fish: a report of 20 cases. Clin Transl Allergy. 2015;5:P55. https://doi.org/10.1186/2045-7022-5-S3-P55.
18. Loo EXL, Sim JZT, Loy SL, et al. Associations between caesarean delivery and allergic outcomes: results from the GUSTO study. Ann Allergy Asthma Immunol. 2017;118:636–8. https://doi.org/10.1016/J.ANAI.2017.02.021.
19. Kuitunen M, Kukkonen K, Juntunen-Backman K, et al. Probiotics prevent IgE-associated allergy until age 5 years in cesarean-delivered children but not in the total cohort. J Allergy Clin Immunol. 2009;123:335–41. https://doi.org/10.1016/J.JACI.2008.11.019.
20. Jensen ET, Kappelman MD, Kim HP, et al. Early life exposures as risk factors for pediatric eosinophilic esophagitis. J Pediatr Gastroenterol Nutr. 2013;57:67–71. https://doi.org/10.1097/MPG.0b013e318290d15a.
21. Nowak-Wegrzyn A, Sampson HA, Sicherer SH. Food protein-induced enterocolitis syndrome caused by solid food proteins. Pediatrics. 2003;111:829.

22. Prematta TR, Fausnight TB. Identical twin Hispanic male infants with nonbilious non-bloody vomiting and diarrhea. Allergy Asthma Proc. 2010;31:111–5. https://doi.org/10.2500/aap.2010.31.3398.
23. Shoda T, Isozaki A, Kawano Y. Food protein-induced gastrointestinal syndromes in identical and fraternal twins. Allergol Int. 2011;60:103–8. https://doi.org/10.2332/allergolint.09-CR-0168.
24. Alexander ES, Martin LJ, Collins MH, et al. Twin and family studies reveal strong environmental and weaker genetic cues explaining heritability of eosinophilic esophagitis. J Allergy Clin Immunol. 2014;134:1084–1092.e1. https://doi.org/10.1016/j.jaci.2014.07.021.
25. Spergel JM, Brown-Whitehorn TF, Beausoleil JL, et al. 14 years of eosinophilic esophagitis: clinical features and prognosis. J Pediatr Gastroenterol Nutr. 2009;48:30–6. https://doi.org/10.1097/MPG.0b013e3181788282.
26. Tan JA, Smith WB. Non-IgE-mediated gastrointestinal food hypersensitivity syndrome in adults. J Allergy Clin Immunol Pract. 2014;2:355–7. https://doi.org/10.1016/j.jaip.2014.02.002.
27. Fernandes BN, Boyle RJ, Gore C, et al. Food protein-induced enterocolitis syndrome can occur in adults. J Allergy Clin Immunol. 2012;130:1199–200.
28. Caubet JC, Ford LS, Sickles L, et al. Clinical features and resolution of food protein-induced enterocolitis syndrome: 10-year experience. J Allergy Clin Immunol. 2014;134:382–389.e4. https://doi.org/10.1016/j.jaci.2014.04.008.
29. Levy Y, Danon YL. Food protein-induced enterocolitis syndrome - not only due to cow's milk and soy. Pediatr Allergy Immunol. 2003;14:325–9. https://doi.org/10.1034/j.1399-3038.2003.00039.x.
30. Sopo SM, Giorgio V, Dello II, et al. A multicentre retrospective study of 66 Italian children with food protein-induced enterocolitis syndrome: different management for different phenotypes. Clin Exp Allergy. 2012;42:1257–65. https://doi.org/10.1111/j.1365-2222.2012.04027.x.
31. Burks AW, Casteel HB, Fiedorek SC, et al. Prospective oral food challenge study of two soybean protein isolates in patients with possible milk or soy protein enterocolitis. Pediatr Allergy Immunol. 1994;5:40–5. https://doi.org/10.1111/j.1399-3038.1994.tb00217.x.
32. Hwang JB, Sohn SM, Kim AS. Prospective follow-up oral food challenge in food protein-induced enterocolitis syndrome. Arch Dis Child. 2009;94:425–8. https://doi.org/10.1136/adc.2008.143289.
33. Jarvinen-Seppo K, Sickles L, Nowak-Wegrzyn A. Clinical characteristics of children with Food Protein-Induced Enterocolitis (FPIES). JACI. 2010;125:AB85. https://doi.org/10.1016/j.jaci.2009.12.335.
34. Ruiz-Garcia M, Díez CE, Sanchez Garcia S, Rodriguez del Rio P. Diagnosis and natural history of food protein-induced enterocolitis syndrome in children from a Tertiary Hospital in Central Spain. J Investig Allergol Clin Immunol. 2014;24:352–3.

Immune Basis of Food Protein-Induced Enterocolitis Syndrome

3

M. Cecilia Berin

Introduction

FPIES is a distinct non-IgE-mediated food allergy that remains an immunologic mystery. The clinical evidence strongly supports the concept that FPIES is an antigen-specific disease, and FPIES is commonly referred to as a cell-mediated food allergy. However, there is a lack of satisfying immunologic explanation for the vomiting, lethargy, and pallor that are commonly observed within 1–4 hours after food ingestion. The objective of this chapter is to review the current evidence supporting the immune pathophysiology of FPIES.

FPIES Reactions Are Associated with Systemic Immune Activation

It has been noted for many years that individuals with FPIES who react to an oral food challenge have an increase in circulating neutrophils as measured 4–6 hours after symptom onset [1, 2]. This increase in neutrophils is a consistent feature and is included in Powell's diagnostic criteria [1]. There is also a growing body of evidence demonstrating eosinophil activation in FPIES. Wada et al. reported that positive FPIES reactions after oral food challenge (OFC) were associated with an elevation of stool eosinophil-derived neurotoxin (EDN) compared to baseline, and baseline samples were slightly but significantly elevated compared to age-matched healthy infants [3]. Eosinophils are resident cells of the small intestine, and it was not clear if this appearance was due to eosinophil activation, intestinal leak, or both. However, IgA in the stool was not elevated post OFC, and presence of elevated

M. C. Berin (✉)
Pediatrics, Icahn School of Medicine at Mount Sinai, New York, NY, USA
e-mail: cecilia.berin@mssm.edu

T. F. Brown-Whitehorn, A. Cianferoni (eds.), *Food Protein Induced Enterocolitis (FPIES)*,
https://doi.org/10.1007/978-3-030-21229-2_3

EDN was not limited to those with diarrhea symptoms [3]. In a follow-up study, Wada and colleagues examined activation markers on eosinophils in the systemic circulation. They found that not only was fecal EDN highly increased after OFC but that circulating eosinophils also had elevated expression of the activation marker CD69 [4].

We have used mass cytometry to simultaneously profile the response of multiple cell types in peripheral blood after oral food challenge in FPIES [5]. Consistent with the observations of Wada and colleagues, we observed activation of eosinophils (increased CD25 expression) in peripheral blood after a symptomatic OFC, but this was not unique to eosinophils. Neutrophils were not only increased in number but also were activated (increased CD25 and CD69). NK cells were activated (increased CD25), and lymphocytes were significantly reduced from the circulation and those remaining had elevated expression of CD69. Monocytes were unchanged in number but were markedly activated (increased expression of the myeloid activation marker CD163). Monocyte activation during a symptomatic FPIES challenge was confirmed by whole blood gene expression that showed elevated expression of arginase 1 and CEACAM1. Cellular assays showed a reduced capacity for activation of monocytes after positive oral food challenge, suggesting that they were in a refractory state. Thus, we found a pan-leukocyte activation in peripheral blood associated with positive food challenges [5]. This suggests that the immune activation is downstream of a mediator released into the systemic circulation, such as a cytokine or other signaling molecule. Cytokines in circulation have been measured and found to be increased after positive food challenges. IL-10 and IL-8 were described as elevated post-challenge by both Caubet et al. [6] and Kimura et al. [7] Kimura et al. also found an elevation in IL-2 in symptomatic patients ($n = 4$) but not in asymptomatic patients ($n = 2$), which also suggests that T cells are activated during symptomatic food challenge. C-reactive protein has been also described as elevated during FPIES reactions [8–10], supporting the concept of systemic inflammation during a positive challenge.

One hypothesis to consider is that severe vomiting may itself result in immune activation. Most studies on FPIES have used control groups that are asymptomatic, such as those with a history of FPIES who have outgrown their disease, and so are not controlled for symptoms. Shimomura et al. investigated the relationship between serum cortisol and circulating neutrophils and eosinophils after FPIES OFC [11]. They found that serum cortisol was elevated in symptomatic but not asymptomatic challenges and that serum cortisol significantly correlated with changes in neutrophil count. Glucocorticoids are known to induce an acute leukopenia and neutrophilia due to altered expression of adhesion molecules, and therefore increased serum cortisol could potentially lead to leukocyte changes. Correlation does not equal causation, but because immune changes have been measured after the onset of symptoms, it is possible that symptoms are responsible for immune activation rather than immune activation being responsible for symptoms. A careful analysis of the kinetics of immune activation in relationship to symptom onset is needed.

Food-Specific Immunoglobulins and FPIES

Although FPIES is a non-IgE-mediated food allergy, up to 30% of FPIES patients may have low levels of IgE against the food [2, 12, 13]. The presence of IgE to the triggering food was found to be associated with persistent FPIES [14], and there are reports of patients with FPIES developing IgE-mediated reactions to the food [14], as well as case reports of FPIES developing after resolution of IgE-mediated allergy to egg or milk [15, 16]. As will be described below, a Th2-biased immune profile has been described for both IgE-mediated food allergy and FPIES, and the presence of IgE may reflect this T cell phenotype. There are conflicting reports of the levels of other immunoglobulin isotypes in FPIES. McDonald et al. reported pre-challenge food-specific immunoglobulin levels in 18 children undergoing food challenge for FPIES [17]. Milk-, egg-, and soy-specific IgA antibodies and egg- and soy-specific IgG antibodies were elevated in symptomatic versus asymptomatic infants. Antibodies were only elevated to the foods which triggered reactions. Konstantinou et al. examined casein-specific IgA responses in patients with milk FPIES, outgrown milk FPIES, non-milk FPIES, and IgE-mediated milk allergy [18]. There was no difference between those with active versus outgrown milk FPIES. Shek et al. observed that patients with milk-induced FPIES had significantly lower milk-specific IgG4 levels than healthy controls, patients with IgE-mediated milk allergy, or patients with allergic eosinophilic gastroenteritis [19]. Although differences in immunoglobulin levels may reflect other underlying mechanisms of pathophysiology, such as altered intestinal permeability or T cell profile, these data do not support a direct role for food-specific antibodies in FPIES.

Food-Specific T Cells and FPIES

FPIES is often described as a cell-mediated response to food proteins. Food-specific proliferation of lymphocytes was reported as increased or unchanged in patients with FPIES [20, 21]. Morita et al. published a comprehensive analysis of T cell cytokine responses in 65 children with non-IgE-mediated milk allergies (comprised of a mix of patients with symptoms consistent with FPIES, food protein-induced enteropathy, and food protein-induced proctocolitis) [22]. Patients were compared to control subjects and those with IgE-mediated allergy to milk. Those with non-IgE-mediated gastrointestinal allergies to milk produced significantly more TNFα, IL-2, IL-3, IL-5, IL-6, IL-10, and IL-13 compared to control subjects, while IFN-γ and IL-17 were not increased. Proliferative responses were noted to α-, β-, and κ-casein and β-lactoglobulin, with minimal proliferative responses to α-lactalbumin. Caubet et al. also examined the proliferation and cytokine response to milk in children with FPIES, IgE-mediated milk allergy, and resolved IgE-mediated milk allergy [6]. As with IgE-mediated milk allergy, there was Th2 cytokine production together with IL-6 and TNFα after in vitro stimulation with caseins. We also examined T cell responsiveness to milk, soy, and rice in children with FPIES to those foods. Using a CD154-based approach that effectively detects antigen-specific T cells in IgE-mediated food allergy [23, 24], we did not find any evidence for increased numbers or altered phenotype of food-specific

CD4+ T cells in FPIES [5]. Therefore, evidence for a pathogenic antigen-specific T cell response in FPIES is lacking, despite the pan-activation of lymphocytes that is observed following oral food challenge.

Future Directions and Challenges in FPIES Research

We now understand that FPIES reactions to foods are associated with a broad systemic inflammatory response, with increased and activated neutrophils, decreased and activated T cells and eosinophils, activated monocytes and NK T cells, increased circulating cytokines, and increased CRP. We are missing an understanding of the trigger. How does a food specifically initiate this systemic inflammatory response when the key elements of antigen recognition – antibodies and T cells – show no evidence for increased food-specific recognition? Perhaps an unconventional antigen is involved in the activation of an invariant or innate cell population (such as intraepithelial lymphocytes in the intestine or NK cells of the liver). A view to events in the local mucosa is needed. The second major unknown is the relationship between symptoms and the systemic inflammatory response. Do symptoms cause inflammation, does inflammation cause symptoms, or do they arise from the same trigger but are unrelated? A high-dimensional immune profiling approach with careful kinetics related to onset of symptoms is needed to place these findings in a network that may indicate causation. These ideas are summarized in Fig. 3.1.

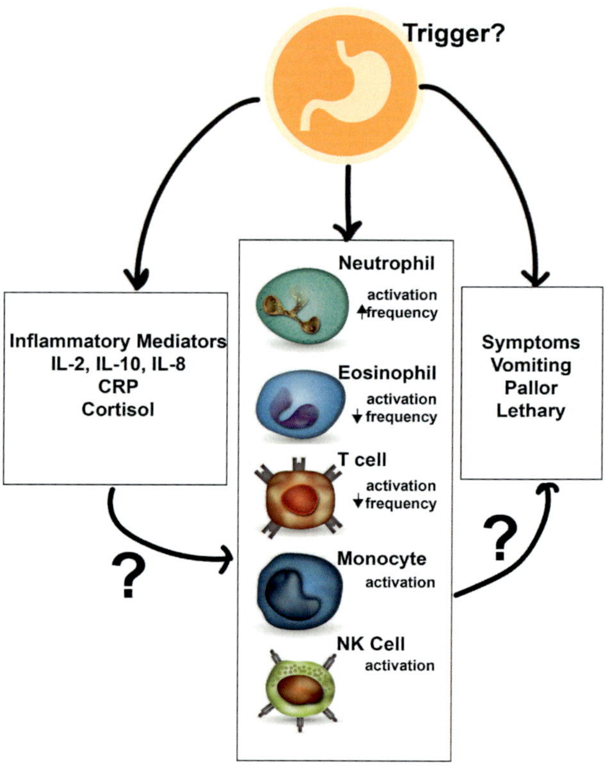

Fig. 3.1 Summary of immune pathways activated in FPIES. Ingestion of the causative food(s) of FPIES results in the development of symptoms after approximately 2 hours. After development of symptoms, systemic immune activation measured by increase in serum inflammatory mediators or changes in blood leukocyte populations is observed. Questions remaining to be answered include identifying the antigen-specific trigger of reactions and determining the relationship between mediators, cells, and symptoms in order to determine causative mechanisms underlying symptoms

Key Points

- Food protein-induced enterocolitis syndrome reactions are associated with systemic immune activation, involving systemic cytokine and chemokine release and activation of monocytes, lymphocytes, NK cells, eosinophils, and neutrophils.
- The mechanism of systemic immune activation in response to specific foods remains unknown, as there is a lack of compelling evidence for antibody or T cell-based pathophysiology.
- Studies of immune events in the gastrointestinal mucosa in response to FPIES trigger foods are needed to elucidate the mechanism of food recognition.

Acknowledgments Thanks to Ms. Lisette Peres for research assistance in the preparation of this manuscript.

References

1. Powell GK. Milk- and soy-induced enterocolitis of infancy. Clinical features and standardization of challenge. J Pediatr. 1978;93(4):553–60.
2. Sicherer SH, Eigenmann PA, Sampson HA. Clinical features of food protein-induced enterocolitis syndrome. J Pediatr. 1998;133(2):214–9.
3. Wada T, Toma T, Muraoka M, Matsuda Y, Yachie A. Elevation of fecal eosinophil-derived neurotoxin in infants with food protein-induced enterocolitis syndrome. Pediatr Allergy Immunol. 2014;25:617–9.
4. Wada T, Matsuda Y, Toma T, Koizumi E, Okamoto H, Yachie A. Increased CD69 expression on peripheral eosinophils from patients with food protein-induced enterocolitis syndrome. Int Arch Allergy Immunol. 2016;170(3):201–5.
5. Goswami R, Blazquez AB, Kosoy R, Rahman A, Nowak-Wegrzyn A, Berin MC. Systemic innate immune activation in food protein-induced enterocolitis syndrome. J Allergy Clin Immunol. 2017;139:1885.
6. Caubet JC, Bencharitiwong R, Ross A, Sampson HA, Berin MC, Nowak-Wegrzyn A. Humoral and cellular responses to casein in patients with food protein-induced enterocolitis to cow's milk. J Allergy Clin Immunol. 2016;139:572.
7. Kimura M, Ito Y, Shimomura M, et al. Cytokine profile after oral food challenge in infants with food protein-induced enterocolitis syndrome. Allergol Int. 2017;66(3):452–7.
8. Kimura M, Ito Y, Tokunaga F, et al. Increased C-reactive protein and fever in Japanese infants with food protein-induced enterocolitis syndrome. Pediatr Int. 2016;58(9):826–30.
9. Kimura M, Shimomura M, Morishita H, Meguro T, Seto S. Serum C-reactive protein in food protein-induced enterocolitis syndrome versus food protein-induced proctocolitis in Japan. Pediatr Int. 2016;58(9):836–41.
10. Pecora V, Prencipe G, Valluzzi R, et al. Inflammatory events during food protein-induced enterocolitis syndrome reactions. Pediatr Allergy Immunol. 2017;28(5):464–70.
11. Shimomura M, Ito Y, Tanaka H, Meguro T, Kimura M. Increased serum cortisol on oral food challenge in infants with food protein-induced enterocolitis syndrome. Pediatr Int. 2018;60(1):13–8.
12. Nomura I, Morita H, Hosokawa S, et al. Four distinct subtypes of non-IgE-mediated gastrointestinal food allergies in neonates and infants, distinguished by their initial symptoms. J Allergy Clin Immunol. 2011;127(3):685–688 e681-688.
13. Nomura I, Morita H, Ohya Y, Saito H, Matsumoto K. Non-IgE-mediated gastrointestinal food allergies: distinct differences in clinical phenotype between Western countries and Japan. Curr Allergy Asthma Rep. 2012;12(4):297–303.

14. Caubet JC, Ford LS, Sickles L, et al. Clinical features and resolution of food protein-induced enterocolitis syndrome: 10-year experience. J Allergy Clin Immunol. 2014;134(2):382–9.
15. Duffey H, Egan M. Development of Food Protein-Induced Enterocolitis Syndrome (FPIES) to egg following Immunoglobulin E (IgE)-mediated egg allergy. Ann Allergy Asthma Immunol. 2018;121:379.
16. Barni S, Mori F, Bianchi A, Pucci N, Novembre E. Shift from IgE-mediated cow's milk allergy to food protein-induced enterocolitis syndrome in 2 infants. Pediatr Allergy Immunol. 2018;29(4):446–7.
17. McDonald PJ, Goldblum RM, Van Sickle GJ, Powell GK. Food protein-induced enterocolitis: altered antibody response to ingested antigen. Pediatr Res. 1984;18(8):751–5.
18. Konstantinou GN, Ramon B, Grishin A, et al. The role of casein-specific IgA and TGF-beta in children with Food Protein-Induced Enterocolitis Syndrome to milk. Pediatr Allergy Immunol. 2014;25:651.
19. Shek LPC, Bardina L, Castro R, Sampson HA, Beyer K. Humoral and cellular responses to cow milk proteins in patients with milk-induced IgE-mediated and non-IgE-mediated disorders. Allergy. 2005;60(7):912–9.
20. Van Sickle GJ, Powell GK, McDonald PJ, Goldblum RM. Milk- and soy protein-induced enterocolitis: evidence for lymphocyte sensitization to specific food proteins. Gastroenterology. 1985;88(6):1915–21.
21. Hoffman KM, Ho DG, Sampson HA. Evaluation of the usefulness of lymphocyte proliferation assays in the diagnosis of allergy to cow's milk. J Allergy Clin Immunol. 1997;99(3):360–6.
22. Morita H, Nomura I, Orihara K, et al. Antigen-specific T-cell responses in patients with non-IgE-mediated gastrointestinal food allergy are predominantly skewed to T(H)2. J Allergy Clin Immunol. 2013;131(2):590–592 e591-596.
23. Berin MC, Grishin A, Masilamani M, et al. Egg-specific IgE and basophil activation but not egg-specific T cells correlate with phenotypes of clinical egg allergy. J Allergy Clin Immunol. 2018;142:149.
24. Chiang D, Chen X, Jones SM, et al. Single-cell profiling of peanut-responsive T cells in patients with peanut allergy reveals heterogeneous effector TH2 subsets. J Allergy Clin Immunol. 2018;141(6):2107–20.

Acute Food Protein-Induced Enterocolitis Syndrome

4

Shyam R. Joshi, Rory E. Nicolaides, and J. Andrew Bird

Introduction

Food protein-induced enterocolitis syndrome (FPIES) is a non-IgE cell-mediated gastrointestinal food hypersensitivity that is now better understood and characterized through research advancements over the past two decades. FPIES is considered a heterogeneous disorder that can vary dramatically in terms of symptomatology and natural history based on a patient's nationality, age of symptoms onset, duration of symptoms, and association with IgE-mediated food allergy.

Patients typically present in their first year of life with recurrent vomiting, diarrhea, and potentially hypovolemic shock. Despite its severity, the condition remains poorly understood, and clinician awareness remains very low. The first international consensus guidelines were published in 2017, which established a more standardized approach to diagnosis and management [1].

FPIES can present in two unique phenotypes: acute and chronic. Acute FPIES is the better classified of the two and involves repetitive vomiting, diarrhea, pallor, dehydration, and in severe cases, shock with metabolic acidosis within 1–4 hours after ingestion of the culprit food [1]. While it can develop at any age, it predominantly occurs in infancy before 12 months of age. The pathophysiology is not currently well understood, but early studies have shown complex interactions between the innate, cellular, and humoral immune systems in the gastrointestinal tract in association with food ingestion. Cow's milk is the most universally implicated food (in up to 40% of cases), but other common FPIES triggers include soy, rice, oats, and

S. R. Joshi
Section of Allergy and Immunology, Oregon Health and Science University, Portland, OR, USA

R. E. Nicolaides · J. A. Bird (✉)
Pediatrics, Division of Allergy and Immunology, University of Texas Southwestern Medical Center, Dallas, TX, USA
e-mail: drew.bird@utsouthwestern.edu

T. F. Brown-Whitehorn, A. Cianferoni (eds.), *Food Protein Induced Enterocolitis (FPIES)*, https://doi.org/10.1007/978-3-030-21229-2_4

fish, which have high geographic correlations [2]. In contrast, chronic FPIES occurs before the age of 3 months and is due to regular ingestion of either cow's milk or soy formula. The typical clinical presentation involves protracted diarrhea, vomiting, hypoalbuminemia, and poor weight gain [2].

Diagnosis of acute FPIES relies on a detailed history taken by the clinician due to the lack of characteristic laboratory, imaging, and endoscopic biopsy findings. Oral food challenge (OFC) is the gold standard for both diagnosis and evaluation for spontaneous resolution of FPIES; however, OFC is not always necessary if the history is convincing. Management revolves around avoidance of the culprit food(s) with most patients usually "outgrowing" it in the first 3 years of life, although it can rarely persist past the first decade of life.

Historical Perspective

In the 1960s–1970s, Goldman et al., Gryboski et al., and Powell each published reports describing the gastrointestinal manifestations of cow's milk allergy [3–5]. Their patients were noted to have vomiting, blood-streaked diarrhea, abdominal distention, septic appearance, and peripheral neutrophilia after ingestion of cow's milk-based formula at a very young age. The symptoms improved with administration of intravenous fluids and transitioning to a hydrolyzed casein-based formula. Recurrence was noted with reintroduction of cow's milk- or soy-based formula within 1–4 hours. Powell proposed the first set of diagnostic criteria and an oral challenge protocol several years later in 1978 [5].

In the 1990s, two larger case series by Burks et al. and Sicherer et al. further characterized this non-IgE-mediated condition with more refined diagnostic criteria and food challenge protocols [6, 7]. The 10th revision of the International Statistical Classification of Diseases and Related Health Problems (ICD-10) provided the first uniform code for FPIES (K52.2) in 2015. More recently, FPIES has become more prominent in pediatric literature; the first international consensus guidelines on the diagnosis and management of FPIES was published in 2017 [1].

Epidemiology

Prevalence

The prevalence of FPIES has yet to be defined, owing primarily to the lack of large-scale epidemiologic studies. In addition, significant selection bias is present due to the majority of cases being reported by large, academic, tertiary referral centers. A recent review of all reported cases suggests that FPIES is more common than was previously thought [8]. This may be due to an actual increase in the disease occurrence or improved awareness and recognition of the disorder in the healthcare community. Katz et al. published the first large-scale, population-based prospective study with a reported prevalence of 0.34% (cumulative incidence of 3 per 1000) of

CM-FPIES in an Israeli cohort over a 2-year period [8]. In the United States and Italy, two series reported a yearly prevalence of approximately 1% when observing FPIES cases presenting in an outpatient pediatric allergy setting [9, 10]. The only large-scale, country-wide study to date was performed in Australia, reporting an incidence of acute FPIES in infants <24 months over a period of 2 years as 15.4/100,000/year [11].

Age of Onset

The age of symptom onset is highly correlated to the age of introduction of foods into the diet. Infants with earlier introduction of CM- or soy-based formula typically have earlier onset compared to those who are initially breastfed. Symptoms often occur after the first or second ingestion of the food trigger in 75% of cases [12]. In comparison, chronic FPIES occurs at a younger age and is considered a disorder of newborns occurring after the introduction and repeated exposure to CM or soy protein formulas. The median age of onset ranges from 1 to 4 weeks of age [3, 5].

The age of onset of FPIES to CM or soy typically occurs at a younger age than FPIES caused by solid foods. The onset of CM-FPIES or FPIES due to soy ranges from the first days of life to 12 months of age (median age 3–5 months) versus the median age of solid food-induced FPIES being 4–7 months [2]. The earlier onset of CM- or soy-induced FPIES is reflective of their earlier introduction compared to solid foods.

Older children and adults can develop acute FPIES de novo most commonly due to crustaceans (shrimp, lobster, prawn, and crab), mollusks (scallop, oyster, and mussel), egg, and fish. This is often associated with a previous history of intolerance or avoidance of the specific food until later in life [13, 14].

Risk Factors

Information on risk factors is limited. The majority of the data is from an Israeli birth cohort study by Katz et al. FPIES was more frequently seen in infants born to Jewish parents and in those born by cesarean section [8]. It has been postulated that cesarean section delivery can disrupt the gut microbiota which may promote the development of FPIES, but additional studies are needed to further elucidate this theory [15]. Other associations evaluated were not found to be significant including gender, gestational age, birth weight, maternal age, number of siblings, maternal daily dairy consumption, and age at CM protein introduction. Mehr et al. noted a slight increase in rate of acute FPIES to multiple foods in infants who are exclusively breastfed for less than 4 months, which needs to be further investigated [11]. Based on this limited data, no specific food introduction or avoidance is recommended in the prenatal or postnatal period [1].

A meta-analysis has shown a slight male predominance of 50–60% [15]. No hereditary or familial association has been evaluated; however, there have been three reports of siblings with FPIES all of whom were twins (two fraternal, one identical). Of these, all pairs reacted to the same food protein (CM in two sets, soy protein in one set) [16, 17].

Although FPIES is a non-IgE-mediated disorder, concurrent atopic disease and family history of atopy are frequent, ranging from 20% to 77% in two cohort studies [10, 16]. Eczema is the most common atopic disorder present at diagnosis around the world, but higher rates are reported in studies from Australia and the United States (Australia 46%, the United States 34%) compared to other countries (Italy 9%, Japan 10%, and Israel 7%) [8–10, 15]. Other atopic disorders have been reported but at less frequent rates likely due to their later onset [9, 12].

Pathophysiology

The immunopathophysiology of FPIES is poorly understood and requires further studies to clarify its underlying mechanisms. In general, FPIES is considered a cell-mediated disorder with involvement of many different cell types and immunomodulating agents leading to inflammation in the gastrointestinal tract, primarily in the colon but also noted in the ileum [2]. It is hypothesized that this inflammation results in increased intestinal permeability and fluid shifts into the gastrointestinal lumen, with a potential serotonin pathway involvement due to the studied effects of ondansetron improving emetic symptoms in acute FPIES [18]. There have been explorations into the relationship between IgE and non-IgE mechanisms in patients with FPIES, mainly due to the fact that some patients with FPIES have specific IgE to their trigger food as well as Th2 responses similar to those occurring in patients with IgE-mediated allergy [16, 19–21]. Table 4.1 offers a summary of the evidence for proposed mechanisms contributing to the pathophysiology of FPIES.

Clinical Presentation

Acute FPIES is a heterogeneous disorder, and its clinical presentation can greatly vary depending on several factors including age of onset, nationality, and association with IgE-mediated sensitivity. It is linked to intermittent, infrequent exposure to the culprit food (in contrast to chronic FPIES which occurs after regular, frequent exposure). Symptoms ensue after ingestion of the offending food in sufficient quantity, and reactions are dependent on the quantity of food allergen ingested. Patients not infrequently report previously tolerating the food in up to 40% of cases [11]. Age of presentation is dependent on when particular foods are introduced into the diet; for example, children who are started on either cow's milk- or soy-based formula from birth can have symptoms as early as the first few days of life. On the other hand, children who are exclusively breastfed and have cow's milk-FPIES may not develop symptoms until later due to delayed introduction of cow's milk protein.

Table 4.1 Proposed mechanisms in the pathophysiology of acute FPIES

Implicated cell type or proposed mechanism	Evidence supporting hypothesis	Potential implications
Cellular mechanisms		
T cells	CD4+ T lymphocytes: Older studies: PBMC stimulation by the causal antigen induced greater cell proliferation in children with FPIES than in children with negative OFC [22] Recent studies: no difference between children with CM-FPIES and controls in the proliferation of T cells or Th2 cytokines after casein stimulation [23] CD4+ CD25+ regulatory T cells: Higher frequency of circulating CD4+ CD25+ regulatory T cells specific for CM-protein in children outgrowing non-IgE-mediated CM-hypersensitivity, compared to children with active CM hypersensitivity [24]	There exists an immunologically mediated response rather than intolerance, with further studies needed to elucidate the precise mechanisms A potential explanation for why infants with FPIES become tolerant to their food trigger over time, in general
Eosinophils	Infants with FPIES have demonstrated clusters of eosinophils on intestinal biopsies FPIES patients with chronic diarrhea show Charcot-Leyden crystals in stool samples [25] Eosinophilia in peripheral blood with increased expression of CD69 [26]	Eosinophils are not only a normal part of the GI tract, but their accumulation is commonly seen in many GI disorders (IgE-mediated hypersensitivity, eosinophilic gastroenteropathies, GERD, IBD, and food-induced proctocolitis), suggesting a potential continuum of eosinophilic GI disorders with similar underlying mechanisms
Neutrophils	FPIES patients had neutrophils in gastric juice aspirates and in stool mucus [27] Peripheral blood neutrophilia and leukocytosis have been demonstrated in patients with acute FPIES [12, 28]	Neutrophilia likely secondary to the secretion of different cytokines and chemokines (e.g., TNF, IL-8) related to the inflammatory reaction
Platelets	Thrombocytosis is found in acute and chronic FPIES, recorded in 63% of episodes in one series [12]	Likely a stress-induced acute phase reactant

(continued)

Table 4.1 (continued)

Implicated cell type or proposed mechanism	Evidence supporting hypothesis	Potential implications
Monocytes	Children with active but unresolved FPIES showed significant activation of cells of the innate immune system via mass cytometry whole blood profiling, as well as pan T-cell activation and redistribution from the bloodstream after positive OFC; not shown in those who had outgrown FPIES [29]	There is systemic involvement of the innate immune system in FPIES reactions
Mast cells	Children with active CM-FPIES compared to those who had developed tolerance but with previous CM-FPIES had (1) higher baseline tryptase levels and (2) no change in tryptase after OFC [1]	Could suggest a potential presence of increased mast cell load or low-grade intestinal mast cell activation
Humoral mechanisms		
IgG, IgG4, IgE, and IgA to casein	Significantly lower levels of serum CM-specific α-, β-, and κ-csIgG4, casein-IgG, and casein-IgG4 were found in children with active CM-FPIES compared to those who tolerated CM [23, 30, 31] Children with a positive OFC versus negative OFC had higher levels of IgA-specific antibodies to CM, egg, and soy and higher IgG antibodies specific to egg and soy [32] The presence of IgE to the triggering food was described as a marker of persistent FPIES; patients with resolved CM-FPIES have been reported to have IgE-mediated reactions to CM [19]	IgE may be locally produced in the intestinal mucosa, but not reaching the serum, and playing a role in food reactions
Cytokines		
IFN-γ, TNF-α, TGF-β1 imbalance and interactions	FPIES patients have been found to have increased TNF-α expression on epithelial and lamina propria cells and decreased expression of TGF-β1 receptors in their intestinal mucosa on duodenal biopsies [33] Deficient T-cell-mediated TGF-β responses to casein were demonstrated in children with active CM-FPIES [31]	Food-allergen stimulated T-lymphocytes secrete pro-inflammatory cytokines IL-4, IFN-γ, TNF-α, which could act synergistically to increase intestinal permeability and subsequently contribute to the influx of antigen into the submucosa [34] TGF-β1 antagonizes IFN-γ to protect the gut epithelial barrier and prevent foreign antigen penetration, making a lower expression of TGF-β1a potential contributor to FPIES reactions

Implicated cell type or proposed mechanism	Evidence supporting hypothesis	Potential implications
Interleukins	IL-8 serum levels were significantly higher in CM-FPIES patients after positive OFC compared to those with negative OFC [1] When compared to children with IgE-CM allergy, children with CM-FPIES had a significantly higher casein-specific IL-9 production [23] IL-10 was significantly increased in the serum of children with CM-FPIES after a positive OFC and not after negative OFC to CM. When studying the supernatant from a PBMC cultured with casein, IL-10 was lower in children with active CM-FPIES compared to resolved CM-FPIES [23] Children with non-IgE-mediated milk allergies (a mix of patients with FPIES, food protein-induced enteropathy, and food protein-induced proctocolitis) produced significantly more TNF-α, IL-2, IL-3, IL-5, IL-6, IL-10, and IL-13 compared to control subjects (children with IgE-mediated allergy to milk) [21]	IL-8 has been implicated in the initiation of inflammatory processes, as a chemoattractant of neutrophils into tissues, and it has been proposed that it is released through IgE-related mechanisms, although with an unclear role in FPIES [35] IL-9 derived from mast cells has been suggested to be involved in intestinal anaphylaxis [36], with further investigation needed regarding its role in FPIES IL-10 may play a role in how FPIES tolerance to CM is developed
IP-10	Patients with active CM-FPIES and positive OFC trended toward an increased level of serum IP-10 [23]	IP-10 is secreted in response to IFN-γ with a role as a chemoattractant for activated T-cells and has been shown to be increased in patients with IgE-mediation food allergy [37]. It may also be involved in mechanisms behind non-IgE-mediated food allergies as well

Abbreviations: *PBMC* peripheral blood mononuclear cell, *OFC* oral food challenge, *GERD* gastroesophageal reflux disease, *IBD* inflammatory bowel disease, *csIgG4* casein-specific IgG4, *IL* interleukin, *IFN-γ* interferon-γ, *TNF-α* tumor necrosis factor-α, *TGF-β1* transforming growth factor -β1, *IP-10* interferon γ-induced protein 10

Classic Acute FPIES

Acute FPIES is characterized by repetitive, forceful emesis (possibly exceeding 20 episodes) that usually begins within 1–4 hours after ingestion (ranges from 30 minutes to 6 hours), decreased level of activity, pallor, and dehydration (Table 4.2). In severe cases, patients can become lethargic with associated hypotension, hypothermia, and/or abdominal distention.

While repetitive protracted vomiting is nearly universal in cases of acute FPIES, other symptoms can be highly variable depending on the specific phenotype of the patient, which can vary over time. Diarrhea is often watery (infrequently with mucus) and occurs in 7–54% of patients [9, 10, 19]. Bloody stools are only present

Table 4.2 Clinical features of mild and severe acute FPIES in relation to ingestion of culprit food [1]

	Mild-to-moderate acute FPIES	Severe acute FPIES
Clinical presentation		
1–4 hours after ingestion	Vomiting onset (can range from 30 minutes to 6 hours): 1–3 episodes of intermittent vomiting, can be bilious Decreased activity level Pallor Mild dehydration, able to rehydrate with oral fluids	Vomiting onset (can range from 30 minutes to 6 hours): ≥4 episodes of forceful, bilious vomiting Decreased activity level, lethargy Pallor Dehydration requiring intravenous hydration Can be present: Hypotension Abdominal distention Hypothermia Hospitalization
4-24 hours after ingestion	Diarrhea onset (typically between 5 and 10 hours): mild watery diarrhea, can be bloody Persistent symptoms from above	Diarrhea onset (typically between 5 and 10 hours): severe watery diarrhea, can be bloody Persistent and/or progressive symptoms from above
More than 24 hours after ingestion	Symptoms typically have resolved after appropriate management and avoidance of culprit food(s)	Symptoms have often resolved after appropriate management and avoidance of culprit food(s) Sequelae from reaction may remain
Between ingestions or after elimination	Asymptomatic Normal growth	Asymptomatic Normal growth
Laboratory findings	Elevated neutrophil count Thrombocytosis Peripheral eosinophilia Elevated CRP Stool positive for leukocytes, eosinophils, or increased carbohydrate content	Elevated neutrophil count Thrombocytosis Peripheral eosinophilia Elevated CRP Stool positive for leukocytes, eosinophils, or increased carbohydrate content Methemoglobinemia Metabolic acidosis

Abbreviations: *FPIES* food protein-induced enterocolitis syndrome

in 4–10% of acute FPIES cases in most of the world; however, up to 47% of infants in Japan have reported bloody stools likely representing a distinct phenotype [38, 39]. Typically, diarrhea develops 5–10 hours after ingestion and can persist for up to 24 hours [8, 12]. Overall, diarrhea has been reported more frequently in children under the age of 2 months and in specific geographic regions such as Japan and South Korea [6, 27, 40].

Other clinical manifestations such as lethargy, pallor, hypotension, hypothermia, and dehydration can be present. Several cohort studies have shown an incidence of hypotension in up to 15% of cases, but this frequency is likely subject to selection bias based on reports from tertiary referral centers [11, 19, 41]. Hypothermia of less than 36 °C has been present in up to 10% of cases. Ileus requiring laparoscopy has also been reported [42]. The discrepancies in the clinical presentations found throughout the literature are likely due to the heterogeneous nature of the disorder.

Reactions typically resolve within 24 hours after ingestion. During the time in-between exposures or after elimination of the culprit food, patients are generally asymptomatic and are observed to grow normally. There have been no reported deaths due to an acute FPIES reaction.

Clinical Variation Based on Age

Clinical presentation can vary considerably based on the age of the patient. While repetitive protracted vomiting is the most common presenting symptom in all types of acute FPIES, diarrhea is much more common in infants less than 2 months of age [6]. In addition, acute FPIES with bloody stools has been found to have an earlier presentation (day 7 of life) compared to acute FPIES with non-bloody stools (day 26 of life) in a single Japanese study [43].

Acute FPIES in adults is not well studied likely due to its relative rarity. Tan and Smith published the largest reported case series of 31 patients with acute non-IgE-mediated food hypersensitivity that shared multiple characteristics with infantile acute FPIES [14]. The main difference in regard to clinical presentation in adult patients was that the predominant symptom was abdominal pain, which was present in 77% of patients, followed by vomiting and diarrhea at 71% and 58%, respectively. The median time to symptoms onset was 60 minutes [14]. While this disorder shares many similarities to infantile acute FPIES, it may represent a distinct disorder with a different pathophysiologic etiology.

Atypical Acute FPIES

While the majority of patients with symptoms consistent with acute FPIES do not have specific IgE (sIgE) sensitivity by serology or skin prick testing to the offending food, there is a subgroup of patients who do have detectable sIgE. The term "atypical FPIES" has been coined to describe this specific disorder. In addition to classic acute FPIES symptoms, these patients can also have symptoms consistent with an acute IgE-mediated hypersensitivity such as urticaria, angioedema, flushing, and wheezing. This condition will be further discussed under *Laboratory Testing* later in this chapter.

Chronic FPIES

The clinical presentation of chronic FPIES is distinct from acute FPIES and is discussed in detail in Chapter 6.

Food Triggers

FPIES can be caused by any food, but the most commonly reported are cow's milk, soy, rice, and oats [8]. There are geographic variations in the prevalence of food triggers, due to genetic factors, population differences, and regional dietary and breastfeeding practices. It should be noted that although most infants and children will react to a single food (usually CM), a portion also react to multiple triggers. Average percentages for reacting to a single or multiple triggers are reported in Table 4.3 [1].

Cow's Milk and Soy

Cow's milk has consistently been the most common food associated with acute FPIES around the world except for Australia where rice is the predominant trigger [8–11, 27, 44]. A likely explanation to the CM's prevalence is that it is often one of the earliest foods introduced into an infant's diet. In the United States, Italy, the United Kingdom, and Australia, the percentage of acute FPIES cases due to CM were as high as 67%, 65%, 46%, and 33%, respectively [10, 11, 15]. While data is very limited, baked milk exposure to children with CM-FPIES appears to be safe, but additional studies are needed before any definitive conclusions can be made [11].

FPIES due to soy or combined cow's milk/soy proteins in formula-fed infants is common in the United States with rates up to 25–50% of total cases, but it is uncommon in other countries such as Israel, Italy, Spain, the United Kingdom, and Australia (Table 4.4) [15, 44]. Up to 40% of infants will react to both CM and soy, notably most in the first 6 months of life with the introduction of formula [27]. This number is similar to other studies conducted in the United States by Ruffner,

Table 4.3 Average percentage of children with acute FPIES with reactions reported to varying numbers of food triggers [1]

Number of food triggers	Percentage of children with acute FPIES reporting reactions
1	60–70%
2–3	20–30%
≥4	10%

Table 4.4 Common food co-allergy in children with acute FPIES [1, 8, 11, 45]

FPIES to:	Clinical cross-reactivity or co-allergy	Observed occurrence
Cow's milk	Soy	<16–40%
	Other animal milk	Unknown[a]
	Lactose-free milk	100%
	Extensively hydrolyzed casein-based formula	<10–21%
	Amino acid-based formula	<4%
	Any solid food	<16–28%
Soy	Cow's milk	<30–40%
	Any solid food	<16%
Solid food (any)	Another solid food	<44%
	Cow milk or soy	<25%
Legumes	Soy	<80%
Rice	Oats	<42%
	Wheat	5%
	Corn	9%
Poultry	Other poultry	<40%
Fish	Other foods (not fish)	42%

This summary should be interpreted with caution as much of this data is derived from single center studies with more severe phenotypes likely over-estimating the risk of co-allergy

Abbreviation: *FPIES* food protein-induced enterocolitis syndrome

[a]While the cross-reactivity/co-allergy is unknown between cow's milk and milk from other animals, goat's milk and sheep's milk should be avoided due to high homology of protein sequences. Milks from donkey, camels, or both might be better options as they are typically well tolerated in IgE-mediated CM allergy

Sicherer et al., Nowak-Wegrzyn and Muraro, and Burks et al. [6, 7, 9, 16]. However, this finding was not seen in Italian and Israeli studies, potentially due to differences in the microbiome or the order of food introduction [8, 10].

Children with CM-FPIES are at a higher risk of having solid food FPIES, most commonly due to grains [1, 11]. Systematic introductions of solids should be considered to minimize risk of a reaction either at home or in a clinical setting. This will be further discussed later in this chapter.

The onset of CM- and/or soy-induced FPIES can occur from the first days of life to 12 months of age (median age 3–5 months) which is significantly earlier than solid food FPIES [2]. The earlier onset is likely reflective of the earlier introduction to CM- or soy-based formula compared to other foods.

Breastfeeding

It has been suggested that there is a protective role of breastfeeding against FPIES because reports of acute FPIES to CM and soy in exclusively breastfed infants are rare [40, 46–48]. A higher report of symptoms during breastfeeding in Japan of up to 30% of infants developing FPIES suggests a potential genetic disposition [39]. Current theories for the protective mechanisms of breast milk include that the food trigger is highly processed, the threshold dose may not be reached in breast milk, and the presence of immunoglobulin A.

Routine elimination of trigger foods from the maternal diet while breastfeeding is not indicated if the infant remains asymptomatic [1]. Conversely, if symptomatic FPIES occurs while exclusively breastfeeding, elimination of the suspected food trigger should be initiated, and allergist consultation is advised. If no improvement were noted, then it would be reasonable to consider discontinuation of breastfeeding while introducing hypoallergenic formula.

Solid Food FPIES

The most common solid food FPIES triggers in the United States and Australia are rice and oats (Fig. 4.1). In these countries, co-reactivity to both rice and oats has been reported in slightly more than one third of patients with rice-induced FPIES (Table 4.5) [9, 11, 19]. Other grains that have been implicated to a much lesser extent include wheat, corn, quinoa, mixed grains, and barley [9, 11].

Reactions to rice may be more severe due to their findings that children with rice FPIES compared to CM or soy were significantly more likely to require intravenous fluid resuscitation than those with milk or soy FPIES (42% vs. 15%, $P = 0.02$) [51]. This is supported by previous findings by Nowak-Wegrzyn et al. which showed that 14 patients with solid food FPIES trended toward more severe reactions such as hospitalization, shock, and sepsis evaluations [16].

There is an ongoing discussion regarding the risk of cross-reactivity between grains (Table 4.4). The majority of this data is gathered from single academic centers with more severe phenotypes, making extrapolations to the general public limited. It is postulated that if there is an increased sensitivity, it may be explained by the shared

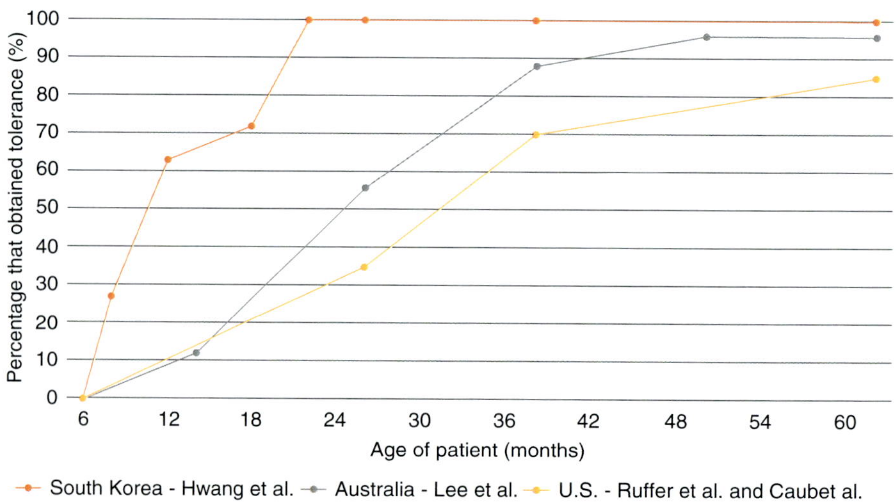

Fig. 4.1 Age at tolerance acquisition for CM-FPIES in South Korea, Australia, and the United States [9, 19, 27, 49]

Table 4.5 Overview of foods implicated in acute FPIES [9, 11, 45, 50]

Milk	Legumes
Cow's milk	Soy
Goat's milk	Green peas
Hen's egg	Kidney beans
Egg white	Green beans
Egg yolk	Lentils
Grains	Vegetables
Rice	Sweet potato
Oat	Potato
Wheat	Carrot
Corn	Squash
Barley	Other[a]
Quinoa	Fruit
Meats	Banana
Chicken	Apple
Turkey	Pear
Beef	Peach
Pork	Plum
Lamb	Strawberry
Seafood	Melon
Hake	Other[b]
Tuna	Peanut
Salmon	Tree nuts
Shellfish (shrimp, crab, lobster, prawn)	Tapioca
Mollusks	
Other[c]	

[a]Other vegetables include tomato, spinach, cauliflower, cucumber, and pumpkin

[b]Other fruits include avocado, blueberry, apricot, grape, cherry, coconut, mango, pineapple, orange, kiwi, and raspberry

[c]Other fish include sole, monkfish, swordfish, sea bass, mackerel, gilthead sea bream, and megrim

taxonomic relationship between rice and other grains (oats, rye, barley, wheat) which are in the same subfamily Festucoidae [51]. Of these, wheat, rye, and barley are more genetically distant from rice and oats because they exist in the same tribe Triticeae. This could suggest that children with rice- or oats-induced FPIES may be less likely to have cross-reactions with these more distantly related cereals, supported by the fact that there have been only three cases in literature of a child having FPIES caused by both rice and wheat [11, 52]. It has been shown in a single center report that the majority of oats FPIES patients will tolerate cow's milk protein [53].

Solid FPIES: Other Foods

There are a number of other foods implicated in causing solid food FPIES including meat (chicken, turkey, lamb, beef, pork), fruit (apples, pears, peaches, bananas), vegetables (sweet potato, white potato, squash), legumes (green pea, lentils), seafood (fish, shrimp, mollusks), egg white, and peanuts [12, 16, 54]. A list of foods that have been implicated is shown in Table 4.5.

It has been observed that older children and adults can develop de novo FPIES reactions to crustacean shellfish (shrimp, crab, and lobster), fish, mollusks, and egg, with a similar syndrome of nausea, abdominal cramps, vomiting, and diarrhea [2].

Solid FPIES: Regional Differences

There are geographic variations in some of these solid food FPIES triggers, similar to the regional differences seen in CM- and soy protein-FPIES occurrences. For example, fish (sole, salmon, tuna, cod) is the most common trigger in infants and toddlers in Spain and Italy, with a typical age of onset older than for cereals and other solid foods [12, 45, 55]. This is likely due to the importance of fish in the diet of these cultures and early age of introduction of fish compared to other countries.

Diagnosis

Diagnostic Criteria

Acute FPIES remains a clinical diagnosis, and recognition of classic symptoms is important to be able to quickly diagnose and manage this potentially serious condition. A detailed history by the clinician is the most important tool in making the diagnosis and should include a comprehensive account of the reaction, specific symptoms involved, timing of symptoms in relation to food ingestion, all possible food triggers, and reproducibility of the reaction with repeated exposures to suspected food(s).

No laboratory or radiologic findings are specific for the diagnosis of FPIES, and routine use of radiologic tests is not recommended. On the other hand, certain laboratory tests can help support the diagnosis of acute FPIES and, more importantly, may be helpful to rule out other conditions that may present with similar symptoms. Laboratory and radiologic testing will be discussed in detail later in this chapter.

Several diagnostic criteria have been proposed over the years, but those outlined by Nowak-Węgrzyn et al. in the "International Consensus Guidelines for the Diagnosis and Management of Food Protein-Induced Enterocolitis Syndrome" are the most widely accepted [1]. Table 4.6 outlines the major and minor criteria. The diagnosis of acute FPIES requires the patient meet the major criterion as well as at least three of the minor criteria. One important difference compared to previously published criteria is the removal of the age limit of less than 9 months of age as more recent literature highlights the fact that while more commonly occurring in infancy, acute FPIES can occur in older children or even adults.

Oral Food Challenge Protocol

While an oral food challenge (OFC) is considered the gold standard in confirming the diagnosis, if an infant presents with a convincing history, an OFC is not indicated and should possibly be avoided as the risk may outweigh the benefit. This is

Table 4.6 Diagnostic criteria for patients presenting with possible acute FPIES [1]

Major criterion	Minor criteria
Vomiting in the 1- to 4-hour period after ingestion of the suspect food and absence of classic IgE-mediated allergic skin or respiratory symptoms	1. A second (or more) episode of repetitive vomiting after eating the same suspect food 2. Repetitive vomiting episode 1–4 hours after eating a different food 3. Extreme lethargy with any suspected reaction 4. Marked pallor with any suspected reaction 5. Need for emergency department visit with any suspected reaction 6. Need for intravenous fluid support with any suspected reaction 7. Diarrhea in 24 hours (usually 5–10 hours) 8. Hypotension 9. Hypothermia

The diagnosis of FPIES requires that a patient meets the major criteri on and ≥3 minor criteria. If only a single episode has occurred, a diagnostic OFC should be strongly considered to confirm the diagnosis, especially because viral gastroenteritis is so common in this age group. Furthermore, although not a criteria for diagnosis, it is important to recognize that acute FPIES reactions will typically completely resolve over a matter of hours compared with the usual several-day time course of gastroenteritis. The patient should be asymptomatic and growing normally when the offending food is eliminated from the diet

especially true if the patient has had ≥ two episodes in the past 6 months and has done well while avoiding the suspected food [19]. If only a single episode has occurred and the diagnosis remains unclear, then an OFC should be strongly considered to confirm the diagnosis as several other conditions, such as infectious gastroenteritis, can present with similar symptoms in this age group. In addition, OFCs can be useful if multiple foods are being considered to reduce the burden of over-restricting the patient's diet.

Multiple OFC protocols have been published internationally, but practices highly vary as the total dose and dosing regimen has not been systematically studied [1, 20, 28, 56, 57]. Figure 4.2 summarizes the recently published "International Consensus Guidelines for the Diagnosis and Management of Food Protein-Induced Enterocolitis Syndrome" by Nowak-Węgrzyn et al. [1]

All protocols emphasize the need for close supervision and that all OFCs should be performed in a clinical setting as up to 50% of positive OFC results require treatment with intravenous fluids [20]. While some reactions can be managed by oral fluid rehydration and/or intramuscular ondansetron, the ability to place an emergent peripheral intravenous line and having immediate access to intravenous fluids are a necessity [1, 8]. In addition, many expert clinicians routinely place peripheral intravenous access prior to all FPIES OFCs.

Dosing practices are highly variable with some protocols providing the entire challenge dose in a single serving, while others separate them over a 30–60-minute period. The current consensus recommends 0.06–0.6 g (typically 0.3 g) of food protein per kilogram of body weight that is administered in three equal doses over 30 minutes. This regimen is used to approximate a serving size and should not generally exceed 3 g of food protein or 10 g of total food (100 mL of liquid). A more conservative approach can be used in patients with a history of severe reactions by

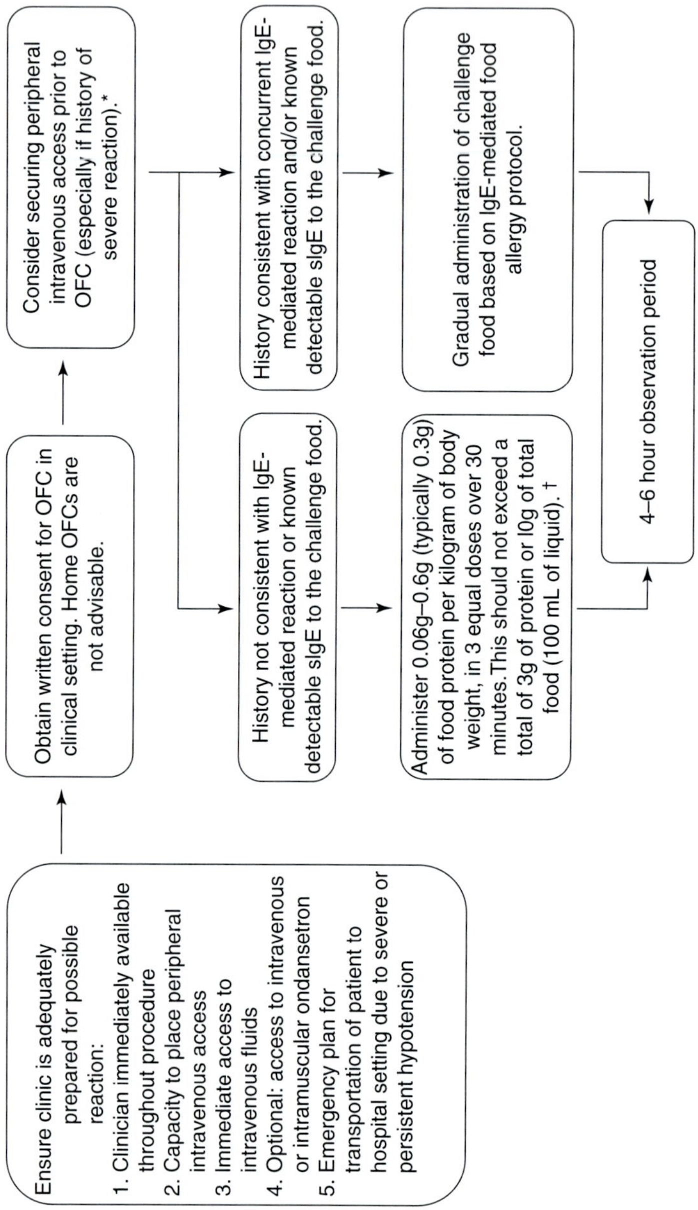

*Optional baseline CBC with differential can be drawn to assist in the interpretation of the OFC and is up to the provider performing the food challenge.

†Lower starting doses, longer intervals between doses, and longer observation period should be considered in patients with a history of severe reactions. If a very low OFC dose is given and tolerated, then a full serving (e.g., 3g of food protein) is to be given after 2–3 hours of observation.

Fig. 4.2 Sample oral food challenge protocol for acute FPIES

reducing the initial dose or by increasing the interval between doses. If a very low dose of food is initially given without a reaction during a 2–3-hour observation period, then a full serving size should be provided with an additional 4–6 hours of observation.

Patients with a history suggestive of a concomitant IgE-mediated food allergy or with known sIgE to the challenge food should undergo an OFC cautiously. A more gradual approach is recommended following protocols used for IgE-mediated food allergy challenges. The main difference in the FPIES challenge compared to a standard OFC for diagnosis of IgE-mediated food allergy is that a longer post-challenge observation of 4–6 hours should be implemented to evaluate for an acute FPIES reaction.

OFCs are, in addition, very useful in determining whether FPIES has been outgrown, which will be discussed later in this chapter under the management section as well as in Chapter 12.

Interpretation of Oral Food Challenge

The diagnostic criteria used for an OFC are slightly different than that used on initial presentation based on history alone. Previous iterations have included regularly evaluating complete blood counts (CBC) and stool studies; however, more recent studies have shown less profound changes in neutrophil counts and frequency of diarrhea leading to a more phenotype-driven approach in interpreting OFCs [19, 27].

The major and minor criteria for OFC interpretation are shown in Table 4.7. A challenge is considered failed (i.e., positive) if the major criterion is met along with ≥ two minor criteria. Notably, the major criterion is the same as the diagnostic criteria used when diagnosing acute FPIES on initial presentation (Table 4.6), but the minor criteria significantly vary. Most remarkably, the OFC diagnostic criteria include the addition of an increase in peripheral neutrophilia by 1500 neutrophils above baseline. While baseline and challenge neutrophil counts are optional in the

Table 4.7 Diagnostic criteria for the interpretation of OFCs in patients with a history of possible or confirmed FPIES [1]

Major criterion	Minor criteria
Vomiting in the 1- to 4-hour period after ingestion of the suspect food and the absence of classic IgE-mediated allergic skin or respiratory symptoms	1. Lethargy 2. Pallor 3. Diarrhea 5–10 hours after food ingestion 4. Hypotension 5. Hypothermia 6. Increased neutrophil counts of ≥1500 neutrophils above the baseline count

The OFC will be considered diagnostic of FPIES (i.e., positive) if the major criterion is met with ≥ two minor criteria

OFC outlined earlier in this chapter, they can be used diagnostically based on clinician preference.

As the use of ondansetron has increased for the management of an acute FPIES reaction, concern has arisen that it may prevent patients from meeting all of the diagnostic criteria during an OFC. In the clinical setting, the treating provider should have the flexibility to decide when its use is appropriate, weighing the risk of misdiagnosis by blunting the reaction early versus the benefit of possibly averting more severe symptoms. The OFC may be considered positive in this setting even if only the major criterion is met. For research purposes, providers should more strictly adhere to the diagnostic criteria to ensure challenge positivity.

Laboratory, Skin, and Radiologic Testing

As mentioned previously, there are no laboratory or radiologic findings that are specific for FPIES. No routine tests are specifically indicated, but in some instances, testing can be useful in ruling out other conditions that have similar presenting symptoms.

Laboratory Findings

While very nonspecific, several laboratory abnormalities have been seen during episodes of acute FPIES reactions including elevated peripheral neutrophils, thrombocytosis, elevated C-reactive protein, elevated peripheral eosinophil counts, and in severe cases, methemoglobinemia. These findings are not considered pathognomonic but may be helpful in supporting the diagnosis (Table 4.2).

Elevated Neutrophil Count

An increase of peripheral neutrophils was first noted by Gryboski in 1967 [4]. Since that first report, several studies have noted a similar increase, which peaked 6 hours after last ingestion of the culprit food [19, 28]. The increase in neutrophils can be quite profound but highly variable, with one study reporting an average increase of 4500 neutrophils/mm^3 (range, 700–15,000/mm^3) after a positive challenge [16]. The elevation is thought to be multifactorial due in part to an increase in IL-8 as well as cortisol [23, 58, 59]. This elevation has historically been an important diagnostic criterion but now is only an optional laboratory value used during an observed OFC [1].

Thrombocytosis

Peripheral thrombocytosis has also been observed in one case series with 63% of patients presenting with a platelet count of >500 × 10^9 platelets/L [12]. This elevated level is thought to be secondary to a stress response leading to a release of platelets from the spleen into the peripheral circulation.

Peripheral Eosinophilia

A Japanese study found a correlation of elevated eosinophilia in patients with acute FPIES during OFC [60]. Infants who were classified as early-onset (≤10 days of age) had a median peripheral eosinophilia of 9.8% compared to late-onset infants at 5.4%. In addition, peripheral eosinophilia was found to have a positive correlation with the incidence of vomiting and bloody stools. This increase is thought to be secondary to Th2-driven inflammation given increased levels of IL-4, IL-5, and IL-13 previously observed [21]. Peripheral eosinophilia has also been negatively correlated with age of tolerance acquisition, which may make it a useful measure of good prognosis, although multiple confounders are present [60].

Elevated C-Reactive Protein

C-reactive protein (CRP) has been closely evaluated in Japanese infants as a possible biomarker for disease activity and severity [61]. CRP was found to be elevated in 55% of infants with FPIES, making it an important tool in differentiating it from food protein-induced proctocolitis (FPIP) in this population of patients [61]. In addition, it was positively correlated with fevers in the FPIES group. A more recent study has shown a correlation with elevated CRP levels during positive FPIES OFC with later age of tolerance acquisition (21 months compared to 12 months, $p < 0.01$) [60]. It is unclear if these correlations can be extrapolated to other patient populations or if they are unique to Japanese infants.

Methemoglobinemia and Acidemia

Methemoglobinemia was first observed by Murray and Christie in a retrospective analysis of US infants when challenged with cow's milk protein [41]. Additional studies have noted this transient elevation in severe cases of acute and chronic FPIES, which was managed with methylene blue [27, 62]. Metabolic acidosis can also be observed due to protracted hypotension.

Food-Specific IgE Testing (Serum Serology and Skin Prick)

Food-specific IgE testing has not been found to be helpful during the initial evaluation of acute FPIES as the majority of patients have undetectable serum IgE to the suspected FPIES food at the time of diagnosis [7, 8, 10, 11, 16, 19]. In addition, negative-specific IgE testing does not rule out acute FPIES.

Nevertheless, food sIgE testing is helpful in specific situations. First, a minority of patients with acute FPIES may have detectable IgE on either serology or skin prick testing to the suspected food. This is termed "atypical FPIES." Based on limited data, children with atypical FPIES to CM may demonstrate slower resolution of their FPIES [7, 19, 49, 63]. This has been consistent in other food groups as well, although with significant lower number of patients studied. Another important caveat is that patients that are sIgE negative at initial diagnosis of FPIES can develop sIgE sensitivity at a rate of 2–20% during follow-up [7, 10, 19, 63]. This is especially important when evaluating for resolution of FPIES with OFC as patients may benefit from a more conservative protocol if sIgE sensitivity is detected. It is recommended that all patients with CM-FPIES should undergo sIgE testing before OFC [1].

Likely due to FPIES association with atopy, approximately 20–40% of patients with FPIES will develop sIgE sensitivity to other common food allergens at some point during their clinical course [7, 19]. Therefore, a careful history needs to be taken at follow-up visits, and appropriate testing should be considered.

Stool Studies

Changes in stool have been noted during acute FPIES reactions including the presence of blood, leukocytes, and eosinophils as well as increased carbohydrate content [28, 64]. While stool studies are not routinely used in the diagnosis of FPIES, they can be useful in supporting the diagnosis or in ruling out other conditions.

Endoscopic Evaluation and Gastric Lavage

Endoscopy is rarely if ever indicated for evaluation of acute FPIES as reactions are episodic and typically completely resolve within 24 hours of ingestion of the culprit food. In a single center study in South Korea, greater than ten leukocytes per high-powered field during gastric juice analysis was associated with a positive acute FPIES OFC to cow's milk [65]. Prior to the establishment of clinical criteria for FPIES, endoscopy was performed not infrequently in patients with chronic symptoms. Earlier studies on chronic FPIES during which endoscopy was performed have shown inflammatory changes in the small and large intestine including jejunal villous atrophy, edema, and increased infiltration of inflammatory cells (lymphocytes, plasma cells, eosinophils, and mast cells), friable colonic mucosa, and minute ulcers throughout the colon [6, 33, 66]. These findings are discussed in further detail in Chapters 6 and 7.

Radiologic Findings

Similar to laboratory testing, no radiologic findings are specific for FPIES, and such testing should not be routinely used in the diagnosis of FPIES [1]. Earlier studies have shown several nonspecific findings in chronic FPIES infants such as air-fluid levels, intramural gas, narrowing and thumb printing of the sigmoid and rectum, and thickening of the plicae circulares in the duodenum [12, 42]. If the patient has an atypical presentation for FPIES, radiologic evaluation may be helpful in ruling out other conditions with similar symptomatology if clinically appropriate.

Atopy Patch Testing

Patch testing has not been thoroughly evaluated as a means to identify the offending food as only two small studies have been performed to date [67, 68]. Fogg et al. showed a sensitivity of 100%, specificity of 71%, positive predictive value of 75%, and negative predictive value of 100% [67]. While this was encouraging, a follow-up study with a slightly older population of patients by Jarvinen et al. showed a sensitivity of 11.8%, specificity of 85.7%, positive predictive value of 40%, and negative predictive value of 54.5% [68]. Based on conflicting data from the two studies, patch testing is not recommended at this time. Additional investigation is needed to further explore patch testing as certain factors may be important in optimizing the quality of this test including age of patient, time since most recent reaction, and the definition of the a positive test.

Differential Diagnosis

Challenges to Diagnosis

It is imperative to keep a high index of suspicion for acute FPIES to avoid misdiagnosis, delays in diagnosis, and unnecessary diagnostic and therapeutic interventions experienced by patients with acute FPIES. This is likely due to the fact that acute FPIES does not have a specific biomarker or a pathognomonic symptom that points to the diagnosis.

Mehr et al. reported that only 2 of 19 children with acute FPIES presenting to the emergency department were discharged with the correct diagnosis in a single tertiary medical center in Australia [12]. Of the patients who presented with acute FPIES in the hospital, they commonly received additional evaluations of abdominal imaging studies (34%), sepsis workups (28%), and surgical consultations (22%). A retrospective Italian review by Fiocchi et al. revealed the time lapse between the first episode and the diagnosis was approximately 8 months, with a median of three acute events before the diagnosis was made [69]. Most recently, Mehr et al. found that only 25% of those children presenting to a health professional after their first acute FPIES reaction were diagnosed correctly [11]. In the same study, only 44% had a correct diagnosis after their second FPIES episode and 30% after their third reaction. A comprehensive summary of differential diagnoses to consider and their distinguishing characteristics from FPIES are presented in Table 4.8.

Infection: Sepsis and Acute Viral Gastroenteritis

The most frequent misdiagnoses seen in patients with acute FPIES are acute viral gastroenteritis and sepsis. The diagnosis of sepsis in FPIES patients has been reported in 20 different publications and is more likely to be diagnosed in younger children (mean age at presentation, 11 months) [69]. Shared symptoms of the two include a sudden onset of weakness, vomiting, tachycardia, hypotension, and signs of end-organ dysfunction including oliguria and neurological impairment, as well as laboratory features of leukocytosis, thrombocytosis, elevated neutrophil count, metabolic acidosis, and methemoglobinemia. The difference in FPIES when contrasted to sepsis is the lack of fever (except in the Japanese population where it can be seen in up to 13% of acute FPIES reactions) which is one of the cardinal symptoms of sepsis, and only normal or slightly elevated inflammatory markers are

Table 4.8 Differential diagnoses to be considered in FPIES and their distinguishing characteristics from FPIES [1, 69–71]

Diagnosis or disease	Distinguishing characteristics from FPIES
Most common	
Sepsis	Cardinal symptom of sepsis is often fever. Also common is elevated inflammatory markers and requires more than fluid resuscitation to improve symptoms
Acute viral gastroenteritis	Usually a single episode of illness, frequently with known sick contacts. Other symptoms including fever and more profuse diarrhea. Etiologic viruses or bacteria identified in stool studies and often less serious and less rapid presentation than FPIES
Presentation typically at younger ages (i.e., *within the first few months of life)*	
Necrotizing enterocolitis	Present in newborns and younger infants. Progression of symptoms even more rapid than FPIES. Shock, bloody stools, and abdominal radiographs with intramural gas. Physical exam with abdominal distention to acute abdomen. Requires more than fluid resuscitation to improve symptoms
Pyloric stenosis	Usually presents between 3 and 6 weeks of life, rarely after 12 weeks. Projectile vomiting, usually of curdled milk from sitting in the stomach. Decreased bowel movements. Physical exam signs of "palpable olive" in the right epigastrum
Hirschsprung disease	Delayed passage of meconium. Physical exam with abdominal distention. Can lead to failure to thrive
Gastroesophageal reflux	Incidence increases between 2 and 6 months of age, decreases after 7 months, resolved in 85% of infants by 12 months. More chronic and not as severe emesis. No lower gastrointestinal symptoms
Presentation typically at later ages (i.e., *beyond the first few months of life)*	
Anaphylaxis	Usually rapid onset of symptoms (within minutes to 2 hours of exposure) and other symptoms present (e.g., urticaria, angioedema, wheezing, stridor, etc.). Positive IgE testing
Food aversion	Physical avoidance of food introduction, such as shutting mouth or turning head from bottle, breast, spoon, or food or taking small amount of food and then rejecting, arching back, crying, or spitting out food
Lactose intolerance	Emesis after ingestion of lactose-containing dairy products or cow's milk and, when severe, also bloating, cramping, diarrhea, and stomach rumbling
Celiac disease	Progressive malabsorption and no relationship between the time of food ingestion and development of symptoms. Laboratory testing positive for celiac serology

Coagulation defects	Does not correlate with ingestion of a specific food. Symptoms of easy bleeding. Abnormal coagulation laboratory testing
Alpha-1 antitrypsin deficiency	Does not correlate with ingestion of a specific food. Present with white stools, pruritis, jaundice, and possible pulmonary involvement. Physical exam with hepatomegaly. Abnormal hepatic laboratory testing. Positive family history of alpha-1 antitrypsin deficiency, emphysema, or unexplained cirrhosis
Ehlers-Danlos syndrome	Does not correlate with ingestion of a specific food. Symptoms of hypotonia, joint hypermobility, easy bruising, fragile vessels, velvety, and hyperextensible skin. Positive family history
Mast cell activation syndrome	Does not correlate with ingestion of a specific food. Other symptoms including flushing, itching, nasal congestion, cough, wheeze, diarrhea, and recurrent abdominal pain. Laboratory testing with mast cell mediators (e.g., N-methyl histamine, prostaglandin D2, or 11-β-prostaglandin F2 α, leukotriene E4)
Neurological disorders (cyclic vomiting)	Does not correlate with ingestion of a specific food. Requires more than fluid resuscitation to improve symptoms
Obstructive problems (malrotation, volvulus, Ladd bands)	Does not correlate with ingestion of a specific food. Requires more than fluid resuscitation to improve symptoms. Abdominal imaging with evidence of obstruction
Other categories of disorders to consider	
Food protein-induced gastrointestinal disorders: IgE-mediated (immediate gastrointestinal hypersensitivity, oral allergy syndrome) Mixed (allergic eosinophilic esophagitis, gastritis, and gastroenterocolitis), Non-IgE-mediated (celiac disease, food protein-induced enteropathy, and proctocolitis)	Eosinophilic gastroenteropathies: usually does not correlate with ingestion of a specific food. More chronic and less severe symptoms of vomiting. Laboratory testing more likely to have positive IgE tests Food protein-induced enteropathy: usually does not temporally correlate with ingestion of a specific food. More chronic and less severe symptoms. Most common associated food are CM, soy, wheat, and egg white
Immune enteropathies Autoimmune enteropathy, immunodeficiency, and inflammatory bowel disease	Less common in infants. Does not correlate with ingestion of a specific food. Requires more than fluid resuscitation to improve symptoms

(continued)

Table 4.8 (continued)

Diagnosis or disease	Distinguishing characteristics from FPIES
Inborn errors of metabolism Most common: urea cycle defects, organic acidemias, hereditary fructose intolerance, hyperammonemic syndromes Also: propionic/methylmalonic aciduria, maple syrup urine disease, hyperinsulinism-hyperammonemia syndrome, mitochondrial disorders, ketothiolase deficiency, and pyruvate dehydrogenase deficiency)	Reactions to fruits and sugars (saccharose, fructose). Symptoms of developmental delay, neurological abnormalities. Physical exam with organomegaly. Laboratory testing abnormalities specific to disorder. Requires more than fluid resuscitation to improve symptoms
Primary immunodeficiencies Common variable immunodeficiency, selective IgA deficiency, agammaglobulinemia, X-linked hyper-IgM syndrome, severe combined immunodeficiency, DiGeorge syndrome, bare lymphocyte syndrome, chronic granulomatous disease, Wiskott-Aldrich syndrome, Hermansky-Pudlak syndrome, and immune dysregulation, polyendocrinopathy, and enteropathy syndrome	Diarrhea is usually the more common presenting gastrointestinal symptom. Also present with recurrent infections and other syndromic-specific associated signs and symptoms. Does not correlate with ingestion of a specific food. Requires more than fluid resuscitation to improve symptoms

Abbreviation: *FPIES* food protein-induced enterocolitis syndrome

observed [40]. Acute viral gastroenteritis has been reported in at least 16 publications. It presents similarly to FPIES with vomiting but has other features that distinguish it including fever, more profuse diarrhea, etiologic viruses or bacteria identified in stool studies, and often less serious or rapid presentation than FPIES. In addition, symptoms from FPIES typically resolve within 24 hours, while gastroenteritis has a clinical course of several days.

Differential Diagnoses by Age Range

Other pathologies mistaken for FPIES that often present in infancy include necrotizing enterocolitis, pyloric stenosis, Hirschsprung disease, and allergic proctocolitis. Some that may present at later ages include anaphylaxis, IgE-mediated food allergy, food aversion, coagulation defects, alpha-1 antitrypsin deficiency, Ehlers-Danlos syndrome, mast cell activation syndrome, neurological disorders (cyclic vomiting), and obstructive problems (malrotation, volvulus, Ladd bands).

Gastrointestinal Disorders and Inborn Errors of Metabolism

There are many greater categories of disease entities that belong in the differential diagnosis of FPIES. The first of these are the food protein-induced gastrointestinal disorders, ranging from IgE-mediated (immediate gastrointestinal hypersensitivity and oral allergy syndrome), mixed (allergic eosinophilic esophagitis, gastritis, and gastroenterocolitis), and non-IgE-mediated (celiac disease, food protein-induced enteropathy and proctocolitis) [70]. Other gastrointestinal disorders to consider are gastroesophageal reflux disease, lactose intolerance, and immune enteropathies (autoimmune enteropathy, immunodeficiency, and inflammatory bowel disease). Additional information is in Chap. 7. Next are the inborn errors of metabolism, most commonly urea cycle defects, organic acidemias, hereditary fructose intolerance, and hyperammonemic syndromes, but can range broadly to include propionic/methylmalonic aciduria, maple syrup urine disease, hyperinsulinism-hyperammonemia syndrome, mitochondrial disorders, ketothiolase deficiency, and pyruvate dehydrogenase deficiency [1]. Chapter 8 provides additional information.

Primary Immunodeficiencies

Finally, there are a host of primary immunodeficiencies that can be included in the differential in which children develop gastrointestinal symptoms, more so for the chronic rather than acute phase of FPIES due to diarrhea as the unifying presenting symptom. These include common variable immunodeficiency, selective IgA deficiency, agammaglobulinemia, X-linked hyper-IgM syndrome, severe combined immunodeficiency, DiGeorge syndrome, bare lymphocyte syndrome, chronic granulomatous disease, Wiskott-Aldrich syndrome, Hermansky-Pudlak syndrome, and immune dysregulation, polyendocrinopathy, and enteropathy syndrome [71].

Natural History

While acute FPIES was initially considered a disorder of infancy, more recent reports have shown that it can begin in or extend into late childhood or adulthood [13, 14, 45]. The age of tolerance to acute FPIES caused by CM and soy is generally thought to be earlier than those caused by solid foods. However, there is substantial variability in these studies including significant geographic influence and likely selection bias. For example, in all three large cohort studies in the United States, no difference was seen in the age of FPIES resolution between CM/soy and solid foods [9, 16, 19]. In contrast, Lee et al. showed that in an Australian cohort, FPIES caused by solid foods tended to have a later age of resolution except for when the trigger was rice [49].

As no clear guidelines exist on how frequently OFCs should be conducted to determine if tolerance has been reached, it could be assumed that the available data is likely overestimating the age of tolerance as parents and clinicians tend to continue avoidance instead of conducting OFCs. A large prospective study with regular challenge intervals is needed to better understand the natural history of acute FPIES.

Tolerance to Acute FPIES Caused by Cow's Milk

US studies have estimated the average age of tolerance for CM-FPIES to be between 2.3 and 5.1 years [9, 16, 19]. Resolution rates for CM- or soy-induced FPIES are 35% by age 2, 70% by age 3, and 85% by age 5. These rates are significantly lower than those from other countries. A large Israeli cohort had CM-FPIES tolerance rates of 50% by 1 year, 89% by 2 years, and 90% by 3 years of age [8]. An Australian study had similar results with tolerance of 88% by 3 years of age [49]. Korean data also showed faster resolution rates at 27% at 6 months, 63% at 10 months, 72% at 14–16 months, and 100% at 18–20 months [27]. The average age of CM-FPIES resolution in the Korean study was 12 months of age. This data is summarized in Fig. 4.1.

It has been postulated that the significantly higher average age of resolution in the United States may be in part due to a higher percentage of patients in this population having a concomitant IgE-mediated allergy to CM [49], but interpretation of the data must also consider that challenges are not offered in a uniform manner or at set intervals in the observational US cohorts. Patients in the Korean cohort, in particular, were challenged every 2 months [27], and patients in the United States are typically told to avoid the allergen for at least 1 year before consideration for a repeat challenge.

Tolerance to Acute FPIES Caused by Foods Other Than Cow's Milk

The natural history of acute FPIES caused by foods other than cow's milk has not been well studied. The average age of soy tolerance is highly variable in the United

States ranging from 28.5 months to 6.7 years; conversely, Korean infants outgrew their allergy by an average of 7.8 months [9, 16, 19, 27]. There are several reported cases of soy-induced FPIES that have persisted into late childhood and early adulthood [9, 19].

In Australia, acute FPIES caused by rice was tolerated in 90% of patients at 3 years of age, compared to 40% and 25% in two large US cohorts [16, 19, 49]. Egg-induced and fish-induced FPIES appears to have a poorer prognosis but data is limited [72].

Variables Effecting Rate of Tolerance Acquisition

Several factors have been associated with a slower rate of tolerance acquisition. Having food sIgE to the culprit food at the time of presentation or during an OFC has been associated with older age of tolerance in multiple studies [7, 19, 49]. Data is limited on other factors, but a recent Australian study did provide some insight. In that study, influences that were shown to have an association with later age of tolerance include older age of initial FPIES episode, older age at diagnosis, and category of trigger food (Table 4.9) [49]. Features that have not been shown to be associated include gender, presence of any atopic disorder, number of food triggers, and severity of initial FPIES reaction.

By better understanding the natural history of acute FPIES through more targeted studies, factors that can influence its clinical course can be identified and manipulated to improve outcomes.

Management

Acute Management

Acute FPIES reactions should be considered a medical emergency and treated aggressively on a case-by-case basis for reactions due to accidental exposure or during an OFC. Episodes can progress quickly and lead to hypovolemic shock in up to 15% of cases, although this may be an overestimation due to selection bias of more severe cases presenting to tertiary referral centers [11, 19, 41]. There have been no reported deaths due to FPIES.

Table 4.9 Factors that may influence the age of tolerance in acute FPIES [49]

Increase age of tolerance	No effect on age of tolerance
Detected sIgE to culprit food	Gender
Later age of symptom onset	Presence of atopic disorder
Older age at diagnosis	Number of food triggers
Category of food[a]	Severity of initial FPIES reaction

[a]Studies have varied on which foods typically have a later age of resolution but not enough data is available to make validated conclusions

Management will differ depending on the location of the patient at the time of reaction. If it takes place outside of a clinical setting, mild symptoms (1–2 episodes of vomiting) can be managed with attempted oral rehydration through breastfeeding or with clear liquids. In the situation of a more severe presentation with ≥ three episodes of vomiting and/or lethargy, then emergency services should be called or the patient should present to the nearest emergency department for evaluation [1]. For patients with a history of severe FPIES reactions, they should immediately seek medical attention after known ingestion, regardless of their symptoms.

Figure 4.3 outlines an algorithm that can be used in a clinical setting. Careful monitoring of the patient including obtaining regular vital signs is advisable until the patient returns to baseline. Initial management should center on obtaining hemodynamic stability with fluid resuscitation, orally for mild reactions or intravenously for more severe reactions. Patients should be observed for at least 4–6 hours from the onset of reaction, be able to tolerate oral fluids, and appear at or near baseline before being considered for discharge home.

For moderate to severe cases, if the patient does not already have intravenous access, placement should be strongly considered. Normal saline bolus for fluid resuscitation is recommended at 20 mL/kg and can be repeated as needed for management of hypotension. Several experts recommend the use of single dose methylprednisolone at 1 mg/kg (maximum 60–80 mg/dose) to theoretically reduce inflammation, although this has not been properly studied and its true benefit is unknown [73]. Correction of electrolyte and acid-base abnormalities may be required. In addition, methylene blue for methemoglobinemia can be used [20, 56, 74]. Patients may require vasopressors, supplemental oxygen, and mechanical ventilation in situations of severe shock. Transferring to a higher level of care would be appropriate.

Ondansetron

Ondansetron is a widely used antiemetic agent for nausea and vomiting that has been used during chemotherapy since the 1990s. It inhibits the serotonin 5-HT_3 receptor that has both peripheral and central actions. While generally a safe medication, it has been shown to cause QT interval prolongation and should be cautiously used in patients with known cardiac abnormalities. Two small case series initially showed promising results of stopping FPIES reactions with the use of parenteral ondansetron [18, 75]. A larger retrospective study by Miceli Sopo et al. retrospectively reviewed 66 acute FPIES cases and compared patient outcomes based on ondansetron use [76]. Of the 37 patients that received ondansetron, 81% had resolution of the vomiting after administration compared to only 7% of those that were managed with traditional therapy. They also noted that ondansetron was effective in resolving pallor and lethargy as well as reducing their risk for hospital admission overnight. There does not appear to be any difference in efficacy based on intramuscular or intravenous administration.

The use of ondansetron is recommended for mild, moderate, and severe acute FPIES reactions, but rigorous studies are lacking on its exact mechanism of action and true efficacy (Fig. 4.3) [1].

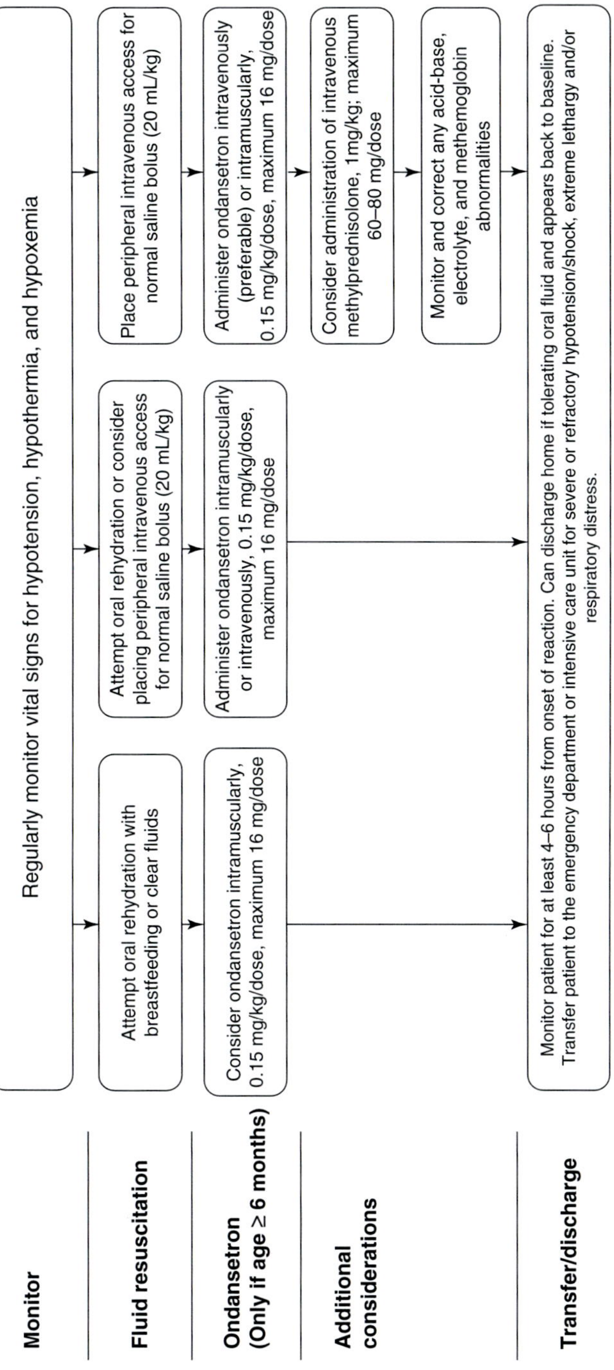

Fig. 4.3 Emergent management algorithm of acute FPIES reaction in a clinical setting

Long-Term Management

Long-term management of acute FPIES revolves around dietary elimination of the suspected foods, adequate nutritional replacement, appropriate planning for possible accidental re-exposure, and regular monitoring for tolerance.

Dietary Elimination

The cornerstone of acute FPIES management is appropriate avoidance of the offending food(s). At this time, an accurate threshold dose has not been established for any food trigger, and no amount is considered safe to ingest [8, 67]. Providers should have the ability to offer appropriate counseling, recommendations on up-to-date resources, and access to a registered dietician that can assist in ensuring adherence to the dietary plan. Nutritional deficiencies can develop in children with food allergies due to dietary restrictions and delayed introduction of new foods into the diet. This will be further discussed in the following sections. Also, Chapter 9 offers additional insight.

Baked Products

At this time, it is recommended that children with FPIES caused by CM or egg should continue avoidance of processed or baked products unless already tolerated in their diet [1]. Data related to baked food exposure in patients with FPIES is scarce compared to that for IgE-mediated allergies. One small case series found several children were able to tolerate baked CM and egg [77]. In addition, a recent large cohort study from Australia showed that all 12 CM-FPIES children with baked CM exposure history were able to tolerate it. In contrast, only one out of five children with egg-induced FPIES tolerated baked egg [11]. A limiting factor in both of these studies is the unknown quantity of baked food ingested as only two cases were performed in a controlled OFC setting.

Breastfeeding and Milk Substitutes

Breast milk remains the optimal nutritional choice for infants and, if possible, should be recommended exclusively for the first 4–6 months of life [78, 79]. FPIES reactions to protein in breast milk remain exceedingly rare in most areas of the world, except for Japan where approximately 10% of acute FPIES reactions are due to breast milk [40]. If breastfeeding is a viable option, children with CM-/soy-induced FPIES should remain on breast milk through the first year of life. In addition, continued breastfeeding beyond the first year should be considered if desired by both the mother and infant [78].

In situations where breastfeeding is not an option, milk substitutes should be chosen based on the risk of reactivity and adequate nutritional value. Table 4.4 outlines the reactivity of milk substitutes in patients with acute CM-FPIES. Partially hydrolyzed casein-based formula should be avoided as this preparation has been shown to have a high degree of reactivity [11, 80]. Extensively hydrolyzed formula (eHF), on the other hand, is generally well tolerated and is recommended in most children [6, 7, 11]. Approximately 10–20% of children will require amino acid-based formula (AAF) due to persistent symptoms with eHF [11, 80, 81]. There is one reported case of persistent acute FPIES symptoms in an infant switched to AAF, although details are not provided [11].

Soy milk may be a suitable alternative but is often avoided in the United States due to the high rate of co-reactivity/cross-reactivity (Table 4.4) [9, 16, 19]. If the provider or parent prefers soy, it should be introduced under close physician supervision [1].

The cross-reactivity/co-reactivity of milk produced from other animals has not been studied in FPIES. Recommendations can likely be accurately extrapolated from data available from IgE-mediated allergy studies. Goat's and sheep's milk should be avoided due to their high homology of protein sequence with CM. Milks from donkey, camels, or both might be better options as they are typically well tolerated in IgE-mediated CM allergy [1].

Food Introduction

Cross-reactive/co-allergy does exist (Table 4.4) in acute FPIES, and instructions should be provided to patients and their families on the safe introduction of age-appropriate foods. Early intervention from the provider will help reduce the risk of an overly restrictive diet and prevent food aversion. Empiric guidelines were published in the international consensus guidelines [1]. These guidelines provide a practical, systematic approach by highlighting less allergenic foods that can be introduced at home. These recommendations are particularly important in populations that are at higher risk for multiple food-induced FPIES – early onset FPIES before the age of 5 months and reactions to fruits and vegetables [11]. Typically, tolerance to a single food in a food group is a good prognostic indicator that the patient will tolerate other foods from the same group [20].

For children with severe reactions to CM or soy, provider supervised introduction of a mixture of several solid foods is an accepted approach to prevent unnecessary avoidance [1]. This should be followed by gradual buildup at home to age-appropriate servings of each solid food.

Epinephrine Autoinjector

Epinephrine autoinjectors are not routinely prescribed for FPIES due to minimal benefit, but they can be considered for patients that have concomitant food sIgE sensitivity and are at risk for anaphylactic reactions [82].

Available Resources

The FPIES Foundation (www.fpiesfoundation.org) and the International FPIES Association (www.fpies.org) are two global organizations that provide resources to patients, caregivers, and providers, promoting advocacy and awareness to the general public.

Timing of OFC to Evaluate for Tolerance

Evaluating for tolerance is an essential component in long-term management of acute FPIES as the majority of patients will outgrow their allergy during childhood [9, 19, 49]. Living with a food allergy drastically decreases one's quality of life (QoL), and removal of this label at the earliest possible date should remain a vital goal [83–85]. QoL measures have been shown to improve in caregivers whose children undergo OFC [86].

There is no consensus agreement regarding the best time to perform an OFC assessing for tolerance in patients with acute FPIES. Cultural and regional social factors along with personal preferences have led to various practices around the world. The current international consensus guidelines do not provide any specific recommendations but do mention that multiple experts in the United States perform OFCs within 12–18 months after the most recent reaction due to slower rates of tolerability seen in the United States [1]. Studies from South Korea and Australia evaluated shorter intervals and suggested that performing challenges at earlier time points may be safe and beneficial [27, 49]. These differences can likely be explained by study design, country-specific approaches to management, provider preferences, and phenotypic differences in patients seen at the providers' practice. Large, systematic, prospective studies with preset intervals are needed to better understand the optimal time to perform OFCs.

Prior to performing an OFC, food sIgE testing should be considered as patients can develop sIgE sensitivity to the culprit food at a rate of 2–20% during follow-up [7, 10, 19, 63]. While considered optional for most foods based on detailed history and provider preference, it is recommended that all patients with CM-FPIES should undergo sIgE testing to CM before OFC [1]. This is discussed in more detail earlier in this chapter under the section, "Food-Specific IgE Testing (Serum Serology and Skin Prick)."

Summary

Acute FPIES is a non-IgE-mediated food allergy that presents with repetitive protracted vomiting, diarrhea, lethargy, and in severe cases, hypotension and shock. It is a heterogeneous disorder that can vary significantly due to multiple factors including age of onset, nationality, and association with IgE-mediated sensitivity. While acute FPIES is mainly a disorder of infancy, more recent literature has shown that it can continue in late childhood and adulthood or occur de novo. While the overall incidence is not known, it appears to be increasingly recognized in clinical practice. Common food triggers vary considerably around the world likely due to cultural differences in early feeding patterns. Recently published international consensus guidelines have established uniform diagnostic criteria and have provided a platform to improve future studies [1]. The natural history of acute FPIES appears to differ markedly by nation, but additional large studies with defined intervals for OFCs are needed to determine the age of tolerance and improve management strategies.

Key Points/Clinical "Pearls"

- Food protein-induced enterocolitis syndrome (FPIES) is a non-IgE cell-mediated gastrointestinal food hypersensitivity that typically present in their first year of life with recurrent vomiting, diarrhea, and potential exacerbation which can lead to shock.
- Acute FPIES can be caused by any food, but the most commonly reported are cow's milk, soy, rice, and oats.
- Acute FPIES is a clinical diagnosis. Laboratory and radiologic testing is nonspecific but may help in supporting the diagnosis.
- Long-term management of acute FPIES revolves around dietary elimination of the suspected foods, adequate nutritional replacement, appropriate planning for possible accidental re-exposure, and regular monitoring for tolerance.
- Evaluating for tolerance is an essential component in long-term management of acute FPIES as the majority of patients will outgrow their allergy within the first 3 years of life.

References

1. Nowak-Wegrzyn A, Chehade M, Groetch ME, Spergel JM, Wood RA, Allen K, et al. International consensus guidelines for the diagnosis and management of food protein-induced enterocolitis syndrome: executive summary-Workgroup Report of the Adverse Reactions to Foods Committee, American Academy of Allergy, Asthma & Immunology. J Allergy Clin Immunol. 2017;139:1111–26 e4.
2. Nowak-Wegrzyn A, Jarocka-Cyrta E, Moschione Castro A. Food protein-induced enterocolitis syndrome. J Investig Allergol Clin Immunol. 2017;27:1–18.
3. Goldman AS, Anderson DW Jr, Sellers WA, Saperstein S, Kniker WT, Halpern SR. Milk allergy. I. Oral challenge with milk and isolated milk proteins in allergic children. Pediatrics. 1963;32:425–43.
4. Gryboski JD, Burkle F, Hillman R. Milk induced colitis in an infant. Pediatrics. 1966;38:299–302.
5. Powell GK. Enterocolitis in low-birth-weight infants associated with milk and soy protein intolerance. J Pediatr. 1976;88:840–4.
6. Burks AW, Casteel HB, Fiedorek SC, Williams LW, Pumphrey CL. Prospective oral food challenge study of two soybean protein isolates in patients with possible milk or soy protein enterocolitis. Pediatr Allergy Immunol. 1994;5:40–5.
7. Sicherer SH, Eigenmann PA, Sampson HA. Clinical features of food protein-induced enterocolitis syndrome. J Pediatr. 1998;133:214–9.
8. Katz Y, Goldberg MR, Rajuan N, Cohen A, Leshno M. The prevalence and natural course of food protein-induced enterocolitis syndrome to cow's milk: a large-scale, prospective population-based study. J Allergy Clin Immunol. 2011;127:647–53 e1-3.
9. Ruffner MA, Ruymann K, Barni S, Cianferoni A, Brown-Whitehorn T, Spergel JM. Food protein-induced enterocolitis syndrome: insights from review of a large referral population. J Allergy Clin Immunol Pract. 2013;1:343–9.
10. Sopo SM, Giorgio V, Dello Iacono I, Novembre E, Mori F, Onesimo R. A multicentre retrospective study of 66 Italian children with food protein-induced enterocolitis syndrome: different management for different phenotypes. Clin Exp Allergy. 2012;42:1257–65.

11. Mehr S, Frith K, Barnes EH, Campbell DE, FPIES Study Group. Food protein-induced enterocolitis syndrome in Australia: a population-based study, 2012–2014. J Allergy Clin Immunol. 2017;140:1323–30.
12. Mehr S, Kakakios A, Frith K, Kemp AS. Food protein-induced enterocolitis syndrome: 16-year experience. Pediatrics. 2009;123:e459–64.
13. Fernandes BN, Boyle RJ, Gore C, Simpson A, Custovic A. Food protein-induced enterocolitis syndrome can occur in adults. J Allergy Clin Immunol. 2012;130:1199–200.
14. Tan JA, Smith WB. Non-IgE-mediated gastrointestinal food hypersensitivity syndrome in adults. J Allergy Clin Immunol Pract. 2014;2:355–7 e1.
15. Mehr S, Frith K, Campbell DE. Epidemiology of food protein-induced enterocolitis syndrome. Curr Opin Allergy Clin Immunol. 2014;14:208–16.
16. Nowak-Wegrzyn A, Sampson HA, Wood RA, Sicherer SH. Food protein-induced enterocolitis syndrome caused by solid food proteins. Pediatrics. 2003;111:829–35.
17. Shoda T, Isozaki A, Kawano Y. Food protein-induced gastrointestinal syndromes in identical and fraternal twins. Allergol Int. 2011;60:103–8.
18. Holbrook T, Keet CA, Frischmeyer-Guerrerio PA, Wood RA. Use of ondansetron for food protein-induced enterocolitis syndrome. J Allergy Clin Immunol. 2013;132:1219–20.
19. Caubet JC, Ford LS, Sickles L, Jarvinen KM, Sicherer SH, Sampson HA, et al. Clinical features and resolution of food protein-induced enterocolitis syndrome: 10-year experience. J Allergy Clin Immunol. 2014;134:382–9.
20. Sicherer SH. Food protein-induced enterocolitis syndrome: case presentations and management lessons. J Allergy Clin Immunol. 2005;115:149–56.
21. Morita H, Nomura I, Matsuda A, Saito H, Matsumoto K. Gastrointestinal food allergy in infants. Allergol Int. 2013;62:297–307.
22. Van Sickle GJ, Powell GK, McDonald PJ, Goldblum RM. Milk- and soy protein-induced enterocolitis: evidence for lymphocyte sensitization to specific food proteins. Gastroenterology. 1985;88:1915–21.
23. Caubet JC, Bencharitiwong R, Ross A, Sampson HA, Berin MC, Nowak-Wegrzyn A. Humoral and cellular responses to casein in patients with food protein-induced enterocolitis to cow's milk. J Allergy Clin Immunol. 2017;139:572–83.
24. Karlsson MR, Rugtveit J, Brandtzaeg P. Allergen-responsive CD4+CD25+ regulatory T cells in children who have outgrown cow's milk allergy. J Exp Med. 2004;199:1679–88.
25. Caubet JC, Nowak-Wegrzyn A. Current understanding of the immune mechanisms of food protein-induced enterocolitis syndrome. Expert Rev Clin Immunol. 2011;7:317–27.
26. Wada T, Matsuda Y, Toma T, Koizumi E, Okamoto H, Yachie A. Increased CD69 expression on peripheral eosinophils from patients with food protein-induced enterocolitis syndrome. Int Arch Allergy Immunol. 2016;170:201–5.
27. Hwang JB, Sohn SM, Kim AS. Prospective follow-up oral food challenge in food protein-induced enterocolitis syndrome. Arch Dis Child. 2009;94:425–8.
28. Powell GK. Milk- and soy-induced enterocolitis of infancy. Clinical features and standardization of challenge. J Pediatr. 1978;93:553–60.
29. Goswami R, Blazquez AB, Kosoy R, Rahman A, Nowak-Wegrzyn A, Berin MC. Systemic innate immune activation in food protein-induced enterocolitis syndrome. J Allergy Clin Immunol. 2017;139:1885–96 e9.
30. Shek LP, Bardina L, Castro R, Sampson HA, Beyer K. Humoral and cellular responses to cow milk proteins in patients with milk-induced IgE-mediated and non-IgE-mediated disorders. Allergy. 2005;60:912–9.
31. Konstantinou GN, Bencharitiwong R, Grishin A, Caubet JC, Bardina L, Sicherer SH, et al. The role of casein-specific IgA and TGF-beta in children with food protein-induced enterocolitis syndrome to milk. Pediatr Allergy Immunol. 2014;25:651–6.
32. McDonald PJ, Goldblum RM, Van Sickle GJ, Powell GK. Food protein-induced enterocolitis: altered antibody response to ingested antigen. Pediatr Res. 1984;18:751–5.
33. Chung HL, Hwang JB, Park JJ, Kim SG. Expression of transforming growth factor beta1, transforming growth factor type I and II receptors, and TNF-alpha in the mucosa of the small

intestine in infants with food protein-induced enterocolitis syndrome. J Allergy Clin Immunol. 2002;109:150–4.

34. Heyman M, Darmon N, Dupont C, Dugas B, Hirribaren A, Blaton MA, et al. Mononuclear cells from infants allergic to cow's milk secrete tumor necrosis factor alpha, altering intestinal function. Gastroenterology. 1994;106:1514–23.
35. Monteseirin J, Fernandez-Pineda I, Chacon P, Vega A, Bonilla I, Camacho MJ, et al. Myeloperoxidase release after allergen-specific conjunctival challenge. J Asthma. 2004;41:639–43.
36. Chen CY, Lee JB, Liu B, Ohta S, Wang PY, Kartashov AV, et al. Induction of interleukin-9-producing mucosal mast cells promotes susceptibility to IgE-mediated experimental food allergy. Immunity. 2015;43:788–802.
37. Barrios Y, Poza-Guedes P, Sanchez-Machin I, Franco A, Armas H, Gonzalez R, et al. IP-10 in pediatric celiac disease and food allergy. Am J Gastroenterol. 2014;109:1085–6.
38. Mane SK, Bahna SL. Clinical manifestations of food protein-induced enterocolitis syndrome. Curr Opin Allergy Clin Immunol. 2014;14:217–21.
39. Nomura I, Morita H, Ohya Y, Saito H, Matsumoto K. Non-IgE-mediated gastrointestinal food allergies: distinct differences in clinical phenotype between Western countries and Japan. Curr Allergy Asthma Rep. 2012;12:297–303.
40. Nomura I, Morita H, Hosokawa S, Hoshina H, Fukuie T, Watanabe M, et al. Four distinct subtypes of non-IgE-mediated gastrointestinal food allergies in neonates and infants, distinguished by their initial symptoms. J Allergy Clin Immunol. 2011;127:685–8 e1-8.
41. Murray KF, Christie DL. Dietary protein intolerance in infants with transient methemoglobinemia and diarrhea. J Pediatr. 1993;122:90–2.
42. Jayasooriya S, Fox AT, Murch SH. Do not laparotomize food-protein-induced enterocolitis syndrome. Pediatr Emerg Care. 2007;23:173–5.
43. Morita H, Suzuki H, Orihara K, Motomura K, Matsuda A, Ohya Y, et al. Food protein-induced enterocolitis syndromes with and without bloody stool have distinct clinicopathologic features. J Allergy Clin Immunol. 2017;140:1718–21 e6.
44. Ludman S, Harmon M, Whiting D, du Toit G. Clinical presentation and referral characteristics of food protein-induced enterocolitis syndrome in the United Kingdom. Ann Allergy Asthma Immunol. 2014;113:290–4.
45. Vila L, Garcia V, Rial MJ, Novoa E, Cacharron T. Fish is a major trigger of solid food protein-induced enterocolitis syndrome in Spanish children. J Allergy Clin Immunol Pract. 2015;3:621–3.
46. Monti G, Castagno E, Liguori SA, Lupica MM, Tarasco V, Viola S, et al. Food protein-induced enterocolitis syndrome by cow's milk proteins passed through breast milk. J Allergy Clin Immunol. 2011;127:679–80.
47. Tan J, Campbell D, Mehr S. Food protein-induced enterocolitis syndrome in an exclusively breast-fed infant-an uncommon entity. J Allergy Clin Immunol. 2012;129:873, author reply -4.
48. Miceli Sopo S, Monaco S, Greco M, Scala G. Chronic food protein-induced enterocolitis syndrome caused by cow's milk proteins passed through breast milk. Int Arch Allergy Immunol. 2014;164:207–9.
49. Lee E, Campbell DE, Barnes EH, Mehr SS. Resolution of acute food protein-induced enterocolitis syndrome in children. J Allergy Clin Immunol Pract. 2017;5:486–8 e1.
50. Bruni F, Peroni DG, Piacentini GL, De Luca G, Boner AL. Fruit proteins: another cause of food protein-induced enterocolitis syndrome. Allergy. 2008;63:1645–6.
51. Mehr SS, Kakakios AM, Kemp AS. Rice: a common and severe cause of food protein-induced enterocolitis syndrome. Arch Dis Child. 2009;94:220–3.
52. Ikola RA. Severe intestinal reaction following ingestion of rice. Am J Dis Child. 1963;105:281–4.
53. Kapoor M, Bird JA. Cow's milk protein is often tolerated by children with oat-induced FPIES. J Allergy Clin Immunol Pract. 2017;5:496–7.
54. Levy Y, Danon YL. Food protein-induced enterocolitis syndrome--not only due to cow's milk and soy. Pediatr Allergy Immunol. 2003;14:325–9.

55. Miceli Sopo S, Monaco S, Badina L, Barni S, Longo G, Novembre E, et al. Food protein-induced enterocolitis syndrome caused by fish and/or shellfish in Italy. Pediatr Allergy Immunol. 2015;26:731–6.
56. Jarvinen KM, Nowak-Wegrzyn A. Food protein-induced enterocolitis syndrome (FPIES): current management strategies and review of the literature. J Allergy Clin Immunol Pract. 2013;1:317–22.
57. Nowak-Wegrzyn A, Muraro A. Food protein-induced enterocolitis syndrome. Curr Opin Allergy Clin Immunol. 2009;9:371–7.
58. Kimura M, Ito Y, Shimomura M, Morishita H, Meguro T, Adachi Y, et al. Cytokine profile after oral food challenge in infants with food protein-induced enterocolitis syndrome. Allergol Int. 2017;66:452–7.
59. Shimomura M, Ito Y, Tanaka H, Meguro T, Kimura M. Increased serum cortisol on oral food challenge in infants with food protein-induced enterocolitis syndrome. Pediatr Int. 2018;60:13–8.
60. Kimura M, Shimomura M, Morishita H, Meguro T, Seto S. Eosinophilia in infants with food protein-induced enterocolitis syndrome in Japan. Allergol Int. 2017;66:310–6.
61. Kimura M, Shimomura M, Morishita H, Meguro T, Seto S. Serum C-reactive protein in food protein-induced enterocolitis syndrome versus food protein-induced proctocolitis in Japan. Pediatr Int. 2016;58:836–41.
62. Anand RK, Appachi E. Case report of methemoglobinemia in two patients with food protein-induced enterocolitis. Clin Pediatr (Phila). 2006;45:679–82.
63. Onesimo R, Dello Iacono I, Giorgio V, Limongelli MG, Miceli Sopo S. Can food protein induced enterocolitis syndrome shift to immediate gastrointestinal hypersensitivity? A report of two cases. Eur Ann Allergy Clin Immunol. 2011;43:61–3.
64. Mizuno M, Masaki H, Yoshinare R, Ito Y, Morita H, Yoshio H. Hematochezia before the first feeding in a newborn with food protein-induced enterocolitis syndrome. AJP Rep. 2011;1:53–8.
65. Hwang JB, Song JY, Kang YN, Kim SP, Suh SI, Kam S, et al. The significance of gastric juice analysis for a positive challenge by a standard oral challenge test in typical cow's milk protein-induced enterocolitis. J Korean Med Sci. 2008;23:251–5.
66. Fontaine JL, Navarro J. Small intestinal biopsy in cows milk protein allergy in infancy. Arch Dis Child. 1975;50:357–62.
67. Fogg MI, Brown-Whitehorn TA, Pawlowski NA, Spergel JM. Atopy patch test for the diagnosis of food protein-induced enterocolitis syndrome. Pediatr Allergy Immunol. 2006;17:351–5.
68. Jarvinen KM, Caubet JC, Sickles L, Ford LS, Sampson HA, Nowak-Wegrzyn A. Poor utility of atopy patch test in predicting tolerance development in food protein-induced enterocolitis syndrome. Ann Allergy Asthma Immunol. 2012;109:221–2.
69. Fiocchi A, Claps A, Dahdah L, Brindisi G, Dionisi-Vici C, Martelli A. Differential diagnosis of food protein-induced enterocolitis syndrome. Curr Opin Allergy Clin Immunol. 2014;14:246–54.
70. Sampson HA, Anderson JA. Summary and recommendations: classification of gastrointestinal manifestations due to immunologic reactions to foods in infants and young children. J Pediatr Gastroenterol Nutr. 2000;30(Suppl):S87–94.
71. Guerrerio AL, Frischmeyer-Guerrerio PA, Lederman HM, Oliva-Hemker M. Recognizing gastrointestinal and hepatic manifestations of primary immunodeficiency diseases. J Pediatr Gastroenterol Nutr. 2010;51:548–55.
72. Gonzalez-Delgado P, Caparros E, Moreno MV, Clemente F, Flores E, Velasquez L, et al. Clinical and immunological characteristics of a pediatric population with food protein-induced enterocolitis syndrome (FPIES) to fish. Pediatr Allergy Immunol. 2016;27:269–75.
73. Sicherer SH. Food protein-induced enterocolitis syndrome: clinical perspectives. J Pediatr Gastroenterol Nutr. 2000;30(Suppl):S45–9.
74. Malin SW, Lutfi R, Friedman ML, Teagarden AM. Food protein-induced enterocolitis syndrome causing hypovolemic shock and methemoglobinemia. Case Rep Crit Care. 2018;2018:1903787.

75. Miceli Sopo S, Battista A, Greco M, Monaco S. Ondansetron for food protein-induced enterocolitis syndrome. Int Arch Allergy Immunol. 2014;164:137–9.
76. Miceli Sopo S, Bersani G, Monaco S, Cerchiara G, Lee E, Campbell D, et al. Ondansetron in acute food protein-induced enterocolitis syndrome, a retrospective case-control study. Allergy. 2017;72:545–51.
77. Miceli Sopo S, Buonsenso D, Monaco S, Crocco S, Longo G, Calvani M. Food protein-induced enterocolitis syndrome (FPIES) and well cooked foods: a working hypothesis. Allergol Immunopathol (Madr). 2013;41:346–8.
78. Baker RD, Greer FR, Committee on Nutrition American Academy of P. Diagnosis and prevention of iron deficiency and iron-deficiency anemia in infants and young children (0–3 years of age). Pediatrics. 2010;126:1040–50.
79. Section on Breastfeeding. Breastfeeding and the use of human milk. Pediatrics. 2012;129:e827–41.
80. Vanderhoof JA, Murray ND, Kaufman SS, Mack DR, Antonson DL, Corkins MR, et al. Intolerance to protein hydrolysate infant formulas: an underrecognized cause of gastrointestinal symptoms in infants. J Pediatr. 1997;131:741–4.
81. Kelso JM, Sampson HA. Food protein-induced enterocolitis to casein hydrolysate formulas. J Allergy Clin Immunol. 1993;92:909–10.
82. Boyce JA, Assa'ad A, Burks AW, Jones SM, Sampson HA, Wood RA, et al. Guidelines for the diagnosis and management of food allergy in the United States: summary of the NIAID-sponsored expert panel report. J Allergy Clin Immunol. 2010;126:1105–18.
83. Antolin-Amerigo D, Manso L, Caminati M, de la Hoz Caballer B, Cerecedo I, Muriel A, et al. Quality of life in patients with food allergy. Clin Mol Allergy. 2016;14:4.
84. Greenhawt M. Food allergy quality of life. Ann Allergy Asthma Immunol. 2014;113:506–12.
85. Muraro A, Werfel T, Hoffmann-Sommergruber K, Roberts G, Beyer K, Bindslev-Jensen C, et al. EAACI food allergy and anaphylaxis guidelines: diagnosis and management of food allergy. Allergy. 2014;69:1008–25.
86. Franxman TJ, Howe L, Teich E, Greenhawt MJ. Oral food challenge and food allergy quality of life in caregivers of children with food allergy. J Allergy Clin Immunol Pract. 2015;3:50–6.

Management of Acute Food Protein-Induced Enterocolitis Syndrome (FPIES) Reactions

5

Alessandro Giovanni Fiocchi and Valentina Pecora

Case Presentation

A male patient was evaluated at the age of 6 months for a possible allergy to rice. The patient was a full-term male infant delivered via cesarean section and breastfed during the first week of life. Subsequently, a cow's milk-based formula with the addition of rice cream was used to replace breastfeeding. The patient developed frequent episodes of diarrhea, and therefore different types of milk-based formula (cow, goat, or donkey) without eliminating the rice cream were used. At 4 weeks of age, the patient was taken to the emergency room for worsening of the clinical condition (he presented about 8 episodes/day of water diarrhea) with weight loss. The patient was transferred to the intensive care unit. Emergency department evaluation included blood, urine, stool, and screening for cystic fibrosis. He showed an increase in inflammation markers (protein C-reactive 5.68 mg/dL, lactate dehydrogenase 411 IU/L, white blood cells 10.3 10^3/uL, and neutrophils 5.57 10^3/uL) and negative stool cultures. During the hospitalization, he received intravenous fluid resuscitation and dual intravenous antibiotic therapy. He was observed in the hospital for 2 weeks and discharged tolerating an extensively hydrolyzed casein formula without rice cream. He did well until the age of 5 months. The patient experienced an acute FPIES reaction after 1 hour from the ingestion of rice. He developed repetitive vomiting (seven episodes of emesis), pallor, lethargy, and water diarrhea. The patient was taken to the emergency room and required intravenous fluid resuscitation. An intravenous dose of ondansetron was administered to stop the vomiting and limit the fluid loss. He was observed in the hospital for 3 days and discharge with the indication to exclude the rice from the dietary regimen and schedule an allergy evaluation.

A. G. Fiocchi · V. Pecora (✉)
Allergy Department, IRCCS Ospedale Pediatrico Bambino Gesù, Rome, Italy
e-mail: valentina.pecora@opbg.net

T. F. Brown-Whitehorn, A. Cianferoni (eds.), *Food Protein Induced Enterocolitis (FPIES)*,
https://doi.org/10.1007/978-3-030-21229-2_5

Introduction

Despite the first formal report of food protein-induced enterocolitis syndrome (FPIES) dating back to the 1970s [1], the first international evidence-based guidelines to improve the diagnosis and management have been published only recently [2]. This consensus statement has proved extremely useful for identifying an appropriate case management model.

The first step to appropriately treat FPIES is its recognition and diagnosis, which often requires a team approach. Indeed, recognition of FPIES symptoms during the first clinical presentation has resulted in significant benefits for patients preventing new reactions and improving management of this condition [3].

The diagnosis of FPIES is still clinical and it is based on an accurate history. The onset of clinical manifestations ascribable to an acute FPIES reaction is always associated with the exposure to the offending food/s also in the case of unexpected food allergen traces. Even if some investigators have reported FPIES reactions in exclusively breastfed infants [4, 5], the reaction often happens after the first-second milk, soy, or solid food introduction. To date, there are no diagnostic biomarkers, but some peripheral blood parameters may help to establish the diagnosis including (i) increased white blood cell count with neutrophilia, (ii) thrombocytosis, and (iii) leukocytes and eosinophils in the stool. In severe reactions, a condition of metabolic acidosis and methemoglobinemia can be observed [2]. Recently, the role of C-reactive protein as a biomarker of acute FPIES reaction was highlighted [6–8]. The serum C-reactive protein level seems to be correlated with the degree of reaction severity, starting to increase at 6 hours from the onset of symptoms with a peak at 24 hours.

The allergists are playing an important role in diagnosing the syndrome (if necessary with an oral food challenge), providing lifestyle advice and an action plan for managing the acute FPIES reaction. However, general pediatricians and ER physician play an essential, critical role as well as they represent the front-line physicians in assessing and managing of FPIES reactions. Their involvement through educational initiatives represents the most suitable way to cut off the delay of diagnosis [9]. Therefore, the cooperation of specialists and general pediatricians is crucial.

Strict avoidance of the trigger food/s is currently the only reliable way to prevent an acute food-induced reaction [2]. The vigilance required for strict avoidance coupled with the ever-present risk of an accidental exposure results in impaired quality of life of affected patients and their families and can have an impact on nutritional status. The complete avoidance of staple foods such as milk, egg, or wheat could negatively affect an adequate, healthy, and nutritionally balanced diet influencing the optimal growth. In the light of these considerations, a specialist dietitian should be part of the multidisciplinary team for the management of FPIES patients providing the appropriate nutritional support.

Clinical Management Approaches of Acute FPIES Reactions

Once the FPIES is diagnosed and the offending food is identified, reactions to accidental exposures can happen and be characterized by different severity degrees. According to the recent international guidelines, the clinical management will involve different approaches depending on the severity of FPIES acute reaction (Table 5.1) [2], with

Table 5.1 Management of acute FPIES reactions

Type of reaction	Symptoms	Management
Mild	1–2 episodes of emesis without lethargy or pallor	1. Attempt oral rehydration (e.g., breastfeeding or clear fluids) 2. Starting from 6 months of life, intramuscular ondansetron administration (0.15 mg/kg/dose, maximum 16 mg/dose) can be considered 3. Monitor for resolution about 4–6 hours after the onset of gastrointestinal symptoms
Moderate	>3 episodes of emesis, mild lethargy, and pallor	1. Starting from 6 months of life, intramuscular ondansetron administration (0.15 mg/kg/dose, maximum 16 mg/dose) can be considered 2. Peripheral intravenous line placement is always recommended 3. If oral hydration is not adequate, an isotonic fluid resuscitation (e.g., 10–20 mL/kg boluses of normal saline) is required 4. Monitor vital signs 5. Transfer the patient to the intensive care unit for managing extreme lethargy, respiratory distress, persistent or severe hypotension even to a hypovolemic shock condition 6. Monitor for resolution at least 4–6 hours after the onset of gastrointestinal symptoms 7. Discharge to home if the patient is able to tolerate clear liquids
Severe	>3 episodes of emesis, severe lethargy, hypotonia, ashen, or cyanotic appearance	1. An emergency transportation is required 2. Detection of vital signs and place a peripheral intravenous line 3. A rapid restoration of stable hemodynamics through aggressive isotonic fluid resuscitation (e.g., 10–20 mL/kg boluses of normal saline), repeated as needed to correct the hypotension 4. Starting from 6 months of life, intravenous ondansetron administration (0.15 mg/kg/dose, maximum 16 mg/dose) is recommended 5. Consider the intravenous administration of methylprednisolone 1 mg/kg (maximum 60–80 mg/dose) 6. Monitor and correct acid-based and electrolyte abnormalities 7. Correct methemoglobinemia if present 8. Monitor vital signs 9. Discharge to home after 4–6 hours from the onset of reaction when the patient's condition is back to baseline tolerating oral clear fluids 10. Transfer the patient to the intensive care unit for managing extreme lethargy, respiratory distress, persistent or severe hypotension even to a hypovolemic shock condition

Adapted from Nowak-Węgrzyn et al. [2]

rehydration being central in all types of FPIES. Oral rehydration at home is recommended in mild reactions, whereas intravenous hydration is mandatory in severe forms characterized by protracted emesis, lethargy, pallor, diarrhea, hypotension, and metabolic acidosis. Acute FPIES can lead to hypovolemic shock; consequently, the priority in management is restoration of hemodynamic stability.

Mild Reaction

When the patients experienced maximum two episodes of emesis in the absence of lethargy or pallor, an oral rehydration at home should be attempted. In any case, it is always advised to notify the clinician regarding the acute reaction. The oral rehydration may include the use of breastfeeding or clear fluids. The suggestion is to drink small amounts of liquid often to replace water and nutrients that have been lost. The best liquids are oral electrolyte solutions or oral electrolyte maintenance solutions, characterized by a right balance of fluids and minerals to replace those lost during emesis. The clinician should provide specific oral rehydration instructions. In the event of a rapid clinical resolution, access to the emergency room can be avoided. The patient should always be monitored closely by the parents and the clinician. Actually, the appearance of acute diarrhea is possible within 24–48 hours after the onset of gastrointestinal symptoms. The oral rehydration at a medical facility, when possible, is preferred. Starting from 6 months of life, intramuscular ondansetron administration (0.15 mg/kg/dose with a maximum recommended dose of 16 mg) can be considered. After 6–8 hours from the resolution of emesis, it is possible to introduce solid foods.

Moderate Reaction

If the acute reaction is characterized by more than three episodes of emesis, mild lethargy, and pallor, the patient has to be transported to the emergency room for the appropriate management. The priority in the moderate FPIES reactions is to perform continuous hemodynamic monitoring as a tool to help maintain patient fluid balance. Fluid therapy is based on an assessment of the degree of dehydration present. If the fluid loss is not excessive, an oral rehydration may be attempted. Peripheral intravenous line placement is always recommended. In subjects over 6 months of age, the intramuscular administration of ondansetron (0.15 mg/kg/dose with a maximum recommended dose of 16 mg) could represent a valid support to contain the fluid losses. In case of poor clinical control coming from oral hydration, an isotonic fluid resuscitation (e.g., 10–20 mL/kg boluses of normal saline) is required. The monitoring and measurement of vital signs is useful for providing real-time data and necessary to assess the clinical situation of the patient. Continuous monitoring might detect clinical deterioration at an earlier stage, which allows clinicians to take corrective actions. Indeed, if a progressive clinical worsening should be highlighted, the patient must be transferred to the intensive care unit for managing extreme lethargy, respiratory distress, persistent or severe hypotension even to a hypovolemic shock condition. Though the clinical manifestations are stable showing a gradual improvement, the indication is to monitor the patient for at least 4–6 hours from the onset of FPIES symptoms. The most important criterion for discharge to home is the patient's ability to tolerate clear liquids.

Severe Reaction

More than three episodes of emesis, severe lethargy, hypotonia, ashen, or cyanotic appearance characterize a severe FPIES reaction. This clinical condition requires an emergency transportation. Once the patient arrives at the emergency department, the most appropriate medical care can be provided. The detection of vital signs and the placement of peripheral intravenous line represent the first steps toward an appropriate clinical management. The severe reactions require a rapid restoration of stable hemodynamics through aggressive isotonic fluid resuscitation (e.g., 10–20 mL/kg boluses of normal saline), repeated as needed to correct the hypotension. In subjects over 6 months of age, the intravenous administration of ondansetron (0.15 mg/kg/dose with a maximum dose of 16 mg) is recommended. If the placement of intravenous line is delayed due to difficult access and the patient's age is suitable, an intramuscular dose of ondansetron may also help limit further fluid loss. FPIES is considered a non-IgE-mediated food allergy, and in order to reduce a presumed cell-mediated inflammation, a single dose of intravenous methylprednisolone (at 1 mg/kg, with a maximum of 60–80 mg) could be administered [2, 10]. If the patient's clinical condition worsens, a transfer to intensive care will be required. Additional precautions must be put in place including supplemental oxygen, mechanical ventilation or noninvasive positive pressure ventilation for respiratory insufficiency, vasopressors for hypotension, bicarbonate for acidemia, and methylene blue for methemoglobinemia. Epinephrine autoinjectors are not routinely prescribed to FPIES patients, because the hypotension occurred during a severe reaction is theoretically nothing but the result of fluid loss from the gastrointestinal symptoms (prolonged vomiting and diarrhea). For this reason epinephrine without intravenous hydration may not be effective. There is no evidence that the administration of antihistamines may play a role in this type of reactions. A possible discharge can occur only when the clinical condition is completely restored and the patient is able to tolerate oral fluids again.

Pharmacological treatment in FPIES has an ancillary role to rehydration but can be useful in the acute setting.

Reports from case series [11, 12] suggest a possible role for parenteral ondansetron in controlling acute symptoms. Ondansetron is a selective 5-hydroxytryptamine3 (5-HT3) receptor antagonist that has been introduced to clinical practice as an antiemetic for postsurgical and cancer treatment-induced nausea and vomiting [13]. In 2016, a systematic review with meta-analysis underlined the usefulness of ondansetron to control vomiting during acute gastroenteritis improving the efficacy of oral rehydration therapy [14]. 5-Hydroxytryptamine (5-HT, serotonin) is a monoaminergic neurotransmitter that modulates several neuronal functions, the contraction and relaxation of smooth muscles in the respiratory and gastrointestinal tracts and blood vessels, platelet plug formation during hemostasis, provocation of pain, and induction of vomiting. Serotonin also stimulates peristalsis, gastric emptying, and secretion of liquid and electrolytes to the intestine. High concentrations of 5-HT3 receptors are found in the central nervous system (CNS) in the area postrema (chemoreceptor trigger zone); nucleus tractus solitarius (vomiting center); substantia gelatinosa (at all levels); nuclei of the lower brain stems, such as the trigeminal nucleus and the dorsal vagal complex; and the spinal cord [15]. The only relevant adverse effect of ondansetron is the risk of prolonged QT interval, which can lead to torsade de pointes, a potentially fatal arrhythmia. As this is a dose-dependent adverse effect, it has been recommended that a single >32 mg intravenous dose should be avoided. Patients with bradyarrhythmias and patients taking concomitant medications that prolong the QT interval are at greater risk [16]. In 2017, Miceli Sopo et al. compared parenteral ondansetron administration with traditional therapy (intravenous fluids and methylprednisolone [1 mg/kg]) during acute FPIES reactions occurred after an oral food challenge (OFC). The authors have found that only 19% of children treated with ondansetron continued vomiting compared with 93% of children treated with traditional therapy ($P < 0.05$, relative risk = 0.2), but with a lower frequency of vomiting episodes. Children treated with ondansetron were less likely to require an admission overnight compared with those who received traditional therapy ($P < 0.05$). Therefore, the authors conclude that parenteral ondansetron is more effective than intravenous corticosteroids for resolution of the acute symptoms of FPIES [17].

What to Do when Someone Is Experiencing FPIES Reaction?

If the child is experiencing symptoms of FPIES after an accidental ingestion of trigger food, the family members must contact the local emergency services or their physician for guidance (Table 5.2). The history of severe FPIES reaction makes necessary to call immediately an ambulance or go to the nearest emergency department. Otherwise, an oral rehydration at home could be attempted only if the vomiting is less than three times overall.

Table 5.2 Useful information on what to do in case of acute reaction

Clinical history	Management
History of severe FPIES acute reaction	Call an ambulance or go to the emergency department if the trigger food was ingested, regardless of the severity or presence/absence of symptoms
No history of severe FPIES acute reaction	In case of 1–2 episodes of emesis likely associated with mild lethargy, an attempt of oral rehydration (e.g., breastfeed or clear fluids) is suggested If the patient experiences more than 3 episodes of emesis combined with moderate or severe lethargy, calling an ambulance or going to the emergency room is recommended

Table adapted from Nowak-Węgrzyn et al. [2]

Key Idea "Pearls"

- FPIES can be a medical emergency due to severe gastrointestinal symptoms including repeated episodes of vomiting accompanied by watery or bloody diarrhea that can lead to severe dehydration and hemodynamic instability.
- The management of acute FPIES reactions is based on rehydration. Oral rehydration at home is recommended in mild reactions, whereas intravenous fluid replacement is mandatory in severe forms characterized by protracted emesis, lethargy, pallor, diarrhea up to hypotension, and metabolic acidosis. Intramuscular or intravenous administration of ondansetron could represent a valid support to stop vomiting and limit fluid losses.
- The history of severe FPIES reaction makes necessary to call immediately an ambulance or go to the nearest emergency department.

References

1. Powell GK. Enterocolitis in low-birth-weight infants associated with milk and soy protein intolerance. J Pediatr. 1976;88(5):840–4.
2. Nowak-Węgrzyn A, et al. International consensus guidelines for the diagnosis and management of food protein-induced enterocolitis syndrome: executive summary-Workgroup Report of the Adverse Reactions to Foods Committee, American Academy of Allergy, Asthma & Immunology. J Allergy Clin Immunol. 2017;139(4):1111–1126.e4.
3. Fiocchi A, Claps A, Dahdah L, Brindisi G, Dionisi-Vici C, Martelli A. Differential diagnosis of food protein-induced enterocolitis syndrome. Curr Opin Allergy Clin Immunol. 2014;14(3):246–54.
4. Monti G, et al. Food protein-induced enterocolitis syndrome by cow's milk proteins passed through breast milk. J Allergy Clin Immunol. 2011;127(3):679–80.
5. Tan J, Campbell D, Mehr S. Food protein-induced enterocolitis syndrome in an exclusively breast-fed infant-an uncommon entity. J Allergy Clin Immunol. 2012;129(3):873.
6. Kimura M, Ito Y, Tokunaga F, Meguro T, Shimomura M, Morishita H, Seto S. Increased C-reactive protein and fever in Japanese infants with food protein-induced enterocolitis syndrome. Pediatr Int. 2016;58(9):826–30.
7. Kimura M, Ito Y, Shimomura M, Morishita H, Meguro T, Adachi Y, Seto S. Cytokine profile after oral food challenge in infants with food protein-induced enterocolitis syndrome. Allergol Int. 2017;66(3):452–7.
8. Pecora V, Prencipe G, Valluzzi R, Dahdah L, Insalaco A, Cianferoni A, De Benedetti F, Fiocchi A. Inflammatory events during food protein-induced enterocolitis syndrome reactions. Pediatr Allergy Immunol. 2017;28(5):464–70.
9. Dahdah L, Fiocchi A, Mazzina O, et al. FPIES: effects of educational intervention in an Italian children hospital. Allergy. 2014;60(Suppl 99):167.
10. Sicherer SH. Food protein-induced enterocolitis syndrome: case presentations and management lessons. J Allergy Clin Immunol. 2005;115(1):149–56.
11. Holbrook T, Keet CA, Frischmeyer-Guerreiro PA, Wood RA. Use of ondansetron for food protein-induced enterocolitis syndrome. J Allergy Clin Immunol. 2013;135(5):1219–20.
12. Miceli Sopo SM, Battista A, Greco M, Monaco S. Ondansetron for food protein-induced enterocolitis syndrome. Int Arch Allergy Immunol. 2014;164:137–9.

13. Cunningham RS. 5-HT3-receptor antagonists: a review of pharmacology and clinical efficacy. Oncol Nurs Forum. 1997;24(7 Suppl):33–40.
14. Tomasik E, Ziółkowska E, Kołodziej M, Szajewska H. Systematic review with meta-analysis: ondansetron for vomiting in children with acute gastroenteritis. Aliment Pharmacol Ther. 2016;44(5):438–46.
15. Bradley PB, Engel G, Feniuk W, et al. Proposals for the classification and nomenclature of functional receptors for 5-hydroxytryptamine. Neuropharmacology. 1986;25:563–76.
16. Doggrell SA, Hancox JC. Cardiac safety concerns for ondansetron, an antiemetic commonly used for nausea linked to cancer treatment and following anaesthesia. Expert Opin Drug Saf. 2013;12(3):421–31.
17. Miceli Sopo S, Bersani G, Monaco S, Cerchiara G, Lee E, Campbell D, Mehr S. Ondansetron in acute food protein-induced enterocolitis syndrome, a retrospective case-control study. Allergy. 2017;72(4):545–51.

Diagnosis and Management of Chronic FPIES

6

Mary Grace Baker and Anna Nowak-Wegrzyn

Introduction

Although poorly understood and often misdiagnosed, the clinical features of chronic FPIES have been recognized for many decades [1–3]. In contrast to acute FPIES in which symptoms are more easily identified as resulting from the ingestion of a trigger food, chronic FPIES occurs when the trigger food is not immediately identified, with continued ingestion resulting in chronic symptoms [4]. The lack of a clear temporal relationship between the ingestion of a culprit food and symptom onset as well as the symptom overlap with many other gastrointestinal and systemic processes can create a delay in diagnosis, contributing to prolonged symptomatology and increased severity of the patient's condition. This is illustrated by the following case:

A female infant presented to our office for a consultation at age 5 months. The baby was carried by a surrogate and was born full-term by normal spontaneous vaginal delivery with no complications. She was started on a cow's milk formula in the nursery. By day 3 of life, she was noted to be fussy and had frequent bowel movements. After discharge from the hospital, her stools contained mucus, so she was switched to an extensively hydrolyzed casein-based infant formula. Although she initially improved, a few days later, she started having two green, mucus-containing stools after each feeding.

M. G. Baker
Pediatrics, Division of Allergy and Immunology, Icahn School of Medicine at Mount Sinai, New York, NY, USA

A. Nowak-Wegrzyn (✉)
Division of Allergy and Immunology, Department of Pediatrics, Elliot and Roslyn Jaffe Food Allergy Institute, Icahn School of Medicine at Mount Sinai, New York, NY, USA
e-mail: anna.nowak-wegrzyn@nyulangone.org

T. F. Brown-Whitehorn, A. Cianferoni (eds.), *Food Protein Induced Enterocolitis (FPIES)*,
https://doi.org/10.1007/978-3-030-21229-2_6

At age 3 weeks, she had been losing weight. One day, she became acutely pale and lethargic. She was taken to the Pediatric Emergency Department, where she underwent a full sepsis workup. Complete blood count revealed a leukocytosis 22,400 cells/mcL (normal range for age 5000–19,500 cells/mcL), thrombocytosis 650,000 cells/mcL (150,000–450,000 cells/mcL), and eosinophilia with an absolute eosinophil count of 1568 cells/mcL (180–525 cells/mcL). A metabolic panel demonstrated a metabolic acidosis with pH 7.25 and a bicarbonate level of 16. A serum lactate of 3.23 was measured. C-reactive protein (CRP) was 17 mg/L (normal range for age <10.0 mg/L). Fecal calprotectin was elevated at 731 (normal range for age not established); a fecal PCR panel revealed no evidence of bacterial or viral pathogens. Blood and urine cultures returned negative. While in the hospital, the baby was fed a different extensively hydrolyzed casein-based infant formula. She initially appeared to tolerate the new formula well; however, on day 4–5 of the hospitalization, she developed vomiting and diarrhea. It was then that the diagnosis of FPIES to cow's milk was considered, and the decision was made to change to an amino acid-based formula. With this change in her diet, her bowel movements normalized to one to two per day with only occasional mucus. She required a proton-pump inhibitor for gastroesophageal reflux symptoms, but she otherwise tolerated feeds well and was growing and developing normally.

Clinical Presentation

Chronic FPIES is diagnosed exclusively in infants, and to date, only cow's milk and soy have been identified as triggers [5]. Symptoms typically begin within the first 4 months of life, with onset within 1–4 weeks of the introduction of cow's milk- or soy-based formula [6, 7]. Affected infants develop watery diarrhea that may contain mucus and/or blood as well as intermittent but progressive vomiting. Infants less than 2 months are significantly more likely to present with diarrhea, blood in the stool, and failure to thrive compared to older infants [4]. Bloody stools are also observed more commonly in Japan compared to western countries [8]. Due to the gradual onset of symptoms and the poor correlation between time of feeding and symptomatology, the relationship between dietary triggers and symptoms often goes unnoticed. As feedings with the culprit formula continue, the infant becomes progressively more ill with failure to thrive, weight loss, and lethargy or irritability [9, 10]. In severe cases, patients may exhibit abdominal distention, dehydration, hypotension, and even shock [11]. In infants diagnosed with chronic FPIES and placed on an avoidance diet, if the culprit food is excluded for a brief period and then re-introduced, affected patients will experience an acute FPIES reaction upon re-ingestion, definitively confirming the diagnosis [2]. The features of chronic and acute FPIES are compared in Table 6.1 [4, 6, 7, 12].

Table 6.1 Comparison of chronic vs. acute FPIES

Feature	Chronic FPIES	Acute FPIES
Age of onset	Following introduction of formula (typically first days or months of life)	Following introduction of solid foods (typically >4 months)
Trigger foods	Cow's milk- or soy-based formula	Cow's milk, soy, rice, oat, egg, fish, legumes
Symptoms	Intermittent but progressive vomiting, watery diarrhea +/– mucus or blood, failure to thrive, lethargy, dehydration, and shock	Repeated, projectile vomiting 1–4 hours (usually 2 hours) after ingestion with possible diarrhea, lethargy, dehydration, and hypovolemic shock
Laboratory evaluation	Leukocytosis with neutrophilia, elevated eosinophils, thrombocytosis, metabolic acidosis, methemoglobinemia, anemia, hypoalbuminemia, hypoproteinemia	Leukocytosis with neutrophilia, elevated eosinophils, thrombocytosis, metabolic acidosis, methemoglobinemia
Management	Avoidance of cow's milk and soy milk formulas Feeding with breast milk, hydrolyzed formula, or elemental formula Solid food introduction at 6 months starting with low risk foods	Avoidance of culprit food Depending on the trigger food, cautious introduction of other solid foods with progression from lower to higher-risk foods
Symptom resolution	Typically between 2 days and 2 weeks after trigger food elimination; in severe cases bowel rest and total parenteral nutrition may be required	Within 24 hours of trigger food elimination
Natural history	Varies by region but typically resolves within one to five years	Reintroduction of the food may be attempted as soon as 6 months after the last known reaction; typically it is delayed for about 12–24 months, depending on the severity of the prior reactions and the nutritional and social importance of the food

Epidemiology

The onset of chronic FPIES has been described only in infancy. The age at diagnosis varies with the timing of the introduction of cow's milk- or soy-based formula, but most patients are diagnosed before age 4–6 months [4, 6]. Chronic FPIES has been reported worldwide, but the exact prevalence is not certain. In one study of patients in Israel by Katz et al., 13,019 infants born at a single institution over a 2-year period were monitored for signs/symptoms of FPIES to cow's milk [13]. Of these infants, 3 in 1000 (0.34%) went on to be diagnosed with FPIES due to cow's milk, although it is not clear how many of them exhibited chronic symptoms prior to a milk challenge. The diagnosis of chronic FPIES does appear to be somewhat more common in Japan and Korea and seemingly has increased significantly over the last several years [14–16]. It is expected that the reported prevalence worldwide may increase as recognition of this diagnosis continues to improve.

Regarding risk factors for chronic FPIES, work by Caubet et al. identified the introduction of cow's milk formula, soy formula, or both within the first few weeks of life as significantly associated with FPIES to these triggers [17]. Breastfeeding has generally been considered protective. A slight male predominance has been observed. In their Israeli cohort, Katz et al. identified birth by cesarean section and Jewish religion as risk factors for FPIES [13]. Although a family history of atopy is common, siblings with FPIES have been reported only in twins, and the contribution of genetics vs. environmental factors remains uncertain [9, 18].

Regarding triggers, chronic FPIES occurs when the culprit food is ingested very regularly and usually at least daily. Cow's milk and soy are the only reported trigger foods to date. Of note, chronic and acute FPIES have rarely been reported in patients exclusively breastfed [15, 19–21]. It seems that this occurs due to the passage of trace amounts of FPIES triggers through the breast milk.

Pathophysiology

The pathophysiology of chronic FPIES remains poorly understood. It is thought that FPIES occurs due to a combination of factors intrinsic to the gut as well as innate and cell-mediated immune pathways. Much remains to be learned about the complex interplay of each of these processes. Nonetheless, a summary of key findings is provided (Table 6.2).

There has recently been interest in the pathophysiology of FPIES in infants with Down syndrome. Wakiguchi et al. reported two cases of prolonged FPIES to cow's milk in children with Down syndrome [22]. Immune dysregulation and reduced levels of IL-10 have previously been reported in children with Down syndrome [23]. Given that IL-10 may be associated with the acquisition of tolerance, this defect may help explain the delay in FPIES resolution. It has also been shown that TNF-α is increased in Down syndrome patients, which may confer some predisposition to FPIES in this population [23, 24].

Diagnosis

Criteria for the diagnosis of chronic FPIES have recently been proposed [4]. The diagnosis is suggested based on a convincing clinical history, including chronic watery diarrhea and intermittent but progressive vomiting that are not attributable to another disease process and resolve within days to weeks following the elimination of the offending food trigger. If the culprit food is re-introduced after a period of avoidance, an acute FPIES reaction will develop. The diagnosis of chronic FPIES is presumptive in the absence of a positive oral food challenge to the suspected trigger

Table 6.2 Major pathophysiologic changes in FPIES

Process	Reported findings in FPIES
Gastrointestinal factors: defects in barrier function [51, 52]	Low expression of TGF-β1 in duodenal biopsy specimens, leading to reduced gut epithelial barrier function Increased TNF-α expression in duodenal biopsy specimens, resulting in increases in gut permeability Increased IL-9 secretion (measured in supernatants) may contribute to increased gut permeability
Innate immune system (peripheral blood) [3, 52–56]	Neutrophils: Increased count and activation Mast cells: Suspected increased activation or accumulation/density as evidenced by increased baseline serum tryptase; no evidence of degranulation in acute FPIES, as tryptase level does not increase following a reactive challenge Lymphocytes: Decreased Monocytes: No change in absolute number of circulating monocytes but enrichment of CD14+ monocytes and increased activation Eosinophils: Decreased peripheral eosinophils during FPIES reactions but evidence of increased eosinophil activation in the blood and GI tract Natural killer cells: Increased activation CRP: Increased and at levels higher than seen in FPIAP
Cell-mediated immunity [53, 57, 58]	Generally skewed toward T_H2 (measured in supernatants) High levels of IL-2, suggesting some T_H1 activity During reactions, there appears to be pan T-cell activation
Eosinophils [53, 59, 60]	Peripheral blood eosinophilia may be noted at diagnosis and can be marked During acute reactions, the peripheral eosinophil count may decrease, although there is evidence of increased circulating eosinophil activation with increased CD69 expression An increase in fecal eosinophil-derived neurotoxin has been observed, suggesting possible increases in activated eosinophils in the gastrointestinal tract
Cytokine profile [8, 52, 58, 59, 61, 62]	Patients with active FPIES demonstrate deficient TGF-β response (measured in supernatant from the peripheral blood mononuclear cell culture) Serum IL-2, IL-8, and IL-10 increase during FPIES reactions and appear to be involved in the antigen-specific response High serum IL-5 levels correlate with peripheral blood eosinophilia Increases in serum IL-10 appear to correlate with the development of tolerance, although elevated serum IL-10 has been observed in active FPIES

food, although a challenge is not considered imperative in the setting of a compelling clinical history [25].

In infants with chronic FPIES due to cow's milk, hypoalbuminemia and weight gain of less than 10 g/d have been reported to serve as independent predictors of this diagnosis [14]. Laboratory evaluations may reveal a leukocytosis with neutrophilia, thrombocytosis, anemia, hypoalbuminemia, metabolic acidosis, and, in severe cases, methemoglobinemia (Table 6.1). Stool studies may show guaiac positivity, polymorphonuclear neutrophils, eosinophils, Charcot-Leyden crystals, and reducing substances [2, 3, 26].

Although now considered unnecessary for diagnosis, prior to the widespread recognition of this condition, radiographic and endoscopic examinations were common [4]. Abdominal radiographs have demonstrated dilated bowel loops with air-fluid levels and rarely intramural gas [2, 4, 7]. Other reported findings include nonspecific narrowing and thumb printing of the rectum and sigmoid colon as well as thickening of the plicae circulares in the duodenum and jejunum with excess luminal fluid [10]. Upper endoscopic evaluation may demonstrate gastric edema, erythema, friable mucosa, and erosions [27]. Biopsy specimens may show villous atrophy and infiltration of inflammatory cells including lymphocytes and eosinophils [28–31]. Lower endoscopy may appear grossly normal or show proctocolitis with friable mucosa, ulcerations, and loss of vascular pattern in the mucosa [1, 32, 33]. Histopathologic examination of biopsy specimens has revealed infiltration of lymphocytes, plasma cells, and polymorphonuclear cells; destruction of the surface epithelium; crypt abscesses; and glandular changes.

As with acute FPIES, no definitive laboratory or imaging test can be performed to confirm the diagnosis of FPIES. As such, it is important to exclude other processes in the setting of diagnostic ambiguity. A review of the differential diagnosis for chronic FPIES symptoms and distinguishing features is included here (Table 6.3). Additional information on differential diagnosis is discussed in Chaps. 7 and 8.

Table 6.3 Differential diagnosis for chronic FPIES

Diagnosis	Features that distinguish from chronic FPIES
Sepsis	Blood cultures may be positive Unlikely to be recurrent
Viral gastroenteritis	Sick contacts are likely to be identified Symptoms are more self-limited Unlikely to be recurrent
Necrotizing enterocolitis	More common in premature infants during their first weeks of life
Intussusception	Evidence of anatomic abnormality on ultrasound or x-ray
Gastroesophageal reflux disease (GERD)	Not associated with abnormalities in stooling Responsive to treatment with antacid medication
Lactose intolerance	Not associated with vomiting or blood/mucus in the stool More likely to exhibit significant gas and borborygmi
Food protein-induced allergic proctocolitis (FPIAP)	Both conditions may include grossly bloody stools Patients with FPIAP are otherwise healthy with no vomiting, lethargy/irritability, failure to thrive, etc. Symptoms more reliably resolve within the first year No acute symptoms following trigger food reintroduction
Food protein-induced enteropathy [FPE]	Chronic diarrhea Malabsorption; stool positive for reducing substances Anemia, hypoalbuminemia, hypoproteinemia Failure to thrive Intestinal biopsy: villous atrophy No acute symptoms following trigger food reintroduction
IgE-mediated food allergy/anaphylaxis	Symptoms are unlikely to be isolated to the gastrointestinal tract; usually skin and respiratory symptoms are present Symptoms typically occur immediately upon ingestion (within a few minutes to 30–60 minutes) and respond to epinephrine and antihistamines
Inborn errors of metabolism	Typically associated with extra-intestinal manifestations including developmental delay, neurologic symptoms, etc. Supported by evidence of associated abnormal laboratory values

Natural History

Symptoms

Following proper diagnosis and dietary modification, complete symptom resolution can be expected in about 2 days to 2 weeks [7]. As with acute FPIES, it is expected that patients with chronic FPIES will develop tolerance to trigger foods during childhood.

The timing of FPIES resolution varies from patient to patient, and the evidence is very limited. In the United States, the median age of resolution for cow's milk FPIES was 3–5 years [9, 17, 34]. Data from the UK have also suggested that symptoms may persist for many years, with up to 25% of patients with non-IgE-mediated gastrointestinal allergy reporting symptoms at 8 years of age [35]. The study by Katz et al. suggested that the time to resolution in Israeli children may be shorter, with tolerance in 60% at 1 year of age, 75% at 2 years, and 85% at 3 years [13]. A shorter time to resolution has also been noted in Korea by Hwang et al. with tolerance in 27% of patients at 6 months of age, 64% at 10 months, and 73% at 14–16 months [36]. All patients in this study were tolerant by 18–20 months of age.

In Japanese studies, various phenotypic and laboratory features have been correlated with prognosis. It has been observed that FPIES infants with bloody stools achieve tolerance more quickly than patients without bloody stools [8]. All children with FPIES with bloody stools achieved tolerance before age 2, while 50% of children without bloody stools achieved tolerance around age 2, and all children eventually achieved tolerance just after age 3. Additionally, a study by Kimura et al. reported that an elevation in CRP at presentation correlated with a more protracted course, while the presence of eosinophilia at presentation correlated with sooner acquisition of tolerance [37].

Tolerance to soy typically develops somewhat later, often between the ages of 3 and 7 years in the United States and Australia [5, 17, 34, 38]. However, a trend toward earlier resolution in Asia has been reported, with 75% of Korean patients tolerant to soy at 6 months, and all patients tolerant by 12–14 months [36]. These differences are likely related to a more delayed and less frequent formal evaluation for resolution in the US and Australia compared to South Korea. There are rare reports of FPIES to both milk and soy persisting into adulthood, and the presence of food-specific IgE to the culprit food has been associated with a more protracted course [5, 9]. It is also thought that children with Down syndrome may have delayed FPIES resolution with symptoms lasting well into childhood [22].

The reason for the significant variation in the reported natural history of FPIES and time to resolution remains uncertain. Possible explanations include differences in genetics, feeding practices, diet, etc. Discrepancies may also be explained by differences in study methods as well as bias related to the composition of the study populations. It should be noted that infants with chronic FPIES to cow's milk and soy may develop acute FPIES to solid foods, with its own trajectory for symptom resolution [39].

FPIES to Additional Food Triggers

In the United States, it was observed early on that patients diagnosed with chronic FPIES often demonstrate co-reactivity to cow's milk and soy-based infant formulas [5, 26, 33]. It is now estimated that up to 20–40% of infants in the United States are co-reactive [4, 9, 17]. The likelihood of cow's milk and soy co-reactivity increases if FPIES symptoms begin in the first weeks of life [4, 17]. This same level of co-reactivity is not observed in other countries, possibly due to differences in the use of soy-based formula in the United States vs. abroad [13, 19, 40].

It has also been observed that infants diagnosed with chronic FPIES may be at risk for acute FPIES to solid foods [9, 17]. Reactions to rice and/or oat appear to be the most common solid foods to cause reactions in these patients [10]. It is thought that delaying introduction of these cereals until age 6–9 months (but not later) may reduce the risk of acute solid food FPIES [6, 41].

Atypical FPIES and the Association with IgE-Mediated Food Allergy

Patients are considered to have atypical FPIES when the clinical history is consistent with FPIES but the patient demonstrates allergic sensitization with positive skin prick testing or food-specific IgE [5, 39]. It has been observed that children with atypical cow's milk FPIES tend to have a more protracted course with increased time to FPIES resolution, sometimes into adulthood. Upon physician-supervised oral food challenge, it may be observed that a subset of these patients exhibits symptoms of IgE-mediated food allergy and remains unable to tolerate the food despite apparent resolution of FPIES. The frequency of atypical chronic FPIES is unknown; overall the estimates of atypical cow's milk FPIES range from 5 to 20%. Additionally, Caubet et al. reported that 30% of children with FPIES had a concomitant IgE-mediated allergy to a different food [17].

Management and Guidelines

If the diagnosis of chronic FPIES is suspected, the affected patient should be stabilized, and the importance of long-term dietary changes must be reinforced. The cornerstone of management is the avoidance of the trigger food [5]. It is generally recommended that parents of affected infants resume exclusive breastfeeding (if the symptoms were induced by a supplemental feeding with an infant formula), consistent with general pediatric guidelines, or switch to casein hypoallergenic formula [4, 5, 41–43]. Although the co-reactivity between cow's milk and soy FPIES is common in the United States, this is less common abroad, and cautious introduction of the alternative formula could be considered. It is generally felt that maternal avoidance of her infant's FPIES trigger while breastfeeding is not necessary. This recommendation should be re-considered if the infant has acute or chronic FPIES symptoms while breastfeeding or demonstrates failure to thrive [44]. Despite the modification in the maternal diet during breastfeeding and/or a hypoallergenic extensively hydrolyzed infant formula, up to 10–20% of infants may have symptoms that require transition to an elemental formula [9, 10, 17, 45]. When managing breastfed infants with FPIES, nutritional consultation is strongly recommended to minimize the risk of nutritional deficiencies in the infant and the mother [4].

For children with a history of FPIES to cow's milk formula, many families inquire about the safety of foods related to cow's milk, including other animal milks, and the use of cow's milk as an ingredient in baked goods. Data are limited, and recommendations are partially extrapolated from studies of patients with IgE-mediated allergy. Due to the significant amino acid sequence homology between animal milks, it is not recommended that infants substitute goat or sheep milk formula [4, 12, 46, 47]. Limited reports suggest that donkey and camel milk may be tolerated, although these generally are not widely commercially available in western countries [20, 48]. Regarding baked milk, Mehr et al. reported that 12 out of 75 patients with FPIES to milk had been exposed to baked milk, and there were no noted reactions [19]. Meyer et al. also reported tolerance of baked milk in some older children who did not yet tolerate natural cow's milk [35]. Miceli Sopo et al. conducted oral food challenges on a small number of children with cow's milk allergy, and three out of four children were tolerant [49]. Due to the limited data and lack of identifiable factors to predict who might tolerate baked milk, it is felt that baked milk can be continued in children who have already been shown to be tolerant but that introduction of baked milk is best done under physician supervision [4]. It is common for children with IgE-mediated allergy to cow's milk to tolerate baked milk before natural milk, but it is not sure if the same applies to children with FPIES [50]. As such, it is recommended that children with FPIES to cow's milk avoid baked milk.

Due to the association between food ingestion and unpleasant FPIES reactions as well as the delay in introducing new foods due to fear of additional reactions, it is not uncommon for infants with FPIES to go on to demonstrate food aversions, food refusal, etc. [41] Unfortunately, when combined with the already restricted diet, this compounds the risk of nutritional and developmental problems. It is strongly encouraged that a nutritionist be consulted for an evaluation and assistance expanding the diet [4]. Additionally, if a family is apprehensive about introducing new foods at home due to fear of a reaction, physician-supervised introduction of these foods should be offered to ensure adequate nutrition, growth, and development [6].

It is recommended that patients with chronic FPIES be evaluated by an experienced allergist at least annually. Depending on the severity of prior reactions and the timing since the last reaction, it is reasonable to begin considering whether the FPIES has resolved within 1–2 years of the last reaction. Due to the possibility of severe symptoms, it is recommended that patients be evaluated for FPIES resolution with a physician-supervised oral food challenge in the office setting [4, 25]. If there is a history of life-threatening signs/symptoms including hypotension, acidosis, etc., additional precautions including peripheral intravenous line placement and preparation of IV fluids may be required. In cases of atypical FPIES with positive

IgE to the food being challenged, antihistamines and self-injectable epinephrine should also be available [17].

Summary

Chronic FPIES remains elusive, and its epidemiology is unknown. In a classic form, chronic FPIES manifests as a severe infantile disorder of watery diarrhea and intermittent vomiting triggered by feeding with cow's milk- and/or soy-based infant formulas that culminates in failure to thrive, hypoalbuminemia, hypoproteinemia, dehydration, metabolic acidosis and shock. Due to the poorly understood pathophysiology and lack of biomarkers, the oral food challenge remains the only reliable diagnostic test. It is unclear whether chronic FPIES can be triggered by solid foods ingested in lower doses and on a more intermittent basis and or manifest with milder symptoms without dehydration and metabolic acidosis. In spite of the severe initial presentation, it appears that the natural history is favorable with the resolution of cow's milk and soy chronic FPIES within the first few years of life.

Key Points

- Chronic FPIES occurs in young infants when the food trigger, cow's milk- or soy-based formula, is ingested on a regular basis.
- Symptoms initially include watery diarrhea, intermittent vomiting, and irritability but will progress to include failure to thrive, lethargy, dehydration, metabolic acidosis, or even shock if unrecognized.
- The diagnosis of chronic FPIES is suggested based on a careful history and definitively confirmed only through provocation of an acute FPIES reaction upon a supervised oral food challenge with the culprit food.
- It is thought that FPIES occurs due to a combination of factors intrinsic to the gut as well as innate and cell-mediated immune pathways.
- Patients are considered to have atypical FPIES when the clinical history is consistent with FPIES but the patient demonstrates allergic sensitization with positive skin prick testing or food-specific IgE.
- The cornerstone of management is the avoidance of the trigger food.
- In spite of the severe initial presentation, the natural history of cow's milk and soy chronic FPIES is generally favorable with resolution within the first few years of life.
- Depending on the severity of prior reactions and the timing since the last reaction, it is reasonable to begin considering whether the FPIES has resolved within one to 2 years of the last reaction. Due to the possibility of severe symptoms, it is recommended that patients be evaluated for FPIES resolution with a physician-supervised oral food challenge in the office setting.

References

1. Gryboski JD. Gastrointestinal milk allergy in infants. Pediatrics. 1967;40(3):354–62.
2. Powell GK. Enterocolitis in low-birth-weight infants associated with milk and soy protein intolerance. J Pediatr. 1976;88(5):840–4.
3. Powell GK. Milk- and soy-induced enterocolitis of infancy: clinical features and standardization of challenge. J Pediatr. 1978;93(4):553–60.
4. Nowak-Wegrzyn A, Chehade M, Groetch ME, et al. International consensus guidelines for the diagnosis and management of food protein-induced enterocolitis syndrome: executive summary-workgroup report of the adverse reactions to foods committee, American Academy of Allergy, Asthma & Immunology. J Allergy Clin Immunol. 2017;139(4):1111–26.
5. Sicherer SH, Eigenmann PA, Sampson HA. Clinical features of food protein–induced enterocolitis syndrome. J Pediatr. 1998;133(2):214–9.
6. Leonard SA, Pecora V, Fiocchi AG, Nowak-Wegrzyn A. Food protein-induced enterocolitis syndrome: a review of the new guidelines. The World Allergy Organization journal. 2018;11(1):4.
7. Weinberger T, Feuille E, Thompson C, Nowak-Wegrzyn A. Chronic food protein-induced enterocolitis syndrome: characterization of clinical phenotype and literature review. Ann Allergy Asthma Immunol. 2016;117(3):227–33.
8. Morita H, Suzuki H, Orihara K, et al. Food protein-induced enterocolitis syndromes with and without bloody stool have distinct clinicopathologic features. J Allergy Clin Immunol. 2017;140(6):1718–1721.e1716.
9. Nowak-Wegrzyn A, Sampson HA, Wood RA, Sicherer SH. Food protein-induced enterocolitis syndrome caused by solid food proteins. Pediatrics. 2003;111(4. Pt 1):829–35.
10. Jarvinen KM, Nowak-Wegrzyn A. Food protein-induced enterocolitis syndrome (FPIES): current management strategies and review of the literature. J Allergy Clin Immunol Pract. 2013;1(4):317–22.
11. Peduto A, Rocca M, De Maio C, Gallarotti F, Pomero G, Gancia P. Metabolic acidosis as food protein induced enterocolitis syndrome (FPIES) onset in a newborn. Ital J Pediatr. 2018;44(1):52.
12. Nowak-Wegrzyn A, Jarocka-Cyrta E, Moschione Castro A. Food protein-induced enterocolitis syndrome. J Investig Allergol Clin Immunol. 2017;27(1):1–18.
13. Katz Y, Goldberg MR, Rajuan N, Cohen A, Leshno M. The prevalence and natural course of food protein–induced enterocolitis syndrome to cow's milk: a large-scale, prospective population-based study. J Allergy Clin Immunol. 2011;127(3):647–53. e643.
14. Hwang JB, Lee SH, Kang YN, Kim SP, Suh SI, Kam S. Indexes of suspicion of typical cow's milk protein-induced enterocolitis. J Korean Med Sci. 2007;22(6):993–7.
15. Nomura I, Morita H, Hosokawa S, et al. Four distinct subtypes of non-IgE-mediated gastrointestinal food allergies in neonates and infants, distinguished by their initial symptoms. J Allergy Clin Immunol. 2011;127(3):685–8. e681-688.
16. Nomura I, Morita H, Ohya Y, Saito H, Matsumoto K. Non-IgE-mediated gastrointestinal food allergies: distinct differences in clinical phenotype between Western countries and Japan. Curr Allergy Asthma Rep. 2012;12(4):297–303.
17. Caubet JC, Ford LS, Sickles L, et al. Clinical features and resolution of food protein-induced enterocolitis syndrome: 10-year experience. J Allergy Clin Immunol. 2014;134(2):382–9.
18. Shoda T, Isozaki A, Kawano Y. Food protein-induced gastrointestinal syndromes in identical and fraternal twins. Allergol Int. 2011;60(1):103–8.
19. Mehr S, Frith K, Barnes EH, Campbell DE. Food protein–induced enterocolitis syndrome in Australia: a population-based study, 2012-2014. J Allergy Clin Immunol. 2017;140(5):1323–30.
20. Miceli Sopo S, Dello Iacono I, Greco M, Monti G. Clinical management of food protein-induced enterocolitis syndrome. Curr Opin Allergy Clin Immunol. 2014;14(3):240–5.
21. Monti G, Castagno E, Liguori SA, et al. Food protein-induced enterocolitis syndrome by cow's milk proteins passed through breast milk. J Allergy Clin Immunol. 2011;127(3):679–80.

22. Wakiguchi H, Hasegawa S, Kaneyasu H, et al. Long-lasting non-IgE-mediated gastrointestinal cow's milk allergy in infants with down syndrome. Pediatr Allerg Immunol. 2015;26(8):821–3.
23. Nateghi Rostami M, Douraghi M, Miramin Mohammadi A, Nikmanesh B. Altered serum pro-inflammatory cytokines in children with Down's syndrome. Eur Cytokine Netw. 2012;23(2):64–7.
24. Sullivan KD, Evans D, Pandey A, et al. Trisomy 21 causes changes in the circulating proteome indicative of chronic autoinflammation. Sci Rep. 2017;7(1):14818.
25. Panel NIAID-SE, Boyce JA, Assa'ad A, et al. Guidelines for the diagnosis and management of food allergy in the United States: report of the NIAID-sponsored expert panel. J Allergy Clin Immunol. 2010;126. (Suppl:S1–5).
26. Burks AW, Casteel HB, Fiedorek SC, Williams LW, Pumphrey CL. Prospective oral food challenge study of two soybean protein isolates in patients with possible milk or soy protein enterocolitis. Pediatr Allergy Immunol. 1994;5(1):40–5.
27. Coello-Ramirez P, Larrosa-Haro A. Gastrointestinal occult hemorrhage and Gastroduodenitis in Cow's Milk protein intolerance. J Pediatr Gastroenterol Nutr. 1984;3(2):215–8.
28. Fontaine JL, Navarro J. Small intestinal biopsy in cows milk protein allergy in infancy. Arch Dis Child. 1975;50(5):357–62.
29. Walker-Smith J, Harrison M, Kilby A, Phillips A, France N. Cows' milk-sensitive enteropathy. Arch Dis Child. 1978;53(5):375–80.
30. Manuel PD, Walker-Smith JA, France NE. Patchy enteropathy in childhood. Gut. 1979;20(3):211–5.
31. Chung HL, Hwang JB, Kwon YD, Park MH, Shin WJ, Park JB. Deposition of eosinophil-granule major basic protein and expression of intercellular adhesion molecule-1 and vascular cell adhesion molecule-1 in the mucosa of the small intestine in infants with cow's milk-sensitive enteropathy. J Allergy Clin Immunol. 1999;103(6):1195–201.
32. Goldman H, Proujansky R. Allergic proctitis and gastroenteritis in children. Clinical and mucosal biopsy features in 53 cases. Am J Surg Pathol. 1986;10(2):75–86.
33. Halpin TC, Byrne WJ, Ament ME. Colitis, persistent diarrhea, and soy protein intolerance. J Pediatr. 1977;91(3):404–7.
34. Ruffner MA, Ruymann K, Barni S, Cianferoni A, Brown-Whitehorn T, Spergel JM. Food protein-induced enterocolitis syndrome: insights from review of a large referral population. J Allergy Clin Immunol Pract. 2013;1(4):343–9.
35. Meyer R, Fleming C, Dominguez-Ortega G, et al. Manifestations of food protein induced gastrointestinal allergies presenting to a single tertiary paediatric gastroenterology unit. World Allergy Organ J. 2013;6(1):1–9.
36. Hwang JB, Sohn SM, Kim AS. Prospective follow-up oral food challenge in food protein-induced enterocolitis syndrome. Arch Dis Child. 2009;94(6):425–8.
37. Kimura M, Shimomura M, Morishita H, Meguro T. Prognosis of infantile food protein-induced enterocolitis syndrome in Japan. Pediatr Inter. 2017;59(8):855–60.
38. Mehr S, Kakakios A, Frith K, Kemp AS. Food protein-induced enterocolitis syndrome: 16-year experience. Pediatrics. 2009;123(3):e459–64.
39. Michelet M, Schluckebier D, Petit LM, Caubet JC. Food protein-induced enterocolitis syndrome - a review of the literature with focus on clinical management. J Asthma Allergy. 2017;10:197–207.
40. Miceli SS, G V, Dello EN II, M F, O R. A multicentre retrospective study of 66 Italian children with food protein-induced enterocolitis syndrome: different management for different phenotypes. Clin Exp Allergy. 2012;42(8):1257–65.
41. Venter C, Groetch M. Nutritional management of food protein-induced enterocolitis syndrome. Curr Opin Allergy Clin Immunol. 2014;14(3):255–62.
42. Kemp AS, Hill DJ, Allen KJ, et al. Guidelines for the use of infant formulas to treat cows milk protein allergy: an Australian consensus panel opinion. Med J Aust. 2008;188(2):109–12.
43. Kleinman RE. American Academy of Pediatrics recommendations for complementary feeding. Pediatrics. 2000;106(5):1274.
44. Vergara Perez I, Vila Sexto L. Suspected severe acute food protein-induced enterocolitis syndrome caused by cow's milk through breast milk. Ann Allergy Asthma Immunol. 2018;121:245.

45. Kelso JM, Sampson HA. Food protein-induced enterocolitis to casein hydrolysate formulas. J Allergy Clin Immunol. 1993;92(6):909–10.
46. Bellioni-Businco B, Paganelli R, Lucenti P, Giampietro PG, Perbornc H, Businco L. Allergenicity of goat's milk in children with cow's milk allergy. J Allergy Clin Immunol. 1999;103(6):1191–4.
47. Shek LP, Bardina L, Castro R, Sampson HA, Beyer K. Humoral and cellular responses to cow milk proteins in patients with milk-induced IgE-mediated and non-IgE-mediated disorders. Allergy. 2005;60(7):912–9.
48. Mori F, Sarti L, Barni S, et al. Donkey's milk is well accepted and tolerated by infants with cow's milk food protein-induced enterocolitis syndrome: a preliminary study. J Investig Allergol Clin Immunol. 2017;27(4):269–71.
49. Miceli Sopo S, Buonsenso D, Monaco S, Crocco S, Longo G, Calvani M. Food protein-induced enterocolitis syndrome (FPIES) and well cooked foods: a working hypothesis. Allergol Immunopathol. 2013;41(5):346–8.
50. Nowak-Wegrzyn A, Lawson K, Masilamani M, Kattan J, Bahnson HT, Sampson HA. Increased tolerance to less extensively heat-denatured (baked) milk products in milk-allergic children. J Allergy Clin Immunol Pract. 2017.
51. Chung HL, Hwang JB, Park JJ, Kim SG. Expression of transforming growth factor beta1, transforming growth factor type I and II receptors, and TNF-alpha in the mucosa of the small intestine in infants with food protein-induced enterocolitis syndrome. J Allergy Clin Immunol. 2002;109(1):150–4.
52. Caubet JC, Bencharitiwong R, Ross A, Sampson HA, Berin MC, Nowak-Wegrzyn A. Humoral and cellular responses to casein in patients with food protein-induced enterocolitis to cow's milk. J Allergy Clin Immunol. 2017;139(2):572–83.
53. Goswami R, Blazquez AB, Kosoy R, Rahman A, Nowak-Węgrzyn A, Berin MC. Systemic innate immune activation in food protein-induced enterocolitis syndrome. J Allergy Clin Immunol. 2017;139(6):1885–1896.e1889.
54. Pecora V, Prencipe G, Valluzzi R, et al. Inflammatory events during food protein-induced enterocolitis syndrome reactions. Pediat Allergy Immunol. 2017;28(5):464–70.
55. Kimura M, Ito Y, Tokunaga F, et al. Increased C-reactive protein and fever in Japanese infants with food protein-induced enterocolitis syndrome. Pediatr Inter. 2016;58(9):826–30.
56. Kimura M, Shimomura M, Morishita H, Meguro T, Seto S. Serum C-reactive protein in food protein-induced enterocolitis syndrome versus food protein-induced proctocolitis in Japan. Pediatr Inter. 2016;58(9):836–41.
57. Morita H, Nomura I, Orihara K, et al. Antigen-specific T-cell responses in patients with non-IgE-mediated gastrointestinal food allergy are predominantly skewed to T(H)2. J Allergy Clin Immunol. 2013;131(2):590–592.e591-596.
58. Kimura M, Ito Y, Shimomura M, et al. Cytokine profile after oral food challenge in infants with food protein-induced enterocolitis syndrome. Allergol Inter. 2017;66(3):452–7.
59. Kimura M, Shimomura M, Morishita H, Meguro T, Seto S. Eosinophilia in infants with food protein-induced enterocolitis syndrome in Japan. Allergol Inter. 2017;66(2):310–6.
60. Wada T, Matsuda Y, Toma T, Koizumi E, Okamoto H, Yachie A. Increased CD69 expression on peripheral eosinophils from patients with food protein-induced enterocolitis syndrome. Int Arch Allergy Immunol. 2016;170(3):201–5.
61. Konstantinou GN, Bencharitiwong R, Grishin A, et al. The role of casein-specific IgA and TGF-beta in children with food protein-induced enterocolitis syndrome to milk. Pediatr Allergy Immunol. 2014;25(7):651–6.
62. Mori F, Barni S, Cianferoni A, Pucci N, de Martino M, Novembre E. Cytokine expression in CD3+ cells in an infant with food protein-induced enterocolitis syndrome (FPIES): case report. Clin Dev Immunol. 2009;2009:679381.

Gastrointestinal Differential Diagnosis of Food Protein-Induced Enterocolitis Syndrome

7

Trusha Patel and Judith R. Kelsen

Gastrointestinal Differential Diagnosis of Acute FPIES

Infectious Gastroenteritis

The most common cause of an acute onset of vomiting and dehydration in any child is infectious gastroenteritis. While most patients with infectious gastroenteritis have a self-limited illness that resolves with supportive care, some patients with infectious gastroenteritis may develop severe dehydration similar to that seen in patients with FPIES. Although infectious gastroenteritis typically causes both vomiting and diarrhea, patients in the early phases of illness may not have yet developed frank diarrhea and the lack of diarrhea does not rule out diagnosis of infectious gastroenteritis. History of sick contacts may help differentiate infectious gastroenteritis from FPIES, but not all patients with infectious gastroenteritis will have evidence of sick contacts. Typically, onset after consumption of a particular trigger food, particularly if similar episodes have occurred previously, can help distinguish FPIES from infectious gastroenteritis. Stool infectious studies may also be helpful to help diagnose infectious gastroenteritis. However, these often do not result immediately, and the two conditions can be indistinguishable at the initial presentation and may only be differentiated over time.

Pyloric Stenosis

The classic history of pyloric stenosis in infancy is postprandial vomiting that progresses in both volume and forcefulness, leading to severe dehydration due to

T. Patel · J. R. Kelsen (✉)
Division of Gastroenterology, Hepatology and Nutrition, Children's Hospital of Philadelphia, Philadelphia, PA, USA
e-mail: kelsen@email.chop.edu

T. F. Brown-Whitehorn, A. Cianferoni (eds.), *Food Protein Induced Enterocolitis (FPIES)*,
https://doi.org/10.1007/978-3-030-21229-2_7

inability to tolerate feeds. The clinical presentation of severe dehydration is often accompanied by hypochloremic, hypokalemic, and metabolic alkalosis. Diagnosis is typically made with pyloric ultrasound. The treatment is surgical, with a pyloromyotomy leading to rapid resolution of symptoms. The dramatic dehydration seen in patients with pyloric stenosis can be similar to the severe dehydration seen in patients with FPIES and the two conditions can thus be quite difficult to distinguish clinically (particularly in an infant whose only food exposure is to cow's milk protein-containing breast milk or formula). However, the ultrasonographic findings in pyloric stenosis definitively distinguish the two entities.

Malrotation with Volvulus

Malrotation results from an arrest of normal rotation of the embryonic gut. In patients with malrotation, the cecum is located in the mid-upper abdomen and is fixed to the right lateral abdominal wall by Ladd bands. Patients with malrotation are at risk for obstruction (either due to extrinsic compression of the duodenum by Ladd bands) or volvulus (torsion of the intestine). Patients with malrotation may have intermittent volvulus, which may lead to a presentation of intermittent vomiting and dehydration, abdominal tenderness and ultimately, bowel ischemia if volvulus is long-lasting. Malrotation warrants surgical correction in nearly all cases to prevent potential volvulus, but malrotation with volvulus is a surgical emergency [1].

Intestinal Atresia

Intestinal atresia refers to complete obstruction of the intestinal lumen due to a congenital defect. While intestinal atresia may impact any portion of the small or large intestine, atresia of the small intestine is much more common than large intestinal atresia, with duodenal atresia being the most common type [2]. Patients with intestinal atresia may be identified with signs of intestinal obstruction on prenatal ultrasound. However, more than half of these patients are not diagnosed until after birth [3]. Patients with intestinal atresia typically present with abdominal distension, bilious emesis and potentially with failure to pass meconium. With repetitive vomiting, patients may become severely dehydrated. Initial evaluation is abdominal radiography and diagnosis is typically confirmed by contrast study such as upper GI with or without small bowel follow-through, depending on the site of atresia. Management of intestinal atresia involves bowel rest, nasogastric or orogastric suction, and intravenous hydration in the immediate period, followed by surgical repair for definitive treatment. Prognosis is favorable with successful surgical repair.

Necrotizing Enterocolitis

Necrotizing enterocolitis (NEC) occurs in the setting of ischemia of the intestinal mucosa, which leads to necrosis, bacterial translocation, and entry of gas into the bowel wall and potentially into the portal venous system. Necrotizing enterocolitis is more frequently seen in premature infants with comorbidities but has also been described in full-term infants who are otherwise healthy [4]. Necrotizing enterocolitis may present with sudden feeding intolerance and vomiting and may appear to initially improve with hydration and bowel rest, which can be a similar clinical presentation to FPIES. However, unlike FPIES, patients with necrotizing enterocolitis typically have abnormal findings on abdominal exam, such as abdominal distension, discoloration, and significant tenderness. They may also have bilious emesis (as opposed to infants with FPIES who typically have non-bilious emesis, which may progress to become bilious after repetitive vomiting) and hematochezia. A diagnosis of NEC is typically confirmed with abdominal radiography, which classically will show pneumatosis intestinalis, portal venous gas or pneumoperitoneum. Laboratory studies may show anemia, thrombocytopenia, leukocytosis, elevated inflammatory markers, lactic acidosis, hyperglycemia, positive blood culture, or evidence of disseminated intravascular coagulation [5, 6]. Patients with mild-moderate NEC are typically managed with bowel rest, gastric decompression, and intravenous hydration (with total parenteral nutrition for patients requiring prolonged bowel rest), as well as empiric antibiotic therapy [7, 8]. Patients require close monitoring, with serial examination, as well as laboratory and radiographic monitoring. Patients with severe cases of NEC may require surgical intervention.

Anaphylaxis

Unlike FPIES, which is a non-IgE-mediated reaction, anaphylaxis is an IgE-mediated acute, severe allergic reaction with multisystem involvement in response to food, medication, or a variety of other exposures. Anaphylaxis and FPIES can be similar in their temporal association with food exposure and presentation with vomiting. However, anaphylaxis must also involve respiratory or cardiovascular compromise in the acute phase, while patients with FPIES do not typically have these features (aside from the sequelae of severe dehydration and ultimately cardiovascular compromise with persistent emesis in FPIES). The treatment of anaphylaxis involves immediate recognition, emergent intramuscular injection of epinephrine, and subsequent management with additional measures that may include supplemental oxygen or more significant airway management, IV fluid resuscitation, and adjunctive agents (including antihistamines and glucocorticoids).

Adrenal Insufficiency with Adrenal Crisis

The presentation of severe dehydration in patients with FPIES can appear similar to adrenal crisis, which can present with lethargy, nausea, and vomiting. In infants, adrenal crisis is most commonly due to congenital adrenal hyperplasia (CAH) [9]. While the presentations of congenital adrenal hyperplasia can be quite varied, based on the specific underlying biochemical defect, several of these biochemical defects leading to CAH (including 21-hydoxylase deficiency and 3-beta-hydroxysteroid dehydrogenase type 2 deficiency) often present with vomiting, dehydration, hyponatremia, and hyperkalemia [9, 10]. Of note, the presence of hyperkalemia may help differentiate this condition from an acute presentation of FPIES. While diagnosis of CAH is confirmed with serum testing of steroid metabolites, acute diagnosis of adrenal crisis is typically made clinically, based on examination, history, and the laboratory parameters mentioned above. Patients with adrenal crisis are managed with fluid resuscitation, administration of steroids (typically both mineralocorticoids and glucocorticoids), and in some cases with electrolyte supplementation as well [11]. Definitive management of congenital adrenal hyperplasia typically involves long-term steroid therapy and gender-appropriate replacement of androgens or estrogens and progestins for pubertal management, as well as surgical management in some cases.

Intussusception

Intussusception is a condition that involves the invagination of one part of bowel into another part of bowel. While intussusception can be seen in patients of any age, it is most commonly a pediatric condition. The majority of cases are seen in infants and toddlers, with more than half of cases occurring in patients under 1 year of age [12]. Although toddlers and older children most commonly present with complaint of abdominal pain, infants with intussusception most often present with emesis, irritability, and heme-positive stools, which can be similar to that seen in patients with FPIES [12]. While intussusception in adults is almost always associated with an identified lead point, the vast majority of cases in children are idiopathic [13, 14]. The most useful diagnostic study for intussusception is abdominal ultrasound, as there is no radiation exposure and sensitivity is nearly 100% in the hands of experienced ultrasonographers [15]. While small bowel intussusception is typically self-resolved, patients with ileocolic or ileo-ileocolic intussusception often require reduction, either by image-guided enema reduction or surgical reduction [16]. After successful reduction, nearly 10% of patients may have recurrence of intussusception at any point [16].

Increased Intracranial Pressure

While there are numerous causes of increased intracranial pressure, all of which are out of the scope of this particular chapter, increased intracranial pressure is a critical cause of vomiting and dehydration that must always be considered in patients who present with recurrent or severe vomiting. Any red flag symptoms, including macrocephaly, focal neurologic deficit, developmental delay, acute onset of vomiting and lethargy, vomiting that awakens the child from sleep or hypertension with heart rate abnormalities, must immediately raise concern for increased intracranial pressure. As this can be a life-threatening cause of vomiting, clinicians must keep a high index of suspicion.

Additional Conditions to Consider in the Differential Diagnosis for Acute FPIES

Other conditions can present with similar signs and symptoms of severe vomiting and dehydration seen in patients with FPIES but are not discussed here in detail, either because they are rarely seen in the young population most affected with FPIES or because they are discussed elsewhere in this text. Some of these conditions include the following:

- Pancreatitis (very rare in this age group in the absence of direct trauma or surgery).
- Inborn errors of metabolism (discussed elsewhere in this text).
- Hirschsprung disease (discussed below).
- Abdominal mass (may cause extrinsic compression and vomiting).
- Cyclic vomiting syndrome (typically a diagnosis seen in older children).

Potential Workup for Acute Severe Vomiting and Dehydration in Infancy

The clinical evaluation and judgment of the team assessing the patient is critical and will guide the workup in the acute setting. Table 7.1 reviews studies that should be considered in this diagnostic workup of a patient who presents with acute, repetitive vomiting in infancy.

Table 7.1 Suggested evaluation of infants with acute, persistent emesis

Imaging and procedures	When to consider	Potential findings
Two-view abdominal radiograph	Abdominal distension or tenderness Bilious vomiting	Bowel obstruction Pneumatosis, pneumobilia, or pneumoperitoneum, consistent with NEC Intussusception (radiography is not as specific as ultrasound)
Pyloric ultrasound	Repetitive vomiting in a young infant (typically non-bilious)	Pyloric stenosis
Abdominal ultrasound	Patients with new-onset vomiting without obvious cause Patients with episodic abdominal pain concerning for intussusception	Intussusception Pneumatosis, pneumobilia, or pneumoperitoneum consistent with NEC Abdominal mass
Upper gastrointestinal series	Episodic vomiting or bilious vomiting Episodic abdominal pain	Malrotation Intestinal atresia External compression of bowel by abdominal mass

(continued)

Table 7.1 (continued)

Imaging and procedures	When to consider	Potential findings
Head CT or MRI	Patients with focal neurologic deficits Patients with unexplained bruises or other historical information leading to concern for non-accidental trauma Patients with papilledema Patients with developmental delay	Variable and may include evidence of traumatic brain injury, stroke, CNS infection, neoplasm, hydrocephalus, etc.
Laboratory studies	**When to consider**	**Potential findings**
Complete blood count	Patients with fever Patients with weight loss Should be considered in most patients in whom there is not a clear cause of vomiting	Anemia should prompt consideration of GI blood loss, dietary deficiency, intracranial bleed Thrombocytosis should prompt consideration of chronic inflammation Thrombocytopenia should prompt consideration of NEC, fungal infection, DIC Leukocytosis should prompt consideration of infection or inflammation Leukopenia or neutropenia should prompt consideration of infection or malignancy
Comprehensive metabolic panel	Patients with repetitive vomiting Should be considered in most patients with clinical evidence of dehydration to evaluate severity of dehydration and to evaluate for potential electrolyte derangements	Hyponatremia with hyperkalemia should prompt consideration of adrenal crisis Hypokalemia with hypochloremia and elevated bicarbonate should prompt consideration of pyloric stenosis or other source of gastric outlet obstruction or upper GI tract obstruction Decreased bicarbonate should prompt consideration of NEC (or other source of intestinal ischemia), metabolic disease or renal disease
Amylase and lipase	Patients with repetitive vomiting and epigastric abdominal tenderness without explanation	Elevated lipase (>3 times the upper limit of normal) can be indicative of pancreatitis, when taken in combination with epigastric abdominal pain/tenderness or evidence of pancreatitis on ultrasound or cross-sectional imaging
Inflammatory markers (C-reactive protein and/or erythrocyte sedimentation rate)	Patients with fever Patients with weight loss Should be considered in most patients in whom there is not a clear cause of vomiting	Elevated CRP or ESR can be nonspecific but may raise concern for infection or inflammation
Metabolic evaluation	Patients with dysmorphia, failure to thrive, or severe presentation with any intercurrent illnesses	Discussed elsewhere in this text in further detail

Gastrointestinal Differential Diagnosis of Chronic FPIES

Food Protein-Induced Proctocolitis

Food protein-induced proctocolitis is typically caused by cow's milk protein intolerance (also referred to as cow's milk allergy) in infancy. Food protein-induced proctocolitis and FPIES are often considered to be on the same spectrum of food protein-induced gastrointestinal diseases in infants, but it should be noted that FPIES typically falls at the most severe end of the spectrum, while food protein-induced proctocolitis typically has a milder, more chronic presentation. Food protein-induced proctocolitis can lead to vomiting and failure to thrive, but is less likely to lead to acute dehydration. Patients may also present with blood in the stools. Diagnosis is made on a clinical basis and can be supported by hemoccult testing of the stools. Endoscopic evaluation is not routinely recommended. However, if it is performed, findings typically include focally increased eosinophils in all mucosal compartments, with preferential aggregation in the vicinity of lymphoid nodules [17]. Treatment involves elimination of milk and soy proteins from the diet, either by maternal elimination of all milk and soy proteins from the diet (for exclusively breastfed babies) or transition to a partially or fully hydrolyzed formula. This condition is typically benign and self-limited. Most patients can be reintroduced to milk and soy proteins by 1 year of age. Interestingly, over the past several years, there have been several studies that have identified cow's milk protein-induced allergic proctocolitis in infancy as a risk factor for later development of functional gastrointestinal disorders in children [18, 19].

Gastroesophageal Reflux Disease

Physiologic reflux infants are extremely common and even healthy infants can have over 30 episodes of reflux in a day. However, infants who have reflux that is complicated by significant pain, failure to thrive, esophagitis, or respiratory complications (including aspiration) are considered to have gastroesophageal reflux disease (GERD) [20]. Severe cases of GERD can present with significant regurgitation that leads to inadequate caloric intake and poor weight gain. These infants can have associated dehydration and weight loss, which may mimic the presentation of patients with a chronic presentation of FPIES. These two entities can be distinguished by the presence of specific trigger foods and less acute presentation that is seen in FPIES. The diagnosis of GERD is most often made clinically, but 24-hour impedance monitoring can be used as a diagnostic tool for patients in whom the diagnosis is in question or who have severe symptoms that may necessitate more aggressive management. Treatment of GERD typically involves change in feeding practice (smaller, more frequent feeds, pacing with feeds for certain patients, upright positioning for 30 minutes after feeds) and may involve thickening of feeds with infant cereal, trial of partially hydrolyzed formulas or initiation of medical therapy, such as histamine type 2 receptor antagonists, proton pump inhibitors, or a variety of other agents. Surgical management, such as fundoplication, is reserved only for the most severe cases and should be used with great caution.

Hirschsprung Disease

Hirschsprung disease is caused by failure or arrest of migration of the neural crest cells during fetal intestinal development and subsequent absence of enteric neurons at the end of the bowel [21]. The portion of the bowel that is aganglionic (does not contain any enteric ganglion cells) is nonfunctional. Depending on the extent of bowel involvement, patients may have a milder presentation, with delayed passage of meconium, constipation and failure to thrive or a more severe presentation of obstruction, which could include vomiting and abdominal distension in addition to the aforementioned symptoms. While rectal biopsy remains the gold standard for diagnosis, abdominal radiographs, barium enema, and anorectal manometry may provide supporting information. In contrast to patients with FPIES, patients with Hirschsprung disease do not always present with symptoms that occur in relation to oral intake and vomiting, and if present, emesis is more likely to be bilious in Hirschsprung disease, due to the functional intestinal obstruction. Definitive treatment of Hirschsprung disease is surgical. There are a variety of surgical approaches available, with very similar outcomes, and the surgical procedure of choice depends on the experience and preference of the surgeon [22].

Eosinophilic Gastrointestinal Disease

Eosinophilic gastrointestinal disease (EGID) encompasses several disorders of the gastrointestinal tract, including eosinophilic esophagitis (EoE), eosinophilic gastritis (EG), eosinophilic colitis (EC), or eosinophilic gastroenteritis (EGE), based on the location and extent of involvement within the GI tract [23]. Eosinophilic esophagitis, the most common EGID, is a chronic esophageal disease characterized clinically by symptoms related to esophageal dysfunction and histologically by eosinophil-predominant esophageal inflammation [24]. While older children and adolescents typically present with abdominal pain, dysphagia and food impaction, infants and toddlers typically present with failure to thrive, feeding difficulties, reflux symptoms, and vomiting [25]. While both EoE and FPIES are generally considered non-IgE-mediated conditions, patients with EoE are more likely to have food-specific IgE antibodies than patients with FPIES [26, 27]. Generally, patients with FPIES have a more severe presentation than patients with EoE and other forms of EGID, who typically have a more indolent presentation. Treatment of EoE may include dietary therapy (food elimination), acid suppression, topical glucocorticoids, systemic glucocorticoids, and potentially esophageal dilation to treat esophageal strictures.

Congenital Diarrheal Disorders

Congenital diarrheal disorders (CDD) are a heterogeneous group of rare conditions that cause chronic diarrhea with onset in the neonatal period. These conditions can be classified as secretory, inflammatory, or malabsorptive [28]. While the underlying etiologies vary immensely and review of this is outside the scope of this text, one useful model classifies these disorders into four categories characterized by the alteration in absorption and transport of nutrients and electrolytes, enterocyte differentiation and polarization, enteroendocrine cell differentiation, and modulation of the intestinal immune response [29]. Most congenital diarrheal disorders are monogenic and the presentation of these processes varies greatly based on the underlying etiology [30]. The most common overlapping symptoms include diarrhea, feeding difficulties, and failure to thrive. The initial evaluation of an infant presenting with diarrhea within the first month of life should include the following studies: stool studies (discussed in further detail in Table 7.2), complete blood

Table 7.2 Suggested evaluation of infants with failure to thrive with chronic vomiting and/or diarrhea

Imaging and procedures	When to consider	Potential findings
Upper gastrointestinal series	Any patient with bilious vomiting Intermittent episodes of vomiting	Malrotation Intestinal atresia (less likely to present with chronic presentation) Any other anatomic obstruction of the upper GI tract
Esophagogastroduodenoscopy	When anatomic causes of vomiting have been ruled out and patient continues with vomiting Patients with vomiting causing poor weight gain Patient with history of severe food allergies or reactions, raising suspicion for eosinophilic gastrointestinal disorders Patients with suspicion for congenital diarrhea (send duodenal biopsies for mucosal disaccharidase activity measurement, as well as electron microscopy evaluation)	Reflux esophagitis Eosinophilic gastrointestinal disorders Celiac disease Various causes of congenital diarrheal disorders
Flexible sigmoidoscopy or colonoscopy	Chronic diarrhea or blood in the stools in the absence of infection	Very early-onset inflammatory bowel disease Eosinophilic gastrointestinal disorders Food protein-induced proctocolitis

(continued)

Table 7.2 (continued)

Imaging and procedures	When to consider	Potential findings
24-hour impedance monitoring	For patients with suspected reflux which cannot be clearly diagnosed clinically Severe cases of reflux which are non-responsive for standard therapies	Gastroesophageal reflux disease (can quantify severity)
Laboratory studies	**When to consider**	**Potential findings**
Stool infectious studies Bacterial culture. Viral polymerase chain reaction tests. Ova and parasite testing. Rapid cryptosporidium and rapid giardia antigen testing. Note: C. difficile Testing is not recommended in patients under 2 years of age due to high incidence of colonization [39, 40].	Diarrhea lasting longer than 48 hours Infants presenting with severe illness Bloody diarrhea, regardless of duration of illness	Bacterial, viral, or parasitic infection on the stool
Stool electrolytes	Any patient with chronic diarrhea	High sodium or chloride may reflect alterations in intestinal ion transport Stool osmotic gap [290 – 2x(stool Na + K)] may indicate secretory diarrhea when there is a negative osmotic gap and osmotic diarrhea when there is high osmotic gap (>160 mosmol) [41]
Stool reducing substances	Any patient with chronic diarrhea Most useful in patients with watery diarrhea	Reducing substances greater than 0.5% indicates malabsorption of monosaccharides
Stool pH	Any patient with chronic diarrhea Most useful in patients with watery diarrhea	Stool pH less than 5.3 may indicate carbohydrate malabsorption
Stool alpha-1-antitrypsin	Any patient with chronic diarrhea Most useful in patients with poor growth and edema	High stool alpha-1-antitrypsin indicates protein-losing enteropathy (note: This can still be due to a variety of infectious, inflammatory or congenital causes)
Quantitative fecal fat (72-hour stool collection)	Any patient with chronic diarrhea Most useful in patients with greasy stools and/or poor growth	High percentage of fecal fat (compared to enteral fat intake, which must be recorded very carefully during collection) indicates fat malabsorption
Fecal elastase	Any patient with chronic diarrhea Most useful in patients with greasy stools and/or poor growth	Low fecal elastase indicates pancreatic insufficiency (however, it should be noted that patients with watery stools or high-output diarrhea may have artificially low fecal elastase due to dilution)

count, serum electrolytes, inflammatory markers, liver function tests, immunoglobulin levels, a lipid panel, fat soluble vitamins, a coagulation profile and zinc level, as well as potential consideration of immunologic investigation if there is suspicion of immune dysfunction [30]. Stool studies are critical in the evaluation of congenital diarrheas, but their utilization in clinical practice can be challenging due to difficulty with sample collection (as there is often urine contamination), importance of precise correlation of oral intake with stool output, and challenges in interpretation. All patients with congenital diarrhea should have stool infectious studies (including testing for viral, bacterial, and parasitic pathogens), as well as testing of stool electrolytes (including sodium, potassium, and chloride) and calculation of stool osmotic gap, stool pH, reducing substances, stool alpha-1-antitrypsin, and 72-hour fecal fat collection. Other studies that should be considered but interpreted with caution (as they can be nonspecific) include stool elastase, fecal occult blood testing, and stool lactoferrin or calprotectin [30].

Very Early-Onset Inflammatory Bowel Disease

Inflammatory bowel disease (IBD) is a chronic inflammatory condition of the GI tract which includes ulcerative colitis, Crohn disease, and indeterminate colitis. While the rate of pediatric IBD continues to rise, the most pronounced increase in incidence is in the youngest patients, less than 6 years of age, and thus categorized as very early-onset inflammatory bowel disease (VEO-IBD) [31, 32]. Patients with VEO-IBD frequently present with a different phenotype and more severe disease than older patients with IBD. The location of disease can be different: it can be panenteric or primarily colonic inflammation, while older patients most often have inflammation in both the terminal ileum and colon. Children with VEO-IBD have poor response to conventional therapies and are more likely to require surgical management. These differences are due to the greater genetic contribution to the disease, including monogenic defects, in the very young patients than in patients with IBD diagnosed at an older age, who have a polygenetic disease [33–35]. Patients with VEO-IBD may present with a variety of symptoms which may overlap with those seen in patients with FPIES, including failure to thrive, diarrhea, blood, or mucous in the stools and vomiting. However, the two conditions can be differentiated on the basis of several features. Symptoms seen in patients with VEO-IBD are not exclusively linked to specific food exposures and supportive measures such as bowel rest and intravenous hydration that can help patients with both conditions acutely will not alleviate the ongoing symptoms associated with VEO-IBD.

Initial studies in the evaluation for IBD should include stool infectious studies (to rule out acute gastrointestinal infection), fecal calprotectin, and complete blood count with differential, comprehensive metabolic panel, C-reactive protein, and erythrocyte sedimentation rate. While both patients with FPIES and VEO-IBD may have anemia, hypoalbuminemia, leukocytosis and thrombocytosis, the degree of laboratory abnormalities is typically more severe in patients with VEO-IBD and these patients will also have objective measures of intestinal inflammation, including elevated fecal calprotectin (which may also theoretically be elevated in patients with FPIES) and greater chronicity of symptoms. If initial history and clinical evaluation lead to suspicion of inflammatory bowel disease, further diagnostic workup should be pursued. Imaging modalities that are often useful in the characterization of IBD include bowel ultrasound (including contrast-enhanced bowel ultrasound at centers where it is available), and for older children, magnetic resonance enterography and video capsule endoscopy. However, while these imaging modalities may be helpful, endoscopic visualization of the gastrointestinal tract (including intubation of the terminal ileum) and multiple biopsies for histologic evaluation remain the gold standard for diagnosis of IBD [36]. The presence of chronic intestinal inflammation on biopsy specimens makes definitive diagnosis of IBD, and thus rules out FPIES.

The treatment algorithm for inflammatory bowel disease varies greatly based on patient age, location and severity of disease, and associated extraintestinal manifestations of disease. Management approaches for pediatric IBD may include oral aminosalicylate therapies, oral antibiotics, nutritional therapies (including exclusive enteral nutrition or elimination diets), immunomodulators, and biologic therapies. However, as discussed above, patients with VEO-IBD often do not have adequate response to these traditional treatment algorithms.

Along with the rapid advances in sequencing technology, our insight into the disease pathogenesis and clinical consequences in these very young patients with IBD has expanded. A subset of these children has monogenic defects, often involving primary immunodeficiency genes, which are responsible for their unique presentation and severe, refractory disease course [35, 37]. Identification of these defects is critical, as this information can be used to target therapy and prevent the use of inappropriate immunosuppressive therapies in cases of underlying immunodeficiency. For example, the primary immunodeficiency chronic granulomatous disease (CGD) can present with intestinal inflammation consistent with IBD and requires a significantly different therapeutic strategy. While hematopoietic stem cell transplantation (HSCT) is curative for CGD, interim therapies are most often necessary and can include antibiotics and steroids that are also routinely used in IBD. However, tumor necrosis factor alpha inhibitors (anti-TNF), an effective therapy to induce and maintain remission in IBD, is contraindicated in CGD, as it may cause an unacceptably high risk of serious fungal infections [38]. Furthermore, while conventional IBD therapies may not be dangerous in patients with VEO-IBD, they may be ineffective, as they do not target the underlying etiology of disease. Therefore, a comprehensive evaluation for underlying primary immunodeficiency in patients with VEO-IBD, including CGD, is critical prior to the initiation of anti-TNF therapy in a very young patient with IBD. In addition to a complete immune evaluation, genetic studies, such as whole exome sequencing, or targeted sequencing panels, may yield a specific monogenic or digenic defect, allowing for targeted therapy. For example, directed therapy can include immunomodulatory therapies, such as rapamycin, T-cell-directed therapy such as abatacept, or agents that target IL-1. For some cases, such as IL-10 pathway defects, T-cell deficiencies, CGD, hyperinflammatory defects, and others, HSCT may be curative [38].

Additional Conditions to Consider in the Differential Diagnosis for Chronic FPIES

- Cyclic vomiting syndrome (typically a diagnosis that affects older children).
- Gastroparesis (more common in older children).
- Opioid withdrawal or other drug withdrawal (either due to in utero exposure or iatrogenic exposure).
- Functional diarrhea (due to inappropriate formula-mixing or administration of other foods).
- Short bowel syndrome (typically due to intestinal resection).

Potential Workup for Failure to Thrive with Chronic Vomiting and/or Diarrhea in Infancy

While the differential diagnosis of failure to thrive is quite broad, the workup should be driven by the severity of malnutrition, as well as associated symptoms. Table 7.2 reviews diagnostic studies to consider in the evaluation of infants with failure to thrive accompanied gastrointestinal symptoms.

As reviewed in this chapter, the gastrointestinal differential diagnosis of FPIES is extensive, and specific workup should be guided by thorough history and physical examination. While we have discussed a variety of conditions here, this does not serve as an exhaustive review of all conditions that may cause similar symptoms in infants, and clinicians should always maintain a broad differential diagnosis, including metabolic, neurologic, allergic, and other conditions, many of which are reviewed in other chapters in this text.

Key Points/Clinical "Pearls"

- The evaluation, diagnosis, and management of FPIES are best performed by a multidisciplinary team of clinicians.
- Gastrointestinal manifestations of FPIES may be acute and episodic or may follow an indolent, chronic course.
- Clinicians evaluating a patient for FPIES should maintain a low threshold to consider alternative diagnoses.
- Signs and symptoms that should prompt clinicians to perform further diagnostic testing to consider alternative diagnoses in the setting of acute vomiting and dehydration include first-time presentation, fever, known sick contacts, lack of clearly identifiable food trigger, bilious emesis, profound dehydration, cardiorespiratory decompensation, abnormal abdominal examination, or focal neurologic deficits.
- All patients presenting with chronic vomiting and/or diarrhea and failure to thrive should undergo further evaluation for consideration of diagnoses other than FPIES, as this is a diagnosis of exclusion in this setting.

References

1. Covey SE, et al. Prophylactic versus symptomatic Ladd procedures for pediatric malrotation. J Surg Res. 2016;205(2):327–30.
2. Best KE, et al. Epidemiology of small intestinal atresia in Europe: a register-based study. Arch Dis Child Fetal Neonatal Ed. 2012;97(5):F353–8.
3. Haeusler MC, et al. Prenatal ultrasonographic detection of gastrointestinal obstruction: results from 18 European congenital anomaly registries. Prenat Diagn. 2002;22(7):616–23.
4. Maayan-Metzger A, et al. Necrotizing enterocolitis in full-term infants: case-control study and review of the literature. J Perinatol. 2004;24(8):494–9.
5. Hallstrom M, et al. Laboratory parameters predictive of developing necrotizing enterocolitis in infants born before 33 weeks of gestation. J Pediatr Surg. 2006;41(4):792–8.
6. Valpacos M, et al. Diagnosis and management of necrotizing enterocolitis: an international survey of neonatologists and pediatric surgeons. Neonatology. 2018;113(2):170–6.
7. Bell MJ, Ternberg JL, Bower RJ. The microbial flora and antimicrobial therapy of neonatal peritonitis. J Pediatr Surg. 1980;15(4):569–73.
8. Kliegman RM, Fanaroff AA. Necrotizing enterocolitis. N Engl J Med. 1984;310(17):1093–103.
9. Guran T. Latest insights on the etiology and management of primary adrenal insufficiency in children. J Clin Res Pediatr Endocrinol. 2017;9(Suppl 2):9–22.
10. White PC, Speiser PW. Congenital adrenal hyperplasia due to 21-hydroxylase deficiency. Endocr Rev. 2000;21(3):245–91.
11. White PC. Update on diagnosis and management of congenital adrenal hyperplasia due to 21-hydroxylase deficiency. Curr Opin Endocrinol Diabetes Obes. 2018;25(3):178–84.
12. Mandeville K, et al. Intussusception: clinical presentations and imaging characteristics. Pediatr Emerg Care. 2012;28(9):842–4.
13. Ntoulia A, et al. Failed intussusception reduction in children: correlation between radiologic, surgical, and pathologic findings. AJR Am J Roentgenol. 2016;207(2):424–33.
14. Blakelock RT, Beasley SW. The clinical implications of non-idiopathic intussusception. Pediatr Surg Int. 1998;14(3):163–7.
15. Daneman A, Navarro O. Intussusception. Part 1: a review of diagnostic approaches. Pediatr Radiol. 2003;33(2):79–85.
16. Daneman A, Navarro O. Intussusception. Part 2: an update on the evolution of management. Pediatr Radiol. 2004;34(2):97–108; quiz 187.
17. Odze RD, et al. Allergic proctocolitis in infants: a prospective clinicopathologic biopsy study. Hum Pathol. 1993;24(6):668–74.
18. Di Nardo G, et al. Allergic proctocolitis is a risk factor for functional gastrointestinal disorders in children. J Pediatr. 2018;195:128–133.e1.
19. Saps M, Lu P, Bonilla S. Cow's-milk allergy is a risk factor for the development of FGIDs in children. J Pediatr Gastroenterol Nutr. 2011;52(2):166–9.
20. Vandenplas Y, et al. Gastroesophageal reflux, as measured by 24-hour pH monitoring, in 509 healthy infants screened for risk of sudden infant death syndrome. Pediatrics. 1991;88(4):834–40.
21. Heuckeroth RO. Hirschsprung disease – integrating basic science and clinical medicine to improve outcomes. Nat Rev Gastroenterol Hepatol. 2018;15(3):152–67.
22. Lall A, Gupta DK, Bajpai M. Neonatal Hirschsprung's disease. Indian J Pediatr. 2000;67(8):583–8.
23. Cianferoni A, Spergel JM. Eosinophilic esophagitis and gastroenteritis. Curr Allergy Asthma Rep. 2015;15(9):58.
24. Liacouras CA, et al. Eosinophilic esophagitis: updated consensus recommendations for children and adults. J Allergy Clin Immunol. 2011;128(1):3–20 e6; quiz 21–2.
25. Spergel JM, et al. 14 years of eosinophilic esophagitis: clinical features and prognosis. J Pediatr Gastroenterol Nutr. 2009;48(1):30–6.
26. Erwin EA, et al. Serum IgE measurement and detection of food allergy in pediatric patients with eosinophilic esophagitis. Ann Allergy Asthma Immunol. 2010;104(6):496–502.

27. Leonard SA, et al. Food protein-induced enterocolitis syndrome: a review of the new guidelines. World Allergy Organ J. 2018;11(1):4.
28. Posovszky C. Congenital intestinal diarrhoeal diseases: a diagnostic and therapeutic challenge. Best Pract Res Clin Gastroenterol. 2016;30(2):187–211.
29. Berni Canani R, et al. Congenital diarrheal disorders: improved understanding of gene defects is leading to advances in intestinal physiology and clinical management. J Pediatr Gastroenterol Nutr. 2010;50(4):360–6.
30. Thiagarajah JR, et al. Advances in evaluation of chronic diarrhea in infants. Gastroenterology. 2018;154(8):2045–2059.e6.
31. Henderson P, et al. Rising incidence of pediatric inflammatory bowel disease in Scotland. Inflamm Bowel Dis. 2012;18(6):999–1005.
32. Benchimol EI, et al. Trends in epidemiology of pediatric inflammatory bowel disease in Canada: distributed network analysis of multiple population-based provincial health administrative databases. Am J Gastroenterol. 2017;112(7):1120–34.
33. Muise AM, Snapper SB, Kugathasan S. The age of gene discovery in very early onset inflammatory bowel disease. Gastroenterology. 2012;143(2):285–8.
34. Levine A, et al. Pediatric modification of the Montreal classification for inflammatory bowel disease: the Paris classification. Inflamm Bowel Dis. 2011;17(6):1314–21.
35. Kelsen JR, et al. Exome sequencing analysis reveals variants in primary immunodeficiency genes in patients with very early onset inflammatory bowel disease. Gastroenterology. 2015;149(6):1415–24.
36. Turner D, et al. Consensus for managing acute severe ulcerative colitis in children: a systematic review and joint statement from ECCO, ESPGHAN, and the Porto IBD Working Group of ESPGHAN. Am J Gastroenterol. 2011;106(4):574–88.
37. Uhlig HH. Monogenic diseases associated with intestinal inflammation: implications for the understanding of inflammatory bowel disease. Gut. 2013;62(12):1795–805.
38. Kelsen JR, Sullivan KE. Inflammatory bowel disease in primary immunodeficiencies. Curr Allergy Asthma Rep. 2017;17(8):57.
39. Bryant K, McDonald LC. Clostridium difficile infections in children. Pediatr Infect Dis J. 2009;28(2):145–6.
40. Larson HE, et al. Epidemiology of Clostridium difficile in infants. J Infect Dis. 1982;146(6):727–33.
41. Shiau YF, et al. Stool electrolyte and osmolality measurements in the evaluation of diarrheal disorders. Ann Intern Med. 1985;102(6):773–5.

8 The Metabolic Differential Diagnosis of Chronic FPIES

Chaya Nautiyal Murali and Rebecca D. Ganetzky

Introduction

The inborn errors of metabolism are a diverse group of disorders that are characterized by the perturbation of normal energy production, processing of waste products, and intracellular trafficking and processing. Most disorders can be traced to dysfunction in a single enzyme or transporter, and are due to biallelic mutations in the genes encoding these proteins. The vast majority of metabolic disorders are inherited in an autosomal recessive fashion. Thus, the diagnosis of an inborn error of metabolism carries important implications for family members of the affected patient, as parents are obligate carriers for the causative genetic change.

Metabolic disorders can generally be organized into three categories, based on pathophysiology [1].

1. Disorders that cause intoxication
2. Disorders of inadequate energy production
3. Disorders involving complex molecules

Intoxication-Type Inborn Errors of Metabolism

The intoxication-type inborn errors of metabolism are generally caused by perturbations in intermediary metabolism, such as the processing of amino acids, organic

C. N. Murali
Molecular and Human Genetics, Baylor College of Medicine, Houston, TX, USA

R. D. Ganetzky (✉)
Pediatrics, Division of Human Genetics, Children's Hospital of Philadelphia, Philadelphia, PA, USA
e-mail: ganetzkyr@email.chop.edu

T. F. Brown-Whitehorn, A. Cianferoni (eds.), *Food Protein Induced Enterocolitis (FPIES)*, https://doi.org/10.1007/978-3-030-21229-2_8

acids, and sugars. Disorders such as Maple Syrup Urine Disease (MSUD), methylmalonic acidemia, hereditary fructose intolerance, and ornithine transcarbamylase (OTC) deficiency fall within this category. They are characterized by episodic crisis-like events presenting with specific laboratory abnormalities, intolerance of certain types of food, and developmental delay or regression.

In all of these disorders, accumulation of a toxic metabolite (e.g., ammonia, leucine) causes end-organ damage and contributes to the acute presentation. Episodic crises often present with emesis and lethargy, which can resemble the acute presentation of FPIES. Further heightening the similarity between FPIES and intoxication-type metabolic disorders is the fact that many patients avoid eating foods containing large amounts of the compound that cannot be metabolized. For instance, many female OTC carriers are lifelong vegetarians because ingesting high-protein foods, such as meat, make them feel sick; hereditary fructose intolerance patients often refuse to eat fruits and other fructose-containing foods, and can be dismissed as picky children. Metabolic disorders causing intoxication most closely resemble FPIES in the acute clinical presentation (Table 8.1).

Disorders of Inadequate Energy Production

The disorders of inadequate energy production include enzymatic and transport defects involved in ATP formation, glycolysis, and fatty acid oxidation, in addition to other metabolic pathways (Table 8.2). Affected patients suffer from a range of symptoms, including hypoglycemia, lactic acidosis, failure to thrive, cardiac and muscular involvement, and rhabdomyolysis. The initial presentation varies depending on the type of defect. Those with mitochondrial disease can present with lactic acidosis, hypoglycemia, developmental delay or regression, and hepatic dysfunction. Those with fatty acid oxidation disorders can have cardiomyopathy, hypoglycemia, and rhabdomyolysis. Those with glycogen storage disorders can have hepatomegaly, cardiomyopathy, lactic acidosis, hypoglycemia, and hyperuricemia.

In general, disorders of inadequate energy production do not present with diarrhea or food avoidance, which distinguishes them from FPIES. However, affected children can have intermittent lethargy and/or vomiting. Thus, while disorders of inadequate energy production are less likely to be confused with FPIES, they should still remain on the differential diagnosis.

Disorders Involving Complex Molecules

The inborn errors of metabolism involving complex molecules include lysosomal storage disorders, congenital disorders of glycosylation, and peroxisomal biogenesis disorders. Each of these categories of disorders encompasses heterogeneous symptomatology and pathophysiology [1].

The lysosomal storage disorders are generally characterized by the accumulation of complex molecules in the lysosomes, resulting in deposition in various tissues.

Table 8.1 Intoxication-type inborn errors of metabolism that can present similarly to FPIES

Disorder	Defective enzyme	Inheritance	Laboratory abnormalities	Toxic metabolites	Foods avoided	Detected on newborn screening
Ornithine transcarbamylase deficiency	Ornithine transcarbamylase	X-linked	Respiratory alkalosis, hyperammonemia	Ammonia	Protein-rich	Rarely
Maple syrup urine disease	Branched chain ketoacid dehydrogenase	Autosomal recessive	Metabolic acidosis (with gap), ketosis	Leucine	Protein-rich	Typically
Methylmalonic acidemia	Methylmalonyl CoA Mutase, MMAA, MMAB	Autosomal recessive	Metabolic acidosis (with gap), ketosis	Ammonia, acid	Protein-rich	Typically
Classical galactosemia	Galactose-1-phosphate uridyltransferase	Autosomal recessive	Coagulopathy, transaminitis, positive urine-reducing substances	Galactose-1-phosphate	Dairy[a]	Always
Hereditary fructose intolerance	Aldolase B	Autosomal recessive	Hypoglycemia, transaminitis, hyperuricemia	Fructose-1-phosphate	Fruits, vegetables, juice, processed foods	Never

MMA methylmalonic acid

[a]Galactosemia symptoms start near-immediately upon initiation of breastmilk or cow's milk-based formulas

Table 8.2 Inborn errors of metabolism that cause inadequate energy production. Note that some can present with lethargy, overlapping with the presentation of FPIES

Disorder	Defective enzyme	Inheritance	Clinical presentation	Laboratory abnormalities	Detected on newborn screening
Mitochondrial disease	Many	Autosomal recessive or mitochondrial	Hypotonia, developmental regression, seizures, liver failure	Hypoglycemia, lactic acidosis, transaminitis	Never
Pyruvate dehydrogenase deficiency	Pyruvate dehydrogenase complex	X-linked > autosomal recessive	Hypotonia, developmental delay, seizures	Lactic acidosis, elevated pyruvate	Never
MCAD deficiency	Medium-chain acyl CoA dehydrogenase	Autosomal recessive	Hypotonia, lethargy, vomiting, hypoglycemia	Hypoglycemia, absent or trace ketosis, low carnitine	Always
VLCAD deficiency	Very long-chain acyl CoA dehydrogenase	Autosomal recessive	Cardiomyopathy, hepatomegaly, hypotonia, rhabdomyolysis	Nonketotic hypoglycemia, elevated CK	Typically
Glycogen storage disease type 1A	Glucose-6-phosphatase	Autosomal recessive	Hepatomegaly, hypoglycemia	Hypoglycemia, hyperuricemia, lactic acidosis	Never

Affected patients have symptoms distinct to the individual diseases. Symptoms commonly seen in many lysosomal storage diseases include hepatosplenomegaly, developmental delay, short stature and other bony changes, unique behavioral phenotypes, cytopenias, and chronic pain. These disorders have little to no overlap with FPIES.

Congenital disorders of glycosylation (CDGs) are caused by enzymatic defects in the post-translational processing of proteins, most often resulting in improper attachments of sugar moieties to protein products. Over one hundred CDGs have been identified. The most common types are PMM2-CDG and MPI-CDG. PMM2-CDG presents with hypotonia, abnormal fat distribution, failure to thrive, protein-losing enteropathy, and developmental delay [2]. The presence of diarrhea offers some overlap with FPIES. MPI-CDG, on the other hand, can closely mimic FPIES, with cyclic vomiting, hypoglycemia, and protein-losing enteropathy [3].

Peroxisomal biogenesis disorders are due to genetic defects in the formation and maintenance of peroxisomes. These disorders constitute a spectrum that can present with various combinations of developmental delay, severe hypotonia, leukodystrophy, and adrenal insufficiency. Like lysosomal storage disorders, they have little to no overlap with FPIES, and thus will not be covered further in this chapter.

Basic Principles of Metabolic Disease

The inborn errors of metabolism can seem a vast and overwhelming group of diagnoses for the physician who is not a metabolist. Many view metabolic disorders as a tedious list of laboratory findings, associated genes, and treatments to memorize.

However, understanding the basic principles of metabolic disease pathophysiology and treatment can render them significantly more approachable. Thus, we present a brief overview of these principles here.

Pathophysiology

Accumulation of Toxic Metabolites

As noted above, there is a group of metabolic disorders characterized by the accumulation of toxic metabolites. Affected individuals present with varied laboratory abnormalities (see Table 8.1), vomiting, and gastrointestinal discomfort upon ingestion of foods containing offending substrates. This category of metabolic disease can closely resemble FPIES. Careful laboratory analysis is important to diagnose these metabolic disorders, many of which are not diagnosed by expanded newborn screening. A high index of suspicion is necessary to prevent long-term deleterious effects of these toxic metabolites, which accumulate with every ingestion of forbidden foods.

Decreased Energy Production

Many inborn errors of metabolism cause illness due to decreased production of energy. Affected enzymes function in the production of energy from stored macromolecules—glycogenolysis, fatty acid oxidation, and gluconeogenesis—or in the mitochondria, which produce ATP through oxidative respiration. Affected individuals develop hypoglycemia, lethargy, and varied laboratory anomalies. Presentation with lethargy could cause confusion with FPIES, but the presence of hypoglycemia would quickly differentiate these patients as having inborn errors of metabolism.

Principles of Treatment

Treatment of most inborn errors of metabolism involves three main principles:

1. Decreased intake of the offending substrate
2. Removal of toxic metabolites
3. Provision of adequate calories and essential substrates

Thus, many children with metabolic diagnoses are on special diets restricted in the intake of specific macronutrients. They often require medical foods to ensure a balanced diet and are on medications aimed at reducing build-up of toxic metabolites. Without this three-pronged approach, patients can develop long-term organ damage and failure to thrive, among other consequences.

Diagnosis and Screening

A common misconception is that the vast majority of metabolic diseases are detected on the expanded newborn screen. While this holds true for many intermediary inborn errors of metabolism, it is false for several others. For instance, ornithine transcarbamylase deficiency, the most common urea cycle defect, is not detected on the newborn screen, nor are hereditary fructose intolerance and congenital disorders of glycosylation. All three of these disorders can be misdiagnosed as FPIES. Thus, it is important to maintain a high index of suspicion for metabolic disorders even in patients with a reassuring newborn screen.

Importance of Diagnosing Inborn Errors of Metabolism

It is crucial to diagnose inborn errors of metabolism early. The majority of inborn errors of metabolism are treatable, especially those that can be easily confused with FPIES. Early diagnosis and initiation of treatment is key to preventing permanent damage to the central nervous system and other organs, including the heart, liver, and muscles.

Making a diagnosis of metabolic disease is doubly important because it carries implications for the family of the patient. Parents can be made aware of their risk of having another child with the syndrome. Many of these conditions can be clinically variable, and it is important to evaluate apparently unaffected but at-risk family members, such as siblings, for the same diagnosis. Extended family members can use the knowledge to guide their own family planning decisions, as can the child himself or herself upon reaching adulthood.

Common Findings and the Diagnostic Approach in Inborn Errors of Metabolism

Though inborn errors of metabolism are a diverse group of diagnoses, there are historical, laboratory, and clinical findings that should raise suspicion for an underlying metabolic diagnosis. We recommend maintaining a high index of suspicion for inborn errors of metabolism in the workup for suspected FPIES. Paying attention to a few salient details can assist in making the diagnosis if a metabolic disorder is present.

Historical Details

Children with undiagnosed metabolic diseases may have a history of developmental delay, developmental regression, seizures, or intellectual disability. They often have a history of poor feeding, failure to thrive, or aversion to certain foods. A detailed dietary and developmental history can lend insights into possible diagnoses. Pay close attention to the foods that are thought to trigger the FPIES episodes. Do they span multiple foods, which all contain high levels of the same macronutrient (e.g., meat, fish, eggs – protein; or fruit, vegetables, baked goods – fructose)? In general, FPIES is rarely triggered by solid foods, especially meat and fish [4]. Thus, when families report such triggers, an underlying metabolic diagnosis should be higher on the differential.

Inquire into the gastrointestinal history. If children have profuse or chronic diarrhea in addition to emesis, consider congenital disorders of glycosylation (specifically PMM2-, MPI-, and ALG6-CDG), which can present with protein-losing enteropathy, as well as occasional emesis [3, 5, 6]. Consider the age of the patient. FPIES typically resolves by age 5 [4]. If the patient has symptoms persisting into school age, an underlying inborn error of metabolism may be the cause.

Attention to the family history is crucial. Since many of these conditions are autosomal recessive, there may be multiple affected siblings in the same family. Mothers of children with ornithine transcarbamylase deficiency may have a history of brothers who died suddenly in the neonatal period. They themselves may have a history of protein avoidance and psychiatric disorders [7]. Patients whose parents are consanguineous have a higher risk of autosomal recessive conditions.

Suggestive Laboratory Findings

Laboratory findings in metabolic disease vary depending on the underlying diagnosis. However, there are many laboratory anomalies that should raise suspicion for a metabolic diagnosis in general. These anomalies, summarized in Table 8.3, include hypoglycemia, lactic acidosis, severe metabolic acidosis, respiratory alkalosis, transaminitis, coagulopathy, ketosis, and hypoglycemia. FPIES patients may present with metabolic acidosis in the setting of severe episodes of emesis and hypotension, but this should resolve without the provision of calories [8]. Children with metabolic disease, on the other hand, will persist in their laboratory abnormalities until the offending substrate is removed from the diet, the toxic metabolite is removed, and there is adequate provision of calories and macronutrients that can be metabolized (see Table 8.4).

Table 8.3 Common laboratory anomalies associated with various inborn errors of metabolism

Laboratory finding	Possible inborn error of metabolism
Respiratory alkalosis	Urea cycle defect
Gap metabolic acidosis	Organic aciduria
Non-gap metabolic acidosis	Hereditary fructose intolerance
Lactic acidosis	Mitochondrial disorder, pyruvate dehydrogenase deficiency
Ketonuria	Organic aciduria, maple syrup urine disease
Ketotic hypoglycemia	Glycogen storage disorders
Non-ketotic hypoglycemia	Fatty acid oxidation disorders
Coagulopathy	Classical galactosemia, congenital disorders of glycosylation
Hyperuricemia	Hereditary fructose intolerance, glycogen storage disorder type 1
Transaminitis	Hereditary fructose intolerance, classical galactosemia, congenital disorders of glycosylation

Table 8.4 Principles of treatment in metabolic disease and examples of each principle

Treatment principle	Example
Decrease intake of offending substrate	Protein-restricted diet
Remove toxic metabolites	Ammonia-scavenging medications
Provide adequate calories and essential substrates	IV dextrose as needed, medical food, supplements

Suggestive Clinical Features

When diagnosed and appropriately managed, many patients with inborn errors of intermediary metabolism, including organic acidopathies, urea cycle defects, and fatty acid oxidation disorders, have no distinctive features on physical examination. However, in their untreated forms, almost all inborn errors of metabolism cause linear growth failure. Untreated urea cycle defects, fatty acid oxidation defects, and organic acidopathies can also cause microcephaly, developmental regression, and spasticity. Children with glycogen storage disorders can have hepatomegaly. hepatomegaly. Those with congenital disorders of glycosylation can have inverted nipples and unusual fat distribution, especially abnormal gluteal fat pads. Patients affected by certain mitochondrial disorders and pyruvate dehydrogenase deficiency can have dysmorphic facial features resembling fetal alcohol syndrome.

FPIES and Inborn Errors of Metabolism: Similarities and Differences

Similarities

Intoxication-type inborn errors of metabolism and FPIES are both characterized by an episode of crisis, such as vomiting, triggered by a particular type of food. As a result, affected children tend to avoid intake of these foods. In both cases, episodes tend to be recurrent and cause symptoms so severe that children come to emergency medical attention. Additionally, children with FPIES and children with inborn errors of metabolism can both experience diarrhea.

Differences

While FPIES and inborn errors of metabolism are similar in the dramatic features of the "episodes" experienced by affected children, there are many differences between the two conditions that can aid in appropriate diagnosis. First, while both intoxication-type inborn errors of metabolism and FPIES can cause affected patients to avoid certain foods, the pattern of triggering foods is distinct in both categories. FPIES is infrequently associated with solid foods, such as meats and vegetables. The most common trigger for FPIES is milk, and initial presentation occurs at around 7 months of age [4]. Milk or formula can cause decompensations in many metabolic disorders, either due to its sugars (galactose in galactosemia; in some

Table 8.5 Initial labwork that can be performed in the outpatient evaluation of suspected FPIES and results suggestive of inborn errors of metabolism

Laboratory test	Finding suggestive of metabolic disorder
Urinalysis	Ketonuria
Glucose	Hypoglycemia
Complete metabolic panel	Gap or non-gap acidosis, transaminitis
Blood gas	Metabolic acidosis or respiratory alkalosis
Coagulation studies	Coagulopathy
Ammonia	Hyperammonemia
Lactate	Elevated lactate

infant formulas, fructose in hereditary fructose intolerance) or its high protein content; however, they cause decompensation nearly immediately upon introduction, usually in the first few weeks of life. Many children with FPIES are triggered by more than one food, which can cause confusion when considering metabolic disorders. In such cases, attention to the macronutrient content of the triggering foods can lend insight.

Another distinguishing feature is the presence of developmental delay or regression. Most of the inborn errors of metabolism if untreated are associated with chronic developmental delay. In some disorders, episodes of crisis are associated with severe developmental regression. Such findings are not associated with FPIES, and if present, should raise high clinical suspicion for an underlying metabolic disorder. Additionally, children with some inborn errors of metabolism can present with seizures when in acute crisis, triggered by cerebral edema (from hyperammonemia or leucine encephalopathy) or hypoglycemia. Still other children with metabolic diagnoses such as mitochondrial disorders can develop seizures as part of the natural history of the disease. In general, the presence of neurodevelopmental anomalies should increase suspicion for inborn errors of metabolism.

Metabolic diagnoses, unlike FPIES, are lifelong. In one large retrospective study, over 85% of children with FPIES had no further episodes after age 5 [4]. In contrast, children with inborn errors of metabolism will continue to experience episodic emesis, lethargy, and laboratory abnormalities whenever they ingest foods that cannot be metabolized due to their enzymatic defects.

The varied laboratory anomalies associated with inborn errors of metabolism have been described elsewhere (section "Suggestive Laboratory Findings", Table 8.3). In contrast to children with metabolic diagnoses, children with FPIES do not present with hypoglycemia or ketosis, though thrombocytosis has been reported [8]. We suggest sending screening laboratory tests for inborn errors of metabolism when assessing children for possible FPIES (Table 8.5).

Overlap and Interaction Between FPIES and Inborn Errors of Metabolism

As evidenced in this chapter, there is considerable clinical overlap between FPIES and inborn errors of metabolism. Careful review of developmental, diet, and family history, in addition to screening labwork, can help distinguish between the two groups of disorders. Here, we present three illustrative cases in which an inborn error of metabolism was misdiagnosed as FPIES, FPIES was misdiagnosed as an inborn error of metabolism, and FPIES unmasked a predisposition to an inborn error of metabolism. The cases underscore the importance of historical, laboratory, and clinical features in making the correct diagnosis.

Lysinuric Protein Intolerance

Lysinuric protein intolerance is a disorder of renal tubular and intestinal transport resulting in defective absorption and reabsorption of dibasic amino acids (lysine, arginine, ornithine), resulting in secondary urea cycle dysfunction. Affected individuals often present at weaning with recurrent vomiting, diarrhea, lethargy or coma, failure to thrive, and hypotonia. Children with this disorder exhibit an aversion to protein-rich foods, and over time can develop progressive kidney disease, hematologic abnormalities, and osteoporosis, among other complications. Acute episodes present with hyperammonemia. Treatment involves lifelong protein restriction and administration of ammonia-scavenging medications [9].

A 2013 case report described a 12-month-old male who presented with repetitive vomiting and diarrhea after consumption of protein-rich foods [10]. A provisional diagnosis of FPIES to solid foods was made. However, the medical team astutely checked plasma and urinary amino acids, which revealed the diagnosis of lysinuric protein intolerance due to low levels of lysine, arginine, and ornithine in the blood, and high levels in the urine.

This case highlights the importance of closely observing the pattern of foods that induce FPIES-like symptoms. In this case, the child's episodes were triggered by intake of meats, fishes, and eggs, all of which are protein-rich foods. When a child presents with "FPIES" to multiple foods with similar macronutrient characteristics, there should be a high index of suspicion for inborn errors of metabolism.

Hereditary Fructose Intolerance

Hereditary fructose intolerance (HFI) is characterized by vomiting, abdominal distress, hypoglycemia, and lactic acidosis triggered by dietary exposure to fructose. Symptoms typically present around 4–6 months of age, when infants are weaned from breastmilk and begin eating solids. Fructose exposure occurs through intake of fruits, vegetables, liquid medications, table sugar, processed foods (including some infant formula), high fructose corn syrup, and some sugar substitutes. Patients then experience acute nausea, vomiting, pallor, abdominal distress, and hypoglycemia. The hypoglycemia often resolves quickly, and can be missed on laboratory workup.

If the condition goes undiagnosed and affected patients continue to ingest fructose, the disease takes a chronic course, characterized by liver dysfunction, proximal renal tubular dysfunction, and failure to thrive. Affected children often subconsciously learn to preferentially avoid all fructose-containing foods, causing parents to perceive the child as picky. Treatment is lifelong strict avoidance of fructose-containing foods [11].

A 2014 case report described an infant who began having episodic vomiting, pallor, and lethargy after ingestion of fruits. Based on the presentation and history, a clinical diagnosis of hereditary fructose intolerance was made, and genetic testing for common mutations in *ALDOB* was sent. An oral fructose challenge induced hypotension, treated as anaphylaxis; at the time, no hypoglycemia, transaminitis, or hyperuricemia were noted. When genetic testing returned negative, review of the case by an allergist led to the diagnosis of fruit-induced FPIES [12].

This case illustrates the substantial overlap in clinical presentation between FPIES and HFI. Both can present with vomiting, gastrointestinal distress, and lethargy after ingestion of certain foods. However, the absence of typical laboratory abnormalities and the presence of hypotension were clues to the true diagnosis of fruit-induced FPIES.

Trimethylaminuria

Trimethylaminuria is a rare disorder of amine metabolism that causes the affected individual to emit a pungent fishy smell. The autosomal recessive disorder is caused by mutations in the gene encoding flavin monooxygenase 3 (FMO3), which is responsible for converting the malodorous trimethylamine (TMA) into the odorless trimethylamine-N-oxide [13]. Diagnosis is established through genetic testing and urinary testing. Treatment involves restriction of trimethylamine-containing foods and use of special soaps, supplements, and antibiotics [14].

A 2013 case report described the case of an infant with FPIES who emitted a strong fishy odor with every acute episode. His odor was normal between episodes. Urinary studies revealed elevated levels of TMA during FPIES episodes, with normalization between episodes. Genetic testing of *FMO3* revealed a heterozygous pathogenic mutation with polymorphisms that slightly reduced activity on the other allele. In this case, the child's genetically decreased activity of FMO3 was able to cope with a normal amount of TMA. However, the intestinal wall inflammation during acute FPIES episodes likely released a large amount of the cell membrane component and TMA precursor, choline. In the setting of this increased TMA load, his FMO3 enzymatic activity was insufficient, resulting in urinary excretion of TMA and fishy odor [15].

This case underscores the possibility of coexisting FPIES and inborn errors of metabolism. When a patient's clinical course does not fit with that of typical FPIES, other contributing diagnoses must be considered.

Conclusion

The food protein-induced enterocolitis syndrome and many inborn errors of metabolism present in early childhood, often causing severe symptoms that necessitate emergency medical management. Both groups of disorders can present with emesis and lethargy; affected children can experience chronic diarrhea and exhibit aversion to certain foods. The clinical overlap can cause confusion or misdiagnosis between the two groups of disorders, as illustrated by the cases in section "Overlap and Interaction Between FPIES and Inborn Errors of Metabolism".

Though FPIES and inborn errors of metabolism share many similarities, there are several distinctions that can assist in making the right diagnosis. First, children with inborn errors of metabolism can have neurodevelopmental complications, including seizures, developmental regression after illness, intellectual disability, and hypotonia. The presence of any of these findings should significantly increase suspicion for an underlying metabolic disorder. Second, the pattern of triggering foods differs between FPIES and inborn errors of metabolism. Children with metabolic disorders will tend to avoid a broad range of foods, all of which contain large amounts of certain macronutrients that cannot be appropriately metabolized. When a child appears to have FPIES to multiple food types, inborn errors of metabolism should be considered.

Detailed assessment of the family history, not often undertaken in routine evaluations, can be useful in the diagnosis of metabolic disease. As these diagnoses often have autosomal recessive or X-linked inheritance, there may be affected but undiagnosed siblings or maternal uncles who died in infancy of unknown causes. Female carriers of OTC deficiency may have a personal history of psychiatric disturbances. The family history can serve as a tool to increase suspicion for metabolic disease, but a negative family history does not rule out the possibility of an inborn error of metabolism. Physical examination can also lend clues, especially if the child exhibits organomegaly, microcephaly, dysmorphic features, or other sequelae of neurologic damage from toxic metabolites.

Laboratory analysis can often lend the greatest insight when working up a child for FPIES and other possible diagnoses. FPIES has been reported to occur with thrombocytosis, leukocytosis, and metabolic acidosis. Inborn errors of metabolism can present with transaminitis, coagulopathy, ketonuria, ketotic hypoglycemia, severe metabolic acidosis with or without anion gap, and lactic acidosis. We recommend sending a number of screening laboratories, as noted in Table 8.5, when working up a child for possible FPIES.

It is important to keep in mind that expanded newborn screening does not detect all inborn errors of metabolism. Indeed, the most common urea cycle defect,

Table 8.6 Findings in FPIES, inborn errors of metabolism, or both

Finding	FPIES	Metabolic disorder
Hypoglycemia		X
Metabolic acidosis	+/–	X
Respiratory alkalosis		X
Ketosis		X
Transaminitis		X
Hyperammonemia		X
Leukocytosis	X	
Thrombocytosis	X	
Emesis	X	X
Diarrhea	X	X
Hypotension	X	
Family history of atopy	X	
Family history of infant death		X
Aversion to all protein-rich foods		X
Aversion to all fructose-containing foods		X
Episodes triggered by meats	Rare	X
Developmental delay or regression		X
Seizures		X
Hepatomegaly		X
Microcephaly		X

ornithine transcarbamylase (OTC) deficiency, is not detected by newborn screening, nor are rarer, but equally serious, diagnoses, such as mitochondrial disorders and glycogen storage disorders. When an inborn error of metabolism is suspected, a normal newborn screen does not obviate these diagnoses.

Prompt recognition and treatment are crucial in both groups of disorders. FPIES and inborn errors of metabolism are compared and contrasted in Table 8.6. For FPIES, children with repeated exposure to offending foods can have repetitive episodes of vomiting and diarrhea, which can lead to hypotension and shock at their most severe. For inborn errors of metabolism, children who are not appropriately treated with removal of toxic metabolites, specialized diets, and provision of adequate calories and nutrients can suffer from lifelong neurological, hepatic, muscular, or cardiac damage. Without appropriate treatment, many children with inborn errors of metabolism can die from the disease.

Our recommendation is to consider inborn errors of metabolism in all cases of FPIES and to screen for them with a detailed family history, diet history, physical examination focused on microcephaly, organomegaly, and dysmorphic features, and by sending screening laboratories. When the index of clinical suspicion is high, refer to a metabolic specialist, who can further assess the patient and send specialized diagnostic testing.

Clinical Pearls

- The acute presentation of FPIES can closely resemble the acute vomiting of intoxication-type inborn errors of metabolism (IEMs), as well as the lethargy of IEMs associated with decreased energy production.
- IEMs can be categorized as (1) disorders that cause intoxication, (2) disorders of inadequate energy production, and (3) disorders involving complex molecules.
- Early diagnosis and treatment of IEMs, with dietary restriction, substrate-reducing medications, removal of toxic metabolites, and provision of adequate energy, are crucial to prevent long-term damage to the central nervous system, heart, liver, muscles, and other organ systems.
- Close history-taking and examination are crucial in diagnosing IEMs. Suggestive historical findings include aversion to all protein-containing foods, aversion to all fructose-containing foods, and family history of infant death. Important findings on examination include microcephaly and hepatomegaly.
- Labwork can be instrumental in distinguishing IEMs from FPIES. Hyperammonemia, metabolic acidosis, lactic acidosis, transaminitis, and respiratory alkalosis are suggestive of IEMs.
- Diagnosis of IEMs is important not only for the patients' medical care but also for family planning and risk counseling for future pregnancies.

References

1. Saudubray JM, Van den Berghe G, Walter J (John H (2012) Inborn metabolic diseases: diagnosis and treatment. Heidelberg Springer.
2. Sparks SE, Krasnewich DM. PMM2-CDG (CDG-Ia). Seattle: University of Washington; 1993.
3. Janssen MCH, de Kleine RH, van den Berg AP, et al. Successful liver transplantation and long-term follow-up in a patient with MPI-CDG. Pediatrics. 2014;134:e279–83. https://doi.org/10.1542/peds.2013-2732.
4. Ruffner MA, Ruymann K, Barni S, et al. Food protein-induced enterocolitis syndrome: insights from review of a large referral population. J Allergy Clin Immunol Pract. 2013;1:343–9. https://doi.org/10.1016/j.jaip.2013.05.011.
5. Westphal V, Murch S, Kim S, et al. Reduced heparan sulfate accumulation in enterocytes contributes to protein-losing enteropathy in a congenital disorder of glycosylation. Am J Pathol. 2000;157:1917–25. https://doi.org/10.1016/S0002-9440(10)64830-4.
6. Schiff M, Roda C, Monin M-L, et al. Clinical, laboratory and molecular findings and long-term follow-up data in 96 French patients with PMM2-CDG (phosphomannomutase 2-congenital disorder of glycosylation) and review of the literature. J Med Genet. 2017;54:843–51. https://doi.org/10.1136/jmedgenet-2017-104903.
7. Lichter-Konecki U, Caldovic L, Morizono H, Simpson K. Ornithine transcarbamylase deficiency. Seattle: University of Washington; 1993.
8. Bingemann TA, Sood P, Järvinen KM. Food protein-induced enterocolitis syndrome. Immunol Allergy Clin N Am. 2018;38:141–52. https://doi.org/10.1016/j.iac.2017.09.009.
9. Nunes V, Niinikoski H. Lysinuric protein intolerance. Seattle: University of Washington; 1993.

10. Maines E, Comberiati P, Piacentini GL, et al. Lysinuric protein intolerance can be misdiagnosed as food protein-induced enterocolitis syndrome. Pediatr Allergy Immunol. 2013;24:509–10. https://doi.org/10.1111/pai.12096.
11. Baker P, Ayres L, Gaughan S, Weisfeld-Adams J. Hereditary fructose intolerance. Seattle: University of Washington; 1993.
12. Fiocchi A, Dionisi-Vici C, Cotugno G, et al. Fruit-induced FPIES masquerading as hereditary fructose intolerance. Pediatrics. 2014;134:e602–5. https://doi.org/10.1542/peds.2013-2623.
13. Messenger J, Clark S, Massick S, Bechtel M. A review of trimethylaminuria: (fish odor syndrome). J Clin Aesthetic Dermatol. 2013;6:45.
14. Phillips IR, Shephard EA. Primary trimethylaminuria. Seattle: University of Washington; 1993.
15. Miller NB, Beigelman A, Utterson E, Shinawi M. Transient massive trimethylaminuria associated with food protein-induced enterocolitis syndrome. JIMD Rep. 2014;12:11–5. https://doi.org/10.1007/8904_2013_238.

9 Nutritional Management of Food Protein-Induced Enterocolitis Syndrome

Amy Dean

Overview

The nutrition goals for a child with food protein-induced enterocolitis syndrome (FPIES) are the same as goals for any baby or toddler. These include age-appropriate or catch-up weight gain and growth; expansion of dietary variety and progression to age-appropriate feeding skills and behaviors to achieve adequate nutrient intake through an age-appropriate combination of food and beverage; and participation in the social component of eating. The additional challenges are slow food introduction through systematic and sometimes lengthy food trials, which are not always successful, and allergen avoidance until possible resolution of the allergy. These factors can certainly complicate efforts to achieve nutrition goals. The goal of healthcare providers taking care of an infant or toddler with FPIES is to help guide the child and caregivers toward a future of enjoying an appropriate, varied diet that meets her nutrient needs for an active and healthy lifestyle.

Introduction to Cases

FPIES can present in more than one way, and each presentation will progress differently, based on a variety of factors, including subsequent reactions and number of overall triggers, severity of reactions, caregiver preference for feeding style and dietary pattern, and the child's attitude toward feeding after what may have been multiple traumatic experiences or extended periods of food avoidance. The vast majority of infants with FPIES will react to one or a few foods and will follow feeding and growth trajectories that are quite similar to their peers without food allergy. We will use two more complex cases that illustrate some common features that can be encountered and how

A. Dean (✉)
Department of Clinical Nutrition, Children's Hospital of Philadelphia, Philadelphia, PA, USA
e-mail: deana@email.chop.edu

T. F. Brown-Whitehorn, A. Cianferoni (eds.), *Food Protein Induced Enterocolitis (FPIES)*,
https://doi.org/10.1007/978-3-030-21229-2_9

they can be addressed. In Case 1, LZ was breastfed and had his first reaction after introduction of complementary foods (solid food-induced FPIES). With guidance around approach to feeding, he eventually progressed to a varied, age-appropriate diet, including cow's milk, and never experienced slow weight gain or linear growth. In Case 2, MJ was also breastfed initially; however, he did not meet growth goals after his first few weeks of life. He was eventually transitioned to an elemental formula after severe acute reactions to extensively hydrolyzed formula (FPIES to cow's milk), accompanied by weight loss. He later had solid food-induced FPIES as well. With support from the elemental formula, and eventually a milk-free alternative, he also achieved appropriate growth and a varied diet. While individual aspects of each case do not always co-present, we hope the discussion will help to illustrate approaches to navigate each.

Case 1: Patient LZ

LZ was born full term and first presented to the FPIES center at 9 months of age. At that time, he was breastfed and had never ingested infant formula. He had normal stools, and no current gastrointestinal symptoms were reported. His weight gain and linear growth were appropriate for age and proportional (see Fig. 9.1). His diet was supplemented with 400 IU vitamin D3 per day. He had never had bloodwork and did not take any medications.

His caregivers reported giving oat cereal at around 5 months of age. He had repetitive vomiting that began 2 hours after ingestion. He was lethargic and pale. He then had diarrhea for 24 hours. He was able to breastfeed. Initial diagnosis was GERD, which was treated with medication that was stopped prior to his initial visit. At 6 months, he had delayed projectile vomiting, pallor, and lethargy on the fourth presentation of banana. He was diagnosed with FPIES based on reaction history, as per Summary

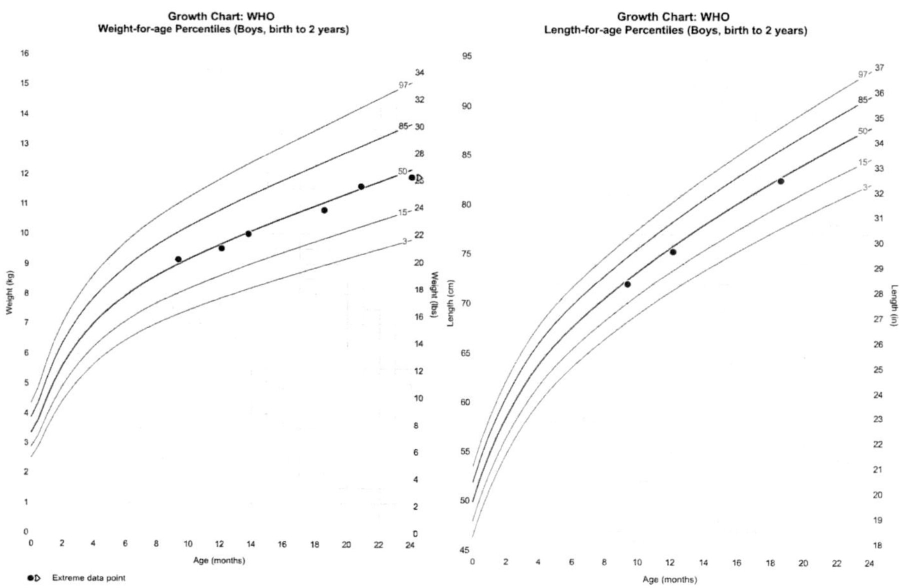

Fig. 9.1 Growth records for patient LZ

Statement 7 (Box 9.1) [1]. No skin or blood testing was recommended, as per Summary Statement (Box 9.2) [1]. After that time, he avoided oat, rice, and banana, as well as rice, cow's milk, and soy, as per Summary Statement 20 (Box 9.3) [1].

Box 9.1
Summary Statement 7: Diagnose FPIES primarily based on a clinical history of typical characteristic signs and symptoms with improvement after withdrawal of the suspected trigger food. From Nowak-Wegrzyn et al. [1]

Box 9.2
Summary Statement 9: Do not routinely perform testing for foods' IgE to identify food triggers of FPIES because FPIES is not an IgE-mediated process. From Nowak-Wegrzyn et al. [1]

Box 9.3
Summary Statement 20: Use dietary elimination of the trigger food or foods for the primary management of FPIES and educate caregivers and other care providers regarding avoidance strategies. From Nowak-Wegrzyn et al. [1]

Initial Visit (9 Months Old)

By the time of his initial visit, the caregiver had gradually added quinoa and a variety of fruits and vegetables to his diet. A few of these he usually refused, and caregivers suspect this was due to texture. He had not had meat, egg, or wheat. His mother was not avoiding any foods in her own diet. He ate 2 ounces of homemade or stage 2 purees at three meals per day, sitting in his high chair during the family meal. He played with finger foods. He was described as a slow eater. He drank water from a sippy cup with meals and nursed between meals and before sleeping. His caregivers' goal foods were meat, berries, and ways to add flavor. They wanted to know when to introduce milk, wheat, and egg.

Plan:

- Start multivitamins with iron.
- Continue to avoid oat, banana, rice, milk, and soy until challenge recommended.
- Food trials (continue for 7–10 days, start with 1–2 teaspoons, and gradually increase portion size): meat, beans/lentils, grain alternatives/potato, berries, spices, and oils (product and recipe suggestions provided).
- Adjust feeding schedule once he has a protein food: three meals with food followed by breast milk.

- Continue to offer finger foods for practice.
- Discuss and give strategies for transitioning from smooth puree to increased textures.
- Milk plan options (based on whether parents are comfortable with home trial or prefer hospital setting):
- Start with yogurt trial, and then he might be able to transition to cow's milk at 12 months.
- Wait until 15 months, and then introduce cow's milk.
- Introduce milk alternative as ingredient, and then transition at 12 months until milk trial at 15 months.

Interim Phone Calls

He reacted to chicken. Since then, feeding is a struggle! Sometimes he enjoys food, but usually he swats spoon, turns his head, and he refuses to open his mouth. He takes breast milk easily from breast or bottle. Caregivers have to force the spoon into his mouth to get him to eat. He eats 2–3 oz. of puree per meal, but it usually takes 30–40 minutes to finish.

Plan:

- Try to give him a spoon to alternate feeding himself, stop forcing him to eat and try to have fun with him at meals while you are enjoying your own food (to take the focus off of his eating), and encourage exploration of soft solids without pressuring him to eat them, in case he's getting tired of purees.
- Consider feeding therapy through early intervention or feeding center if concerns continue.

Follow-Up Visit #1 (12 Months Old)

New foods: egg (baked and then scrambled), berries, quinoa, peanut butter, olive oil, beef (he does not really like), turkey, and several vegetables. He just started yogurt.

Reactions since last visit: chicken (plain – made with chicken stock without other ingredients).

Started multivitamins with iron.

Eating is better! He is using spoon, finger feeding, biting, and chewing. He is now eating 3 meals per day (including protein: quinoa cereal, meat, egg), he eats thick chunky purees and finger foods on his tray, and then he takes breast milk from breast or bottle.

Plan:

- Continue yogurt trial, and then trial whole milk, if tolerated, can transition from breast milk to 4 oz. whole milk after meals. Then, wean breastfeeding when baby and mother are ready.
- Trials: corn and avocado.

- Daily pattern:
- Continue 3 meals per day: offer a protein (meat, fish, egg, yogurt) + starch (corn, quinoa, potato) + fruit/vegetable.
- Include a fat source at each meal: olive oil, vegetable oil, avocado, butter, egg yolk, almond butter, etc.
- Offer 4–6 oz. whole milk after meals.
- Offer finger foods at 2 snacks per day: try dipping when he is ready.

Interim Phone Calls

The caregiver decided to do rice challenge in the hospital instead of a trial at home. Then he ate several pieces of rice cereal from his brother's snack (in the morning and again in the afternoon) without reaction. He is scheduled rice challenge anyway due to small amount ingested. He passed rice challenge and increased serving sizes at home.

Follow-Up Visit #2 (18 Months Old)

He reacted to accidental chicken exposure and reacted to lamb during trial.

He eats table foods, only: Now, he is eating the same foods as his family! (family has changed what they eat somewhat – e.g., turkey instead of chicken).

The caregiver is now giving foods with multiple ingredients, avoiding main triggers, but not worrying about every minor ingredient.

A variety of foods includes many fruits (avoid banana), vegetables, quinoa, wheat, corn, rice, farro, bulgur, peanut, egg, small amounts of meat and fish (avoid chicken, lamb), cow's milk, and oils.

He has weaned from breast milk.

Portions at some meals are small for age. He drinks 4–5 sippy cups of milk per day (up to 30 oz.).

Plan:

- Consider challenges at hospital: oat and banana at age 2 years.
- Decrease milk intake to 12–16 oz. per day to encourage food intake.
- Review age-appropriate meal pattern.
- At the next visit, you can discuss stopping multivitamins if milk intake decreases and food portions increase.
- Trials: continue shrimp and then raspberries and beans (recipes and product ideas provided).

Case 1 Discussion

As per Summary Statement 21 (Box 9.4), routine avoidance of foods that trigger a reaction via infant's direct ingestion is not currently recommended for most infants because FPIES reactions via breast milk are uncommon. A maternal elimination

Box 9.4
Summary Statement 21: Do not recommend routine maternal dietary elimination of offending triggers while breastfeeding if the infant is thriving and remains asymptomatic

diet is rarely required. If reactions to proteins carried in breast milk are suspected, start with a 2-week elimination of cow's milk. If symptoms do not resolve, consider trial elimination of soy, followed by grains or other foods, depending on which are included in mother's diet.

Every breastfeeding mother of an infant with FPIES should be asked about her diet, weight trend, and any recent lab work. Some mothers eliminate many foods in an effort to stop or avoid reactions in their infants. This can leave the mother at risk for nutrient deficiency, excessive weight loss, and decreased milk supply, often without clear improvement in the infant's symptoms. Reintroduction of removed foods should be encouraged if no improvement has been observed. Basic nutrition advice for the mother can be offered as part of the care of the infant, including encouragement to consume protein sources, add fat, eat to satisfy appetite, and start supplementation with multivitamins and calcium (in the case of milk avoidance). Mothers avoiding multiple foods or who are experiencing ongoing weight loss or symptoms of nutrient deficiency, including pallor, fatigue, and hair loss, should be encouraged to seek evaluation by their primary care provider and a dietitian specializing in women's health and lactation.

A common question during initial or early clinic visits regards how to introduce foods. In order to avoid ambiguity in the event of a reaction, it is best to trial one food at a time. Specific protocols vary between institutions and providers; however, a reasonable schedule would be to start with one to two teaspoons of a new single-ingredient food on the first day and to continue to offer increasing portions of the trial food (allowing the baby to eat as much as she wants on the last day or two) for 7–10 days before starting the next trial. All tolerated foods should be continued in the diet during future trials, allowing the child's repertoire to grow. After a successful trial, each food should be offered daily or several times per week in order to avoid future reactions that sometimes occur after extended breaks from consuming a food. Some families shorten or extend trials based on their child's typical reaction pattern. For example, if the baby usually reacts within the first 3 days of the trial, caregivers might switch to a schedule of five-day trials. If symptoms are often unclear after 7 days, longer trial schedules might be adopted. Longer trials result in slower expansion of the diet, however, so the shortest cycle that accommodates clear results should be followed. Communication is a crucial component of trials. Caregivers should be educated to expect stool changes with diet changes, which should stabilize over the course of the trial period. If caregivers are uncomfortable interpreting symptoms, they should contact the child's medical providers to discuss their observations prior to ending a trial due to minor symptoms or due to symptoms that are likely related to a cause other than food, such as teething or acute illness.

Caregivers also need guidance regarding what foods to introduce. The goal is to expand variety and advance textures gradually, using foods from the family's typical diet to meet the child's nutritional needs. Appropriate food choices are unique to the child's reaction history and other factors specific to a given child. There are many ways to think about which foods to trial, in addition to the risk for reaction that may be the most common concern among caregivers. Some properties to consider when choosing foods for any infant, especially those with a limited diet and a cautious food introduction schedule, include nutrition, the family's usual pantry, risk for reaction, and versatility, availability, practicality, and affordability of foods (see Fig. 9.2).

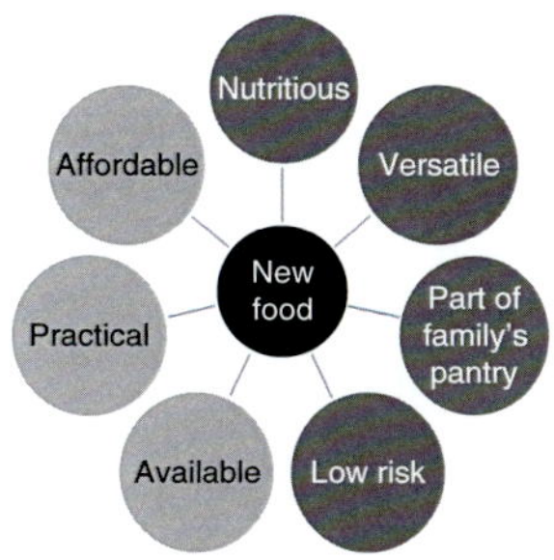

Is it Available?	**Is it Nutritious?**
What's in season? Consider local shopping options, ability to order online **Is it Practical?** Consider whether acquiring, storing, and preparing is reasonable for the family. Example: avocado might not be practical if other family members do not eat it (can be expensive, spoils quickly once it is cut, and is much larger than a single serving for an infant) **Is it Affordable?** Discuss lower-cost options (examples: frozen fish, in-season produce, buying in bulk or by the case) Consider foods that are part of the WIC package Give strategies for limiting waste (example: freeze coconut milk ice cubes) **Caregiver preference** Prioritizing a food that is a parent or child priority can • Increase buy-in in overall plan • Decrease stress over other restrictions when key foods are included in the diet • be emotional/symbolic reflection of the child as a member of the family when a child starts to eat certain traditional foods or staples	Is it a good source of key/missing nutrient(s) or similar to the staple food that it replaces (example: milk)? This is more important for infants and toddlers who do not drink a fortified formula **Is it Versatile?** Consider texture/culinary uses • Critical to supporting development of feeding skills with diet based on few foods • Also contributes to the development of the social component of eating because child has something appropriate to eat in a variety of settings • Focus on creative uses of each food - empowering to frustrated caregivers of children with few safe foods • Tip: Start by considering currently consumed foods in terms of their versatility and assess gaps **Is it already in the pantry?** The goal is to share the same diet as family, especially siblings, or find foods that can be consumed in similar fashion, for now • Develops the social component of eating, makes parental and peer role-modeling possible • Also capitalizes on any benefit from taste preference acquisition from maternal diet via breast milk by continuing exposure to, and familiarity with, the family's staple foods **Is there a Low risk of reaction?** Based on FPIES Consensus guidelines [1] and CHOP data [2]. Also consider susceptibility to cross-contamination.

Fig. 9.2 Properties to consider when choosing foods to introduce

Of primary concern to caregivers and the medical team is how to limit the risk of additional reactions during the process of introducing new foods to the diet. The most common food triggers vary depending upon where in the world people live. For example, rice is a common trigger in Australia, and fish is common in Italy. In the United States, reactions to cow's milk and soy are seen most frequently, while rice and oat are the most common solid food triggers [1]. There is increased incidence of coallergy to these foods. Subsequently, initial avoidance of all of these foods is typically recommended when an infant presents with history of reaction to any of these foods. The incidence of reaction to other foods is lower (see Fig. 9.2), and relationships between history of reaction to one food and risk for reaction to another are not well-defined, although successful introduction of a food does favor the likelihood of tolerance of other foods in the same group [1]. These general facts should be discussed with caregivers and can be a source of reassurance and confidence to move forward with making selections of next foods for trial. Foods that don't typically need food trials as they are tolarterd by most FPIES patients are listed in Box 9.5. Table 9.1 can be used as a guide for introducing foods based on relative risk for reactions, as well as key nutrients and appropriate texture. Foods that are not included in the table should be discussed individually with the family, taking the child's specific history and food environment into account.

Studies have shown that a child's risk for nutrient deficiency, as well as poor weight gain and growth later on, increases proportional to the number of food allergy triggers [3]. Table 9.2 shows common FPIES trigger foods and the nutrients that might be missing from the diet when they are avoided, as well as suggestions to replace them.

For breastfed infants with FPIES, several nutrients are commonly inadequate in the diet. Supplementation with 400 IU of vitamin D is recommended from birth; however, it is often avoided due to parental fear of reaction to product ingredients. Drops with minimal ingredients, such as olive oil or coconut oil, are commercially available. Breast milk is no longer an adequate source to maintain infant iron stores by 6 months; however, fortified cereals are often avoided and meats delayed in favor of lower-risk fruit and vegetable introduction. Guidance to introduce lower-risk meats, fortified lower-risk grains, and suggestions for multivitamins with iron should be provided. Older infants need food sources of protein, fat, and a variety of vitamins and minerals. Table 9.1 can be used to guide expansion of variety. A multivitamin should be considered for infants with limited variety or volume of intake. An emphasis should be placed on inclusion of fat sources at meals, especially when there is concern for adequate weight gain or when meals are low-calorie. The calorie density of meals can be reduced due to delays in texture progression from puree to table foods or when fruits and vegetables make up a large part of the volume consumed. Adding fats may take creativity, as the most commonly suggested sources of extra calories and fat tend to be from high-fat dairy products; however, some suggestions are presented in Box 9.6. There are also many allergen-free analog products available that can be appropriate substitutes for additives like butter and mayonnaise. For infants and toddlers who need a supplemental calorie and protein source in addition to vitamin and mineral supplementation, hypoallergenic formula should be considered, as this can provide macro- and micronutrients together. Access to insurance coverage should be discussed when this option is presented, due to the high cost associated.

Table 9.1 Empiric guidelines for selecting weaning foods in infants with FPIES [1]

Ages and stages	Lower-risk foods[a]	Moderate-risk foods[a]	Higher-risk foods[a]
4–6 mo (as per AAP, CoN)	Vegetables		
If developmentally appropriate and safe and nutritious foods are available: Begin with smooth, thin purees and progress to thicker purees. Choose foods that are high in iron. Add vegetables and fruits.	Broccoli, cauliflower, parsnip, turnip, pumpkin	Squash, carrot, white potato, green bean (legume)	Sweet potato, green pea (legume)
6 mo (as per WHO)	Fruits		
Complementary feeding should begin no later than 6 mo of age: In the breastfed infant, high-iron foods and supplemental iron (1 mg/kg/d) are suggested by 6 mo of age. Continue to expand a variety of fruits, vegetables, legumes, grains, meats, and other foods as tolerated.	Blueberries, strawberries, plum, watermelon, peach, avocado	Apple, pear, orange	Banana
8 mo of age or when developmentally appropriate	High-iron foods		
Offer soft-cooked and bite-and-dissolve textures from around 8 mo of age or as tolerated by infant.	Lamb, fortified quinoa cereal, millet	Beef, fortified grits and corn cereal, wheat (whole wheat and fortified), fortified barley cereal	Higher-iron foods: Fortified, infant rice and oat cereals
12 mo of age or when developmentally appropriate	Others		
Offer modified tolerated foods from the family: Table-chopped meats, soft cooked vegetables, grains, and fruits.	Tree nuts and seed butters[a] (sesame, sunflower, etc.) [a]thinned with water or infant puree for appropriate infant texture and to prevent choking	Peanut, other legumes (other than green pea)	Milk, soy, poultry, egg, fish

View Table in HTML

This table should be considered in the context of the following notes:

A. Exclusive breastfeeding until 4–6 months of age and continuing breastfeeding through the first year of life or longer as long as mutually desired by both mother and child (Baker et al. [4])

B. If an infant tolerates a variety of early foods, subsequent introduction can be more liberal. Additionally, tolerance to one food in a food group (green pea) is considered a favorable prognostic indicator for tolerance of other foods from the same group (legumes; Sicherer [5])

AAP, CoN American Academy of Pediatrics, Committee on Nutrition, *WHO* World Health Organization

[a]Risk assessment is based on the clinical experience and published reports of FPIES triggers

Box 9.5: Safe Foods and Ingredients to Watch

- *Safe foods (no trial required)*: cane sugar, salt, baking soda (baking powder contains starch – usually corn/potato), refined oils, other oils (not expeller pressed), artificial colors, flavors, and sweeteners.
- Ingredients to watch (may trigger reaction): starch (grain-derived; processing will determine whether protein is present), gum (legume and plant-derived), pectin (fruit-derived).

Table 9.2 Foods commonly implicated in food protein-induced enterocolitis syndrome and their nutrients [6]

Main foods implicated in FPIES	Common food sources	Nutrients
Milk	Butter/most fat spreads, cheese, cow/sheep/goat milk evaporated/condensed milk, cream, ghee, yoghurt, ice creams, custard, dairy desserts, and manufactured foods using milk or butter in their ingredients	Protein, carbohydrate, fat, vitamin A, vitamin D, riboflavin, pantothenic acid, vitamin B12, calcium, magnesium, phosphate [7]
Soy	Soy sauce, soy products, meat substitutes, breads, vegetarian/vegan foods, processed meat, for example, hot dogs, foods labelled as "diet" and "high protein"	Protein, thiamin, riboflavin, pyridoxine, folate, calcium, phosphorus, magnesium, iron, zinc, protein, and fiber [7]
Egg	Egg white and yolk, cakes, biscuits, speciality breads, and mayonnaise	Protein, riboflavin, biotin, protein, vitamin A, vitamin B12, vitamin D, vitamin E, pantothenic acid, selenium, iodine, and folate [7]
Fish and seafood	All types of white and fatty fish, anchovy (Worcester sauce), aspic, caviar, surimi, Caesar salad, Gentleman's relish, kedgeree, fish sauce, paella, bouillabaisse, and gumbo	All fish: Protein, iodine
	Some people may tolerate canned fish	Fish bones: Calcium, phosphorus, and fluoride
	Fish oil capsules may cause reactions in highly sensitized individuals	Fatty fish: Vitamins A and D, omega-3 fatty acids
	Crayfish, crab, lobster, shrimp, prawns	Shellfish and mollusks: Zinc, selenium, copper, iron [7]
	Clams, mussels, oysters, octopus, squid, snails, scallop	
Grains: Wheat/barley/oats	Bread, breakfast cereals, pasta, cakes, biscuits, crackers, cold cooked meat, pies, batter, flour, semolina, spelt, couscous, bottled sauces and gravies, barley water, soup, flapjacks or cereal bars, porridge	Carbohydrate, fiber, thiamine, riboflavin, niacin, calcium, iron, and folate if fortified [7]
Rice	Rice-based dishes: Sushi, paella, curries, gumbo, and risotto	Carbohydrate, calcium, iron, phosphorus, potassium, thiamine, riboflavin, niacin, folate, and pantothenic acid
	Rice cereal	

Table 9.2 (continued)

Main foods implicated in FPIES	Common food sources	Nutrients
	Rice pudding	
Chicken, Turkey, lamb	Any meat-containing dishes	Protein, (fat), selenium, phosphorus, potassium, zinc, iron
		Vitamin B6 and niacin
Sweet potato	Sweet potato and dishes containing sweet potato such as curries or vegetarian meals	Beta-carotene (vitamin A), pantothenic acid, thiamine, niacin, riboflavin, magnesium, manganese, and potassium
Peas	Vegetarian meals	Folic acid, pantothenic acid, niacin, thiamine, pyridoxine, ascorbic acid, vitamin K, vitamin A, calcium, iron, copper, zinc, and manganese

FPIES food protein-induced enterocolitis syndrome

Box 9.6: Thinking of Food Introduction in Terms of Food Group

Fruits and Vegetables:

- Low risk for reaction.
- Introduce a variety of colors: dark green and bright orange indicate high nutrient content.
- Safest to buy fresh and prepare yourself, but frozen can save money and texture is good for puree/mash/soft finger food.

Grains:

- Choose grain alternatives (similar to grains in terms of nutrients and culinary uses) such as quinoa, millet, sorghum, amaranth, buckwheat, and corn.
- Many recipe blogs and alternative products are available (e.g., pasta).
- Look for iron-fortified products.

Meat/protein:

- Texture can be challenging. Try cooking techniques that result in soft, moist meat.
- Beef is a good source of iron – for poultry, dark meat offers increased fat and minerals.
- Give plain form – processed forms (egg sausage) can include allergenic ingredients.
- Eggs are good texture for babies and useful for baking with alternative grains.

- Baked egg/cow's milk has not been studied in FPIES but is sometimes tolerated by children who react when they drink milk and eat cheese, yogurt, and other dairy products or eat egg dishes.

Dairy/alternatives:

- For babies with solid food FPIES, avoidance of milk and soy typically is recommended for the first year unless the baby is already consuming at the time of the first reaction.
- For infants, elemental and extensively hydrolyzed formulas are recommended.
- Milk alternatives (see Table 9.3).
  - Used in recipes in late infancy or as beverage after the first birthday, when food intake provides adequate nutrition.
  - Products are not equivalent in terms of nutrient content (see Table 9.3).
  - Yogurt, cheese, and dessert items are usually less fortified or not fortified at all.

Fats/oils:

- Oils, except expeller-pressed, typically have very low-protein content and are low risk.
- Tree nuts, peanuts, and seeds.
- Avocado.
- Coconut cream.
- High-fat meat and meat drippings.
- Egg yolk.

Table 9.3 Milk alternative product comparison

(8 fl oz)	Calories, protein, fat	Calcium, vitamin D	Caution with
Whole milk	150 kcal, 8 g pro, 8 g fat	300 mg, 120 IU	Cow's milk, soy, legume, or grain allergy
Soy	70–170 kcal, 3–10 g pro, 0–5 g fat	0–450 mg, 0–120 IU	
Pea	100 kcal, 8 g pro, 4.5 g fat	450 mg, 120 IU	
Oat	130 kcal, 4 g pro, 2.5 g fat	300–350 mg, 100 IU	
Rice	110–130 kcal, 1 g pro, 2–3 g fat	0–300 mg, 100 IU	
Hemp	70–160 kcal, 2–4 g pro, 5–6 g fat	300–500 mg, 100–120 IU	
Coconut	45–100 kcal, 0–1 g pro, 4.5–5 g fat	100–450 mg, 100–140 IU	
Almond	30–120 kcal, 1–5 g pro, 2–3 g fat	0–450 mg, 100–120 IU	Tree nut allergy

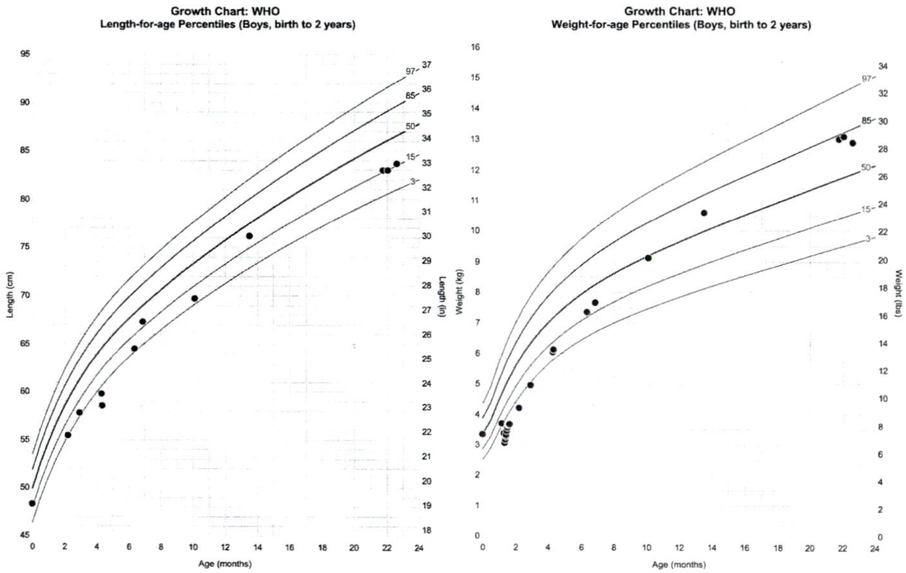

Fig. 9.3 Growth records for patient MJ

Case 2: Patient MJ

Patient MJ was born full term and was breastfed until 5 weeks of age, when an intact cow's milk protein formula was introduced. He was brought to the emergency department for repeated vomiting and inconsolable crying and was discharged with diagnosis of reflux. His pediatrician noted weight loss 2 days later and diagnosed milk-protein allergy. He was transitioned to an extensively hydrolyzed cow's milk infant formula; however, he returned to the emergency department 2 days after that, with continued forceful vomiting and watery diarrhea with feeds as well as lethargy. Profound weight loss was also noted (see Fig. 9.3). He was admitted for severe dehydration and metabolic acidosis into pediatric intensive care unit and was made NPO (nothing by mouth) while rehydrated on intravenous fluids (IVF) and then oral rehydration solution. When extensively hydrolyzed formula was reintroduced (clinicians felt he had infection or, less likely, metabolic condition), severe vomiting and dehydration recurred, and he was ultimately diagnosed with chronic FPIES to cow's milk and started on an elemental formula following fluid resuscitation. He tolerated the formula and was discharged.

After discharge, he was followed outpatient by a gastroenterologist, where he was noted to be symptom-free with good weight gain and growth. His parents began to introduce foods at 6 months, starting with fruits and vegetables, and successfully added a variety. He did have diarrhea with mucus and increased fussiness with banana, carrot, and pear, and these foods were stopped. He was referred to the FPIES center for guidance with food introduction.

Initial Visit (7 Months Old)

He was taking elemental formula in a bottle six times a day and happily ate a 4 oz. container of fruit or vegetable puree once daily. He had continued good growth and weight gain. At parents' request, he had negative skin testing to milk and soy.

Plan:

- Continue elemental formula.
- Avoid milk, soy, oat, rice, wheat, banana, carrot, and pear.
- Continue food introduction with 7-day trials: introduce a variety of colors of fruits and vegetables, grain alternatives, meat, legumes, avocado, and olive oil.
- Products, recipes, and texture suggestions are provided.
- Parents are encouraged to offer two foods per meal and increase to two meals per day when ready.

Interim Phone Calls

Mother reported reaction to squash, which was confirmed by provider based on symptoms and timing. She was also concerned that he reacted to sweet potato, however it was determined to be viral gastroenteritis, as symptom onset was 12 hours after ingestion and he had been eating sweet potato for several weeks prior to the episode.

Plan:

- Encourage to be firm with family members and friends who want to feed him more liberally.

Follow-Up Visit #1 (10 Months Old)

Diet now included several fruits and vegetables, quinoa, turkey, and elemental formula.

He is reacting within 2 days of a new food and parents would like to shorten trials. His food intake has increased to two foods twice daily, but he was having some trouble increasing texture, with frequent gagging. He was drinking less formula and was not meeting vitamin D needs anymore. He continues to show catch-up weight gain and linear growth.

Plan:

- Continue elemental infant formula: the caregiver will discuss transition to pediatric formula or milk alternative at next visit.
- Start vitamin D supplement.
- Shorten trials to 3 days: try fruits and vegetables, almond, peanut, corn, egg, other meats, milk alternatives (hemp, pea protein).

- Food ideas and texture suggestions are provided: give opportunity to explore textures daily.
- Consider evaluation for feeding therapy.

Interim phone calls:

- Start vitamin D.
- Add egg, peanut butter, chickpeas, and coconut (sugar, flour, planning to try milk).
- Seek birthday cake and icing recipes.
- Use vegan cheese, not calcium source, but this is helpful to make pizza.
- Seek macaroni and cheese: clarify flour ingredients and discuss bean- and quinoa-based products with vegan cheese added.

Follow-Up Visit #2 (13 Months Old)

He continues with appropriate weight gain and linear growth.

He continues to avoid milk, soy, oat (during visit, it was discovered that he eats oat-based cereal often), rice, carrot, squash, and banana.

Wheat was added, in addition to foods noted in the interim.

He became more interested in table foods as a variety of safe foods increased: he has stopped purees.

He eats three meals, including protein, starch, fruit/vegetable, and fat source.

He has decreased formula intake to 9 oz. per day and is eating milk-free (pea protein) yogurt daily.

Plan:

- Continue milk, soy, and rice avoidance: soy challenge in hospital at 2 years.
- Food trials: corn, almond, and milk alternative: hemp or pea protein-based milk (he tolerates yogurt made by same company) and fruits and vegetables that caused mucus in stools (wait until 12 months after the last exposure).

Case 2 Discussion

The scope of the factors affecting decision between breast milk and formula is broader than the context of FPIES. Mothers have many reasons for a baseline preference to formula feed from birth or after a period of weeks to months before a diagnosis is ever made. Reasons for formula use within the context of FPIES include maternal nutritional risk or dissatisfaction due to maternal diet restriction, continued symptoms in the infant despite maternal restriction, poor growth, and increased stress, which may also result in decreased breast milk supply.

Some infants with solid food FPIES do tolerate cow's milk or soy formula prior to their first reaction and should be advised to continue. For infants with a pre-existing FPIES diagnosis, extensively hydrolyzed or elemental (free amino acid) formulas are recommended. Goat's milk formulas are not recommended due to the likelihood of cross-reactivity with cow's milk. Homemade formulas also are not recommended, due to risk for excessive renal solute load, difficulty achieving appropriate nutrient composition, and risk for reaction to the component ingredients. For those who need to continue formula past the first birthday due to inadequate nutrition from solid foods, it is appropriate to continue extensively hydrolyzed formula using an infant or toddler product. Elemental products are available in formulations appropriate and marketed for older children and teenagers. There is also a semi-solid elemental product available, which can be used for spoon feeding and fortifying purees. Hydrolyzed and elemental formulas typically have strong aromas and distinct flavor profiles. They are often better accepted when introduced early and served in a bottle or other closed cup (such as a sippy or straw cup). Some children preferred flavored products, which are available commercially or can be created by adding sweeteners and flavor extracts and by blending with fruit or juices.

Adequate protein, vitamin D, and iron are typically supplied by commercial formula that is meeting calorie needs. For this reason, food introduction in the setting of formula use can be liberalized compared with the recommendations appropriate for exclusively breastfed infants. Food introduction choices should be shaped according to other food properties outlined previously in this chapter.

As infants become toddlers, the first phase of food introduction and establishment of complementary feeding gives way to meals that begin to resemble the family meal, transition away from reliance on breast milk or formula as a primary source of nutrition, and exploration of the food landscape outside the controlled home environment.

As a child's food repertoire expands and reactions move further into the past, it is appropriate to transition gradually from strictly single-ingredient products to commercial products with incidental minor ingredients that have not been trialed individually. Packaged foods and introduction of recipes that contain more elaborate flavors will help the child assimilate into the family's eating pattern, make more convenience items accessible, and create interest and enjoyment of foods, which can be helpful during stages when increased food selectivity is common.

In addition to an expanded variety on the plate, the child's beverage will transition around or sometime after the first birthday. As the volume and variety of foods consumed becomes more adequate, beverages should be consumed after food, rather than before. Small amounts of water can be introduced. Timing of the transition from breast milk or infant formula to a milk alternative will depend on mother's preference for weaning, as well as the child's nutrient needs. Some toddlers and children need to continue a fortified formula in order to meet nutrition needs. Typically, around two-thirds of calorie needs [8] should be met by food prior to transition from formula to cow's milk or a milk alternative. A growing variety of commercial milk alternatives are available, based on a rapidly expanding number of plant-based protein sources. These are not nutritionally equivalent to cow's milk, or to one another, with composition depending on the protein source, recipe, and fortification with vitamins and minerals such as calcium, vitamin D, and vitamin B12. See Table 9.3 for a comparison of various product ranges that highlights nutrients of particular concern. Some families prefer to make milks at home in order to avoid ingredients that are often added for texture purposes. Homemade milks can be supplemented or fortified with added nutrients under the guidance of a dietitian. Additional factors that impact the milk chosen include the child's allergy triggers, taste and texture preference, as well as cost and availability. Some products are shelf-stable and can be purchased in bulk or ordered online, which can help reduce cost and increase convenience.

Sharing responsibility and control over the food consumed by a child with food allergies can be a source of stress but can eventually provide a sense of community, relief, and even empowerment to a child taught to navigate his food allergies. Initially, parents may choose to provide all food and beverages consumed outside the home. Gradually, through oral communication, education regarding label reading and cooking methods, and clear documentation, foods from other sources, such as daycare, school, restaurants, and friends and family, should be safely included. Organizations such as FARE (www.foodallergy.org) and Kids With Food Allergies (www.kidswithfoodallergies.org) offer a variety of resources to facilitate these communications and relationships.

Key Points/Clinical Pearls

- The nutrition goals for a child with food protein-induced enterocolitis syndrome (FPIES) are the same as goals for any baby or toddler her age.
- The vast majority of infants with FPIES will react to one or a few foods and will follow feeding and growth trajectories that are quite similar to their peers without food allergy.
- Caregivers work with the nutrition and medical team to expand variety and advance textures gradually, using foods from the family's typical diet to meet the child's nutritional needs. Some children will require fortified formula or vitamin/mineral supplements.
- In order to avoid ambiguity in the event of a reaction, it is best to trial one food at a time. Appropriate food choices are unique to the child's reaction history and other factors specific to a given child.
- Most breastfeeding mothers do not need to eliminate foods from their diets, but most formula-fed babies require a hypoallergenic formula. Timing and selection of a nutritious beverage for transition from breast milk to formula depend on many factors, including nutrition status, food variety, and family preferences.

References

1. Nowak-Wegrzyn A, et al. International consensus guidelines for the diagnosis and managements of food protein-induced enterocolitis syndrome: executive summary—workgroup report of the Adverse Reactions to Food Committee, American Academy of Allergy, Asthma & Immunology. J Allergy Clin Immunol. 2017;139:1111–26.

2. Ruffner M, et al. Food protein-induced enterocolitis syndrome: insights from review of a large referral population. J Allergy Clin Immunol Pract. 2013;1(4):343–9.
3. Robbins KA, et al. Milk allergy is associated with decreased growth in US children. J Allergy Clin Immunol. 2014;134(6):1466–8.
4. Baker RD, Greer FR, Committee on Nutrition American Academy of Pediatrics. Diagnosis and prevention of iron deficiency and iron-deficiency anemia in infants and young children (0–3 years of age). Pediatrics. 2010;126:1040–50.
5. Sicherer SH. Food protein-induced enterocolitis syndrome: case presentations and management lessons. J Allergy Clin Immunol. 2005;115:149–56.
6. Venter C, Groetch M. Nutritional management of food protein-induced enterocolitis syndrome. Curr Opin Allergy Clin Immunol. 2014;14(3):255–62.
7. Venter C, Meyer R. Session 1: allergic disease: the challenges of managing food hypersensitivity. Proc Nutr Soc. 2010;69:11–24.
8. Christie L. Food hypersensitivities. In: Pediatric nutrition. 4th ed. Sudbury: Jones & Barlett Learning LLC; 2012. p. 127–46.

Feeding and FPIES

10

Sherri Shubin Cohen and Colleen Taylor Lukens

Case

K.V. is now a 7-year-old boy who breastfed in infancy but had colic and frequent spitting up. He stopped breastfeeding at 3 months old and was tried on multiple formulas but developed severe eczema and profuse diarrhea. He had vomiting, diarrhea, and lethargy when solid foods were introduced. He was subsequently diagnosed with FPIES and required inpatient management at 16 months of age. He was placed on a restricted diet of elemental formula and no foods. His symptoms improved and were followed closely by gastroenterology and allergy. He willingly drank his elemental formula and never required tube feeds. He tolerated the introduction of some foods, such as strawberries, blueberries, grapes, and avocado, but did not tolerate other foods, such as chicken and cucumbers. At 4 years of age, he would no longer participate in food trials, so was referred to a multidisciplinary feeding team. At that time, he was accepting small amounts of strawberries, blueberries, grapes, bananas, turkey, watermelon, and potatoes. Elemental formula was providing 90% of his total calories. He was evaluated by a physician, dietitian, speech language pathologist, occupational therapist, and psychologist to assess for factors across those domains that could be contributing to his food refusal. Recommendations included outpatient feeding therapy with the goals of increasing his dietary variety, increasing the volume of food he would eat, and decreasing his reliance on formula. He made progress in outpatient therapy for the next 2 years

S. S. Cohen (✉)
Gastroenterology, Hepatology, and Nutrition, Children's Hospital of Philadelphia, Philadelphia, PA, USA
e-mail: cohens@email.chop.edu

C. T. Lukens
Department of Child and Adolescent Psychiatry and Behavioral Sciences, Children's Hospital of Philadelphia, Philadelphia, PA, USA

T. F. Brown-Whitehorn, A. Cianferoni (eds.), *Food Protein Induced Enterocolitis (FPIES)*,
https://doi.org/10.1007/978-3-030-21229-2_10

until he became sick with *Clostridium difficile* colitis and started to refuse foods again. His refusal adversely impacted his nutritional status, which necessitated intensive interdisciplinary feeding therapy at 6.5 years old. His allowed foods at that time were strawberries, apples, watermelon, bell peppers, white potatoes, salmon, turkey soup, pea soup, bananas, almonds, blueberries, peas, oat, avocado, turkey, sweet potatoes, and chicken. When therapy began, he was eating small volumes of only eight of these allowed foods, and elemental formula was providing 80% of his total calories. A variety of therapeutic strategies were used during the intervention program, including appetite manipulation, behavior management, and child directed exploratory play with novel foods. When he completed intensive therapy, he had learned to eat age-appropriate portions of all of his allowed foods at three meals per day. This resulted in decreased dependence on elemental formula from 80% to 20% of his total calories. His parents were integral members of the treatment team and were able to continue his mealtime success at home.

Typical Feeding Development

In order to understand how pediatric feeding disorders develop in the child with FPIES, it is important to recognize typical feeding milestones and to appreciate the range of feeding behaviors that fall within the spectrum of normal development. Feeding skill development follows a predictable progression, but when a child's feeding experiences are atypical, we expect that progression to be interrupted. Interruption anywhere along that progression can alter the child's feeding trajectory.

Feeding behaviors are driven by the hunger-satiety cycle. While the neurological circuitry and hormonal pathways underlying this cycle are in place prenatally, the rewarding aspects of feeding are learned postnatally when fetal continuous feeding changes to infant bolus feeding. In normal development, the hunger-satiety cycle is shaped in early infancy upon the introduction of breastmilk or formula feeds. After this is established, feeding behavior is fairly stable for the first 4 to 6 months of life. In this period, breastmilk or formula is the sole source of nutrition, and the hunger-satiety cycle is reinforced by child-led demand for increased food volumes driven by higher caloric needs associated with rapid weight gain and linear growth.

Oral-motor coordination in early feeding is dependent on key infant reflexes. The first of these is the rooting reflex, which helps an infant locate a food source. When the infant's cheek or lips are touched, she will open her mouth and turn toward the stimulus. The second key reflex is the sucking reflex, which supports breast and bottle feeding by eliciting a suck pattern when the tongue and/or roof of the mouth are touched. Of note, sucking behavior is not only necessary for feeding but will also help an infant to calm and organize herself, and therefore, it is important to provide frequent non-nutritive sucking opportunities in addition to nutritive sucking experiences. The third key reflex is the extrusion or tongue thrust reflex, which causes an infant to push or expel solids out of her mouth with her tongue. This effectively precludes spoon feeding. These primitive reflexes are typically in place for the first 4 months of life, after which point the infant will transition to more volitional or controlled oral patterns. During this early developmental stage, babies should be fed on demand. A variation in volume consumed and in timing of feeds is normal.

The next major milestone in normal feeding is the introduction of spoon feeding. One sign of spoon feeding readiness is the loss of the extrusion reflex. It is also important to consider other developmental readiness signs, such as motor, cognitive, and oral-motor skills, including the ability to maintain an upright sitting posture in a high chair, interest in other people's eating, and mouthing hands and toys. Most babies are not developmentally ready to start spoon feeding until around 6 months of age. Earlier introduction can lead to frustration for both the baby and the caregivers. If the introduction of spoon feeding does not go well, then waiting 1 to 2 weeks before reintroduction may lead to increased success. Spoon feeding at this age is for practice and skill acquisition, not as a significant source of nutrition. Smooth purees, including infant cereal, homemade purees, and commercially prepared purees, are the easiest texture for early spoon feeders.

Defined mealtimes may be introduced between 6 and 8 months of age. Spoon feedings can be offered one, then two, and then three times per day, similar to common mealtimes. The feeding schedule thereby transitions from a child-led, on demand schedule, to a caregiver-led mealtime routine. New foods should be introduced every 3 to 4 days to monitor for allergic reactions in children without FPIES. For children with FPIES, new foods are introduced more slowly, starting with small amounts and gradually increasing to full serving sizes over 7 to 10 days.

Feeding is a sensory-based experience. Smell is a critical element of taste, and children also learn about food from its visual presentation. Purees should be presented on a spoon so children are exposed to these components. If pouched purees are used, they should be squeezed onto a spoon and then offered to the child so she can experience the smell and sight of the food.

At about 8 to 10 months of age, babies are often ready to be offered dissolvable solid foods and soft solid foods. Dissolvable solids include puffs, melts, crackers, cereals, and rice rusks. Soft solids include small pieces of soft-cooked vegetables, avocados, bananas, pancakes, bread, pasta, cheese, tofu, or anything the family eats that can be prepared in a soft cube shape. Children are often able to explore these foods with their hands with increasing success and may begin to bring these items to their mouths. Children may use a variety of grasp patterns to pick up foods at this age, but are often inefficient at feeding themselves. Mashed table foods can be helpful in making the transition between smooth purees and soft solids. Mixed textures (such as most stage 3 baby foods) are difficult for many children and are not necessary for texture progression.

At this stage of development, the baby's oral and pharyngeal (throat) structures are becoming more like those of an adult. Fat pads previously present in the cheeks will diminish, the tongue will occupy less space in the mouth as it grows, and the structures of the airway will lower. Coupled with these anatomical changes, a baby is now able to move her tongue independently from her jaw. This allows for tongue lateralization, or the ability to move pieces of solid food on and off of the teeth and gum surfaces. This is the beginning of chewing pattern development.

At 10 to 12 months, babies are ready for more independence at mealtimes. As their hand-eye coordination develops, they become more efficient at finger feeding and are exploring utensil use. They are developing a more mature, vertical-type chewing pattern. Cup drinking can be introduced at this age. At around 1 year of age, many typically developing children are eating their family foods and are weaning off the bottle. They are more mobile as they start crawling and walking, and they orally explore items throughout their environment, so particular care should be taken to avoid exposure to choking hazards including nuts, whole grapes, popcorn, and hotdogs. Infant formula can be transitioned to whole milk, limiting to 24 ounces per day, or to a higher calorie nutritious beverage for children who are having difficulty gaining weight. The World Health Organization supports continued breastfeeding for the first 2 years of life or as desired by mother and child.

Toddlers are often picky and their eating becomes more variable. They desire increasing independence in general, including at mealtimes. Fear of things that are new (neophobia) is protective for children who have increased independent mobility. While picky eating can be frustrating for families, it helps to decrease children's ingestion of dangerous substances. Most children, therefore, require repeated exposure to a new food before they will add it to their dietary repertoire. It is normal for toddlers to stop eating foods they used to enjoy. Toddler pickiness is within the range of normal when the child replaces those foods with new foods, when she accepts at least one food from every food group, and when her weight gain and growth are age-appropriate. Toddlers generally meet their nutritional needs over longer timespans, for example, over a week instead of a day. It is critical to maintain a consistent mealtime routine by offering food and fluids at 3 meals and 2 snack times per day while the child is seated in an appropriately sized chair at a table. It is important to avoid feeding the child while she is walking around and with distractions such as screen time. Offering healthy food choices, having family meals, limiting mealtimes to 20 to 30 minutes, minimizing grazing between meals, restricting juice to 4 ounces per day, and limiting milk to 24 ounces per day all support toddlers meeting their nutritional needs despite their pickiness and inconsistent acceptance. Toddlers model their behavior from their caregivers, so caregivers should make sure they are eating nutritionally well-balanced meals. Using food as a reward, or withholding it as a punishment, interferes with the establishment of positive mealtime experiences.

When these feeding developmental milestones have been met, the child is likely to continue her trajectory toward independent eating in the school-aged and adult years. She will have established the ability to support her nutritional needs through a varied diet. Ongoing caregiver supervision and guidance helps to strengthen the transition to independent healthy eating. If this development is interrupted at any point, however, children are at risk for developing pediatric feeding disorders.

Pediatric Feeding Disorders

Although there is currently no uniformly utilized set of criteria for diagnosing pediatric feeding disorders, and they have been defined differently for research studies and clinical use, there is growing consensus on how to conceptualize these disorders

[1]. Feeding disorders are associated with nutritional, medical, skill, and psychosocial deficits. For example, feeding disorders can manifest as slow weight gain, impaired linear growth, and micronutrient deficiencies or can lead to a medical condition such as constipation. Feeding disorders can also emerge as deficits or delays in the development of skills associated with eating and feeding, including chewing, swallowing, and utensil use. Finally, feeding disorders can present as behavioral or psychosocial problems in the caregiver, child, or dyad, with persistent refusal to eat as a hallmark sign of a pediatric feeding disorder. Specifically, children may present with refusal to eat certain foods or picky eating, refusal to eat enough food to gain weight and grow, or other disruptive behavior that is incompatible with eating. As well, feeding disorders can manifest as stress or distress in children and their caregivers. In addition, caregivers often engage in compensatory behavior at mealtimes with goals of optimizing their child's nutrition and health (e.g., feeding the school-age child that will not feed themselves, allowing children access to snack foods throughout the day, providing formula via infant bottle to a toddler).

Development of Feeding Disorders

Factors in the same areas in which feeding disorders manifest can influence the development of pediatric feeding disorders. Medical contributors include gastroenterological, respiratory, cardiac, and neurological problems, food allergies and intolerances, and conditions associated with prematurity. Delays in skill development, such as oral-motor deficits that impact a child's ability to chew and swallow or fine motor delays that affect a child's ability to feed himself, can impact the development of pediatric feeding disorders. Finally, psychosocial factors such as behavioral health conditions in the caregiver or child, temperamental qualities, developmental status, and environmental influences can contribute to and maintain pediatric feeding disorders. It is rare for any of these factors to act in isolation; rather, it is the interaction among these factors that leads to the development of pediatric feeding disorders.

What the child learns about food and feeding as a result of these interacting factors influences the trajectory of his feeding development. When children make pleasurable associations with eating from birth, feeding behavior develops in a predictable sequence. A child learns that eating in response to hunger cues leads to satisfaction and comfort. This cycle repeats itself multiple times daily and, in conjunction with physical and cognitive development, drives the child to progress through stages of feeding development. However, if feeding and eating are associated with pain or discomfort rather than satisfaction of hunger, a child's learning about feeding is quite different. The positive associations with feeding that most children learn are interrupted; rather than learning that eating is enjoyable, a child who experiences pain or discomfort learns that eating is uncomfortable, and they begin to avoid the feeding situation. By avoiding food, a child experiences comfort, and a cycle of food refusal, rather than food consumption, is reinforced.

For example, in a child with developmental delay, oral-motor skills may not develop commensurate with a child's chronological age. The well-meaning caregiver presents food that is appropriate for a child of that age. If the child is not equipped with the oral skills necessary to consume that food, he will experience discomfort (e.g., gagging, coughing). This discomfort can quickly become associated with food and the feeding situation, leading to increasing refusal to eat over time. This persistent refusal of food can develop into a pediatric feeding disorder if underlying causal factors are not identified and addressed.

Feeding Disorders in Children with FPIES

For the child with food allergy or FPIES, discomfort and pain associated with food reactions can adversely impact a child's learning about feeding. These negative associations can develop early in infancy as the child experiences his first food reactions. Some food reactions occur relatively closely in time to eating, and as a result, pain and discomfort essentially punish eating behavior. Sustained discomfort associated with chronic food reactions can also adversely impact a child's eating. When this pattern repeats itself, the child's interest in and likelihood of eating in the future decreases substantially. Over time, the entire feeding situation becomes associated with pain, and the child gradually begins to avoid food, caregivers, specific locations in the home, and utensils. When the child with FPIES successfully avoids food and the feeding situation, he experiences feelings of relief and comfort that serve to reinforce the refusal of food. As this cycle repeats, refusal to eat is further strengthened.

Caregivers are left to decide how best to manage a child's refusal to eat while maintaining the child's health and nutrition. Typically, in response to food refusal behavior, caregivers remove food, assuming that the child does not want to eat. As well, caregivers often replace the food with a more preferred, and often less nutritious, food. As refusal behaviors persist over time, and caregivers repeatedly remove and replace food, a child's learning about food is substantially altered. The child learns that engaging in food refusal behavior leads to the removal and replacement of food and that removal of food leads to feelings of relief, further reinforcing food refusal behavior. This ongoing cycle can lead to nutritional instability and the development of a feeding disorder.

Components of the medical treatment of FPIES can indirectly influence the development of a feeding disorder. For example, nutritional supplementation via a high-calorie beverage or supplemental tube feeding may be required during phases of treatment for FPIES. This supplementation decreases a child's appetite, subsequently impacting interest in eating at mealtimes. As well, food elimination may be recommended as part of the course of treatment. Children on elimination diets from a young age miss crucial opportunities to experience a variety of foods and due to this limited exposure become increasingly hesitant to try foods during the re-introduction phase of treatment. During this phase, providers should be aware that additional food reactions could further worsen the food aversion.

Elimination diets associated with FPIES and other food allergic conditions can adversely influence the development of the skills necessary for typical feeding progression, which can further impact the development of a feeding disorder [2].

Many of a child's feeding skills typically develop between birth and 24 months of age. If FPIES is identified during this time and the child's diet is restricted, this can interrupt the typical progression of feeding. For example, if during the transition from bottle or breast feeding to solid food feeding the child is placed on an elimination diet, his opportunities for spoon feeding become increasingly limited, which can delay the development of oral-motor skills necessary for feeding development [2]. Further, a well-meaning caregiver may inadvertently limit a child's experiences with food due to fear of exposure and concern about the impact of future food reactions, and this can ultimately limit skill development.

Finally, food allergies and feeding disorders have been identified as chronic stressors for children and caregivers, which can also contribute to the maintenance of feeding disorders in children with FPIES [3–7]. Caregivers report high levels of stress associated with management of the allergic condition as well as worry about the impact of accidental exposure to allergens. This ongoing stress can alter a caregiver's response to a child in a feeding situation, inadvertently reinforcing problematic mealtime behavior. As well, anxiety in children can have a negative impact on their willingness to engage in food trials and may increase their reluctance to participate in social activities related to food and eating, ultimately fostering the ongoing avoidance of food seen in pediatric feeding disorders.

Epidemiology

Research indicates that feeding disorders are seen in 40–60% of children with chronic medical conditions. The research on prevalence of feeding disorder in children with FPIES is limited. However, a few retrospective studies examining pediatric feeding disorders in children with food allergy have been conducted.

Mukkada and colleagues [8] identified a high prevalence of feeding dysfunction in children with eosinophilic gastrointestinal disease (EGID). The authors note that of 200 children seen over 12 months in their eosinophilic disease program, 17% presented with feeding dysfunction. In a second retrospective study, Yeung et al. [9] found that over 5 years, 40% of children presenting to a center for treatment of pediatric feeding disorders presented as possibly (18%), likely (6%), or very likely (16%) having food allergy based on the presence of eczema, allergic rhinitis, or asthma paired with report of food reaction, RAST, and endoscopy/biopsy. This is higher than the estimated prevalence of 8% in the general population [10].

Similarly, Pentiuk, Miller, and Kaul [11] documented the presence of feeding problems in a subset of children with eosinophilic esophagitis (EoE). The authors found that a sample of children diagnosed with EoE who were referred to an interdisciplinary feeding program for evaluation and treatment of a feeding disorder presented with symptoms commonly associated with pediatric feeding disorders including food refusal, oral aversion, and failure to gain weight.

Finally, in examining contributors to pediatric feeding disorders, Field, Garland, and Williams found that approximately 20% of children evaluated by a multidisciplinary feeding team presented with food allergy or intolerance [12]. Although this is not specific to FPIES, it is suspected that feeding disorders develop similarly in children with FPIES as children with food allergies and EoE.

Multidisciplinary Intervention

Once FPIES is identified and all known triggers are avoided, it is assumed that pain and discomfort are resolved. Despite this, the maladaptive feeding behaviors often persist, reflecting a new learned atypical feeding trajectory and resulting in worsening nutrition and health. In conjunction with treatment of FPIES, the child requires treatment for the pediatric feeding disorder. The standard of care for assessment and treatment of pediatric feeding disorders is multidisciplinary in nature, as it is important for children with pediatric feeding disorders to be evaluated in all realms where contributing factors might exist. As well, intervention in all contributing areas is necessary for improvement.

In addition to management of FPIES, the management of other common sources of discomfort associated with feeding disorders is crucial. For example, in the child that experiences pain associated with gastroesophageal reflux disease (GERD), minimizing the underlying source of discomfort is critical to optimizing the success of therapy to address the pediatric feeding disorder and preventing the worsening of food aversion. Physicians and nurse practitioners are important in identifying and treating these contributors.

It is also important to address delays or interruptions in skill development. Speech language pathologists and occupational therapists along with other developmental interventionists are uniquely trained to identify these delays and help the child resume the typical progression of feeding skill acquisition. This can be achieved within the limits of a child's restricted diet by presenting allowed foods prepared in a variety of shapes and textures. Addressing feeding skill deficits is particularly important for the child with FPIES who may have missed critical windows for acquisition of feeding skills as a result of elimination diets or food avoidance.

If nutrition is compromised as a result of food elimination interventions and food avoidance, nutritional supplementation may be needed. In conjunction with a multidisciplinary team of interventionists, dietitians specializing in the treatment of pediatric feeding disorders are able to identify deficits and generate ideas for safe supplementation that the child is likely to accept.

To address persistent psychosocial factors contributing to the development of pediatric feeding disorders, behavioral health specialists, including psychologists, counselors, and social workers, are integral participants in the child's treatment. These specialists can address stress and distress as well as other mental health difficulties observed in the child, caregiver, and dyad.

Behavioral health specialists are also vital providers in addressing ongoing mealtime behavioral difficulties once medical factors, nutrition, skill development, and other psychosocial contributors are addressed. Ensuring the optimization of these other factors prior to this type of intervention prevents the worsening of food aversion.

Behavioral intervention involves modifying environmental conditions to alter mealtime behavior. For example, hunger at mealtimes can be optimized by decreasing calories provided via supplemental nutritious beverages and maintaining a regular and consistent mealtime routine and schedule. This manipulation of appetite increases the likelihood of success of other behavioral interventions [13]. Altering environmental conditions that maintain food refusal behavior (e.g., attention to disruptive mealtime behavior, removal of food in response to refusal to eat) is another important component of behavioral intervention [14]. By changing how caregivers respond to mealtime behavior, the interventionist attempts to change the likelihood of a particular behavior occurring at future mealtimes (i.e., increasing the likelihood of a child engaging in positive and decreasing the likelihood of a child engaging in maladaptive mealtime behavior).

Conclusion

Feeding development follows a predictable course that allows eating to become associated with pleasurable experiences and satisfaction of hunger. Children with FPIES experience disruptions in that sequence secondary to altered learning about eating that results from a combination of negative associations between pain and eating and limited experience with a variety of foods. For some children, this can develop into a pediatric feeding disorder. As with any other pediatric feeding disorder, children with FPIES are ideally evaluated and managed by a multidisciplinary team of clinicians that facilitates the identification of contributing factors in multiple domains (nutritional, medical, skill development, and psychosocial) and allows for intervention in all realms.

Key Ideas/Pearls

- Feeding skill development follows a predictable progression.
- Negative experiences with feeding, such as from allergic reactions, can disrupt typical feeding progression.
- Pediatric feeding disorders are multifactorial and are ideally evaluated and treated by multidisciplinary teams.

References

1. Goday PS, Huh SY, Silverman A, Lukens CT, Dodrill P, Cohen SS, Delaney AL, Feuling MB, Noel RJ, Gisel E, Kenzer A, Kessler DB, de Camargo OK, Browne J, Phalen JA. Pediatric feeding disorder: consensus definition and conceptual framework. JPGN. 2019;68(1):124–9.
2. Haas AM. Feeding disorders in food allergic children. Curr Allergy Asthma Rep. 2010;10:258–64.
3. Cummings AJ, Knibb RC, King RM, Lucas JS. The psychosocial impact of food allergy and food hypersensitivity in children, adolescents and their families: a review. Allergy. 2010;65:933–45.

4. Garro A, Thurman SK, Kerwin ME, Ducette JP. Parent/caregiver stress during pediatric hospitalization for chronic feeding problems. J Pediatr Nurs. 2005;20(4):268–75.
5. Greer AJ, Gulotta CS, Masler EA, Laud RB. Caregiver stress and outcomes of children with pediatric feeding disorders treated in an intensive interdisciplinary program. J Pediatr Psychol. 2008;33(6):612–20.
6. Shanahan L, Zucker N, Copeland WE, Costello EJ, Angold A. Are children and adolescents with food allergies at increased risk for psychopathology? J Psychosom Res. 2014;77:468–73.
7. Taft TH, Balou S, Keefer L. Preliminary evaluation of maternal caregiver stress in pediatric eosinophilic gastrointestinal disorders. J Pediatr Psychol. 2012;37(5):523–32.
8. Mukkada VA, Haas A, Maune NC, Capocelli KE, Henry M, Gilman N, Petersburg S, Moore W, Lovell MA, Fleischer DVM, Furuta GT, Atkins D. Feeding dysfunction in children with eosinophilic gastrointestinal disease. Pediatrics. 2010;126(3):e672–7.
9. Yeung KA, Taylor T, Scheimann A, Carvalho R, Reinhardt E, Girolami P, Wood R. The prevalence of food allergies in children referred to a multidisciplinary feeding program. Clin Pediatr. 2015;54(11):1081–6.
10. Gupta RS, Springston EE, Warrier MR, Smith B, Kumar R. The prevalence, severity, and distribution of childhood food allergy in the United States. Pediatrics. 2011;128:e9–e17.
11. Pentiuk SP, Miller CK, Kaul A. Eosinophilic esophagitis in infants and toddlers. Dysphagia. 2007;22:44–7.
12. Field D, Garland M, Williams K. Correlates of specific childhood feeding problems. J Paediatr Child Health. 2003;39(4):299–304.
13. Linscheid TR. Behavioral treatments for pediatric feeding disorders. Behav Modif. 2006;30(1):6–23.
14. Fischer E, Silverman AH. Behavioral conceptualization, assessment, and treatment of pediatric feeding disorders. Semin Speech Lang. 2007;28(3):223–31.

Resources

World Health Organization Health Topics: Nutrition. http://www.who.int/topics/nutrition/en/.

American Academy of Pediatrics. HealthyChildren.org. https://www.healthychildren.org/English/Pages/default.aspx.

Natural History of FPIES

11

François Graham, Sophia Tsabouri,
and Jean-Christoph Caubet

Abbreviations

CM	Cow's milk
CMP	Cow's milk protein
FPIES	Food protein-induced enterocolitis syndrome
FU-OFC	Follow-up oral food challenge
OFC	Oral food challenge

Introduction

The natural history of food allergy has been mainly studied for IgE-mediated food allergy. Cow's milk (CM), egg, wheat, and soy IgE-mediated food allergies all have a high likelihood of resolution during early to late childhood, whereas tree nuts, peanut, and seafood IgE-mediated food allergies have a less favourable evolution and often persist into adulthood [1, 2]. On the other hand, data on the natural history of food protein-induced enterocolitis syndrome (FPIES) remain limited, although major advances have been made these past years. As in IgE-mediated food allergy, the natural history of FPIES to CM and soy has a favourable course in the majority of cases, with a resolution before the age of 5 in most populations studied [3, 4]. Data concerning solid FPIES is more variable, with certain foods such as fish, meats, and poultry persisting later in childhood. However, resolution rates vary

F. Graham · J.-C. Caubet (✉)
Pediatric Allergy, University Hospitals of Geneva, Geneva, Switzerland
e-mail: Jean-Christoph.Caubet@hcuge.ch

S. Tsabouri
Department of Pediatrics/Paediatric Allergy, University Hospital of Ioannina,
Ioannina, Greece

T. F. Brown-Whitehorn, A. Cianferoni (eds.), *Food Protein Induced Enterocolitis (FPIES)*,
https://doi.org/10.1007/978-3-030-21229-2_11

widely among countries and food triggers and may depend on the nature of the population studied (general versus referral), dietary habits, frequency of coexisting atopic diseases [4–8], phenotype (i.e. chronic versus acute, mild versus severe), and genetic factors. It is important to note that inherent differences in study designs and variable length between initial reaction and date of tolerance assessment make comparison of data very difficult when assessing the natural history of FPIES. Most studies report the date at which parents reintroduce foods at home and/or data from oral food challenge (OFC) outcomes, which are performed after a defined period of time since the initial reaction (generally around 12–18 months [9, 10]). In both cases, these data may overestimate the age of resolution, since tolerance could occur at an earlier undefined date. In addition, parents are more disposed to reintroduce earlier crucial foods at home (eggs, milk, grains) compared to easily avoided foods such as fish, which can have an impact on reported resolution rates.

This chapter will discuss data in the current literature on the natural history of FPIES to different type of foods as well as the potential evolution to an IgE-mediated food allergy, the factors that might influence the natural history, and the evolution of eliciting doses in FPIES.

Natural History of FPIES to Milk and Soy

CM and soy FPIES are the most prevalent causes of FPIES in most cohorts, affecting up to 69% of patients [9]. The natural resolution of CM FPIES is population dependent and varies from 65% at 10 months in South Korea [8] to only 20% by age 3 in the United States (USA) [9]. Similarly, tolerance to soy varies from 92% at 10 months in South Korea [8] to 27% by age 3 in the USA [4]. We outline below the major studies addressing the natural history of FPIES to CM and soy, and these data are summarized in Table 11.1.

Table 11.1 Resolution rates of FPIES by country and age

Food	Country	Study	n	6 m	8 m	10 m	1 y	2 y	3 y	4 y	5 y
Milk	USA	Nowak-Wegrzyn [4]	25						60%		
		Caubet [9]	70						20%		53%[a]
	Italy	Miceli Sopo [13]	44					63%			
	ROK	Hwang [8]	23	27%	42%	64%					
	Spain	Vazquez-Ortiz [15]	21					50%[b]		75%[b]	
	Israel	Katz [5]	36				50%	89%	94%[b]		
	Australia	Lee [12]	25				12%	56%	88%	96%	96%
Soy	USA	Nowak-Wegrzyn [4]	22						27%		
		Caubet [9]	66						20%		32%[a]
	Australia	Mehr [11]	6						83%		

Table 11.1 (continued)

Food	Country	Study	n	6 m	8 m	10 m	1 y	2 y	3 y	4 y	5 y
	ROK	Hwang [8]	23	75%	91%	92%					
Grains	USA	Caubet [9]	70								65.5%
Rice	USA	Nowak-Wegrzyn [4]	10						40%		
		Caubet [9]	13						28%[a]		
	Australia	Mehr [11]	5						80%		
		Lee [12]	27				0%	63%	87%	100%	
Oat	USA	Caubet [9]	14						30%[a]		
		Nowak-Wegrzyn [4]	6						66%		
Barley	USA	Nowak-Wegrzyn [4]	2						100%		
Egg	Italy	Miceli Sopo [13]	2								100%[c]
	Spain	Vazquez-Ortiz [15]	8						50%[b]		75%[b]
	Australia	Lee [12]	8				0%	12.5%	12.5%	12.5%	25%
		Hsu [35]	2					50%			
Meats	USA	Nowak-Wegrzyn [4]	1						0%		
Poultry		Caubet [9]	6								50%
Fish	USA	Caubet [9]	1								0%
Shellfish	Spain	Ruiz-Garcia [14]	5						20%		
		Gonzalez-Delgado [23]	16								19%
		Vazquez-Ortiz [15]	44							25%[b]	75%
	Australia	Lee [12]	4				0%	25%	25%	25%	25%
V	USA	Nowak-Wegrzyn [4]	3						67%		
L + S	USA	Ruffner [10]	462					35%	70%	80%	
	Spain	Vazquez-Ortiz [15]	81						25%[b]	50%[b]	75%

L liquids, *m* months, *n* number of patients with FPIES to specified food, *ROK* Republic of Korea, *S* solids, *V* vegetables, *y* year

[a]Extrapolated from Kaplan-Meier survival curves in study [9]

[b]Rounded to the nearest year (e.g. 25% resolution rate at 3.8 years placed in the 4-year column)

[c]Extrapolated from figure 6 in study [13]

Data taken from studies where specific resolution rates by age are mentioned

Most tertiary medical centres evaluating the evolution of FPIES to liquids (CM and soy) have found a favourable resolution, with mean ages of tolerance varying between 2 and 3 years [10–15]. Ruffner et al. performed the largest study to date with a total of 462 patients with FPIES in the USA [10]. Sixty-seven percent (310/462) of patients had CM FPIES and 41% (189/462) soy FPIES. Mean age of tolerance to CM and soy were, respectively, 2.7 and 2.8 years [9]. Of note, tolerance rate for CM and soy at 3 and 5 years was not mentioned. In Australia, Mehr et al. [11] performed a retrospective review of 35 children who presented with acute FPIES, of which 20% (7/35) were triggered by CM and 34% (12/35) by soy. The mean age of tolerance was not specified for CM or soy. The authors reported a high resolution of symptoms on OFC in 83% (5/6) of patients with soy FPIES by 3 years of age. They did not specifically comment on the resolution rate of the seven children with CM FPIES. More recently, Lee et al. from the same centre described 25 children with CM FPIES. Mean age of tolerance was not specified. They found a CM FPIES resolution rate of 12% by 1 year, 56% by 2 years, 88% by 3 years, and 96% by 4 years [12]. In Italy, Miceli Sopo et al. performed a retrospective study including 66 children diagnosed with FPIES, of which 67% (44/66) had CM FPIES [13]. Mean age of tolerance to CM was 2 years, as assessed by OFC 1 year after the last reaction. Sixty-three percent achieved tolerance to CM by the age of 18–24 months. In Spain, Ruiz-Garcia et al. conducted a retrospective study comprised of 16 children with FPIES [14], of which CM was the trigger in 44% (7/16) and soy in 6.25% (1/16). Five out of seven patients (71%) tolerated CM at a mean age of 2.3 years, as documented by OFC after a mean time of 10.2 months since the last reaction. Mean age of tolerance for liquids was 2.19 years. Tolerance rate at 3 years was not specified. More recently, Vazquez-Ortiz et al. evaluated 21 patients with CM FPIES and performed OFCs to determine tolerance rate 18 to 24 months after the last known reaction [15]. They found a CM tolerance rate of 50% at 29 months. To summarize data from these studies, the percentage of resolution of CM FPIES varies between 50% [15] and 63% [13] at 2 years to 96% [12] at 5 years.

Two major studies have reported faster tolerance rates for CM and soy FPIES [5, 8]. One of the highest resolution rates was seen in a birth cohort by Katz et al., who performed a large-scale population-based prospective study and evaluated 13,019 Israeli infants, of which 44 children were diagnosed with CM FPIES [5]. Fifty percent (18/36) of patients with CM FPIES recovered by the age of 1 year, 75% (27/36) by 1.5 years, 89% (32/36) by 2 years, and 94% (34/36) by 2.5 years [5]. The second study was a Korean study of 23 patients with infantile milk and soy FPIES diagnosed by OFC and prospectively followed until 2 years of age [8]. First follow-up OFC (FU-OFC) was performed at 6 months, and patients were then allocated randomly to receive CM ($n = 12$) or soy ($n = 12$) formula in a crossover manner at 2-month intervals. CM tolerance rate was 27.3% at 6 months, 41.7% at 8 months, and 63.6% at 10 months. Soy formula tolerance rate was earlier with 75% at 6 months, 90.9% at 8 months, and 91.7% at 10 months. The frequent follow-ups in these studies may have detected patients with earlier resolution of symptoms compared to the US cohorts where tolerance evaluation was performed after 12–18 months [9, 10]. In addition, genetic and dietary factors may play a role.

On the other hand, a study performed by Caubet et al. in a large referral centre in the USA reported a much later tolerance age for liquids [9]. One hundred and sixty patients with FPIES were recruited, of which 44% (70/160) had CM FPIES and 41% (66/160) soy FPIES. The median ages of tolerance to CM and to soy were 13.8 and 6.67 years, respectively. However, this includes patients with atypical FPIES (positive specific IgE). If we exclude these patients, the median age of tolerance decreases to 5.1 years for CM, which is still higher than other studies. CM and soy FPIES resolved in 20% by 3 years and in 55% by 5 years, as assessed by OFC or clinical history. These late resolution rates may be explained by more severe phenotypes and a higher proportion of atopic patients than other studies.

Natural History of Solid FPIES: Specific Foods

Isolated solid FPIES affected 31% of patients in one US study [9] and coexists with liquid FPIES in 50 [10] to 64% of patients [16]. Solid FPIES generally has a later median onset than CM and soy FPIES, varying from 5.5 [4] to 12 months [10], which is likely related to the natural sequence of introduction of foods [10, 11, 14, 17]. Based on the current literature, median age of resolution of solid FPIES varies from 2 years in the USA [4] to 5.5 years in Spain [14].

Grains

FPIES to grains are considered the first cause of FPIES in Australia [16] and the third most common cause of FPIES in other cohorts in North America [9, 10]. Caubet et al. was the only centre to specify the mean age of tolerance to all grain types, with a resolution rate of 65.5% at 5 years [9].

- More specifically, rice FPIES is the most common cause of FPIES after CM and soy in North America [9, 10] and the primary cause of FPIES in Australia [16]. The age of tolerance varies from 3.61 years (mean, n = 88) [10] to 4.7 years (median, n = 36) in the USA [9] and 3.33 years (n = 1) in Italy [13]. Resolution of rice FPIES by age 3 varies between 28% (extrapolated from Kaplan-Meier survival curve) [9] in the USA and 87% (22/27) [12] in Australia. In Spain (n = 6) [15], 25% resolution rate was seen at 3.7 years, 50% at 4.2 years, and 75% at 4.75 years.
- Oat FPIES was the fourth most common food in Caubet et al.'s [9] and Ruffner et al.'s cohorts [10], affecting, respectively, 8.7% (14/160) and 16% (74/462) of patients. The respective mean and median age of tolerance varied from 3.1 years [10] to 4 years [9]. Nowak-Wegrzyn et al. found that 66% (4/6) of children were tolerant to oat by the age of 3 years [4].
- Wheat FPIES affected 10% (46/462) of FPIES patients in Ruffner et al.'s cohort [10], and mean age of resolution was 2.6 years.

- Corn FPIES affected 8% (37/462) of patients in Ruffner et al.'s cohort [10], and mean age of resolution was 5 years. On the other hand, a Spanish cohort had a median age of resolution for corn FPIES ($n = 2$) of 8 months [15].
- Barley FPIES is less common. In Ruffner et al.'s cohort, 11 patients had barley FPIES with a mean age of tolerance at 4.6 years. In Nowak-Wegrzyn's study [4], 100% (2/2) of children with barley FPIES became tolerant by the age of 3.

Egg

Egg is a fairly common trigger of FPIES affecting 4–13% of cohorts [10, 15, 16, 18], although less frequent than CM, soy, and grains. Mean age of resolution varies from 3.5 years ($n = 51$) in the USA [10] to 4.8 years ($n = 2$) in Italy [13]. Egg tolerance varies between 25% (2/6) at 5 years in Australia and 75% (6/8) at 5.25 years in Spain [15]. In the UK, only 29% (2/7) of patients passed OFCs to cooked and baked eggs at, respectively, 3.4 and 4.9 years [18]. Finally in Spain, Vazquez-Ortiz et al.'s cohort of eight patients with FPIES to egg had a 25% resolution rate at 30 months, 50% resolution rate at 41 months, and 75% resolution rate at 63 months [15].

Peanuts and Tree Nuts

Data on the natural history of peanut FPIES is lacking, although cases have been reported in the USA ($n = 9$ [10], $n = 1$ [19]) and Australia ($n = 1$) [16]. Unfortunately, age of tolerance was not reported in these studies.

Poultry and Meats

FPIES to poultry and meats affects 6.3–10% of patients with FPIES [10, 16] depending on the population studied. Chicken was the most common cause in both the USA (21/462) [10] and Australia (19/230) [16]. In Ruffner et al.'s cohort, mean age of tolerance was 2.8 years for chicken and 2.75 years for turkey [10]. In other studies with a limited amount of patients, tolerance to meats varies between 0% (0/1) at 3 years [4] and 50% (3/6) by 5 years [9]. Thus, the number of patients is too small, and further studies are required to draw solid conclusions about the natural history of poultry and meat FPIES.

Fish and Shellfish

Fish FPIES is relatively rare in Australia and North America, affecting 5% [16] and 6.3% [10] of patients, respectively. However, it is the most common cause of FPIES in Spain [20, 21] and second most common cause in Italy [13]. Median age of tolerance to fish is higher than CM [13], varying from 4 to 8.8 years [13, 20–22], with resolution rates between 0% at 5 years the USA [9] and 75% at 5 years in Spain [15].

The largest cohort to date in Spain described 80 patients with fish FPIES; median age of tolerance was 5 years [21]. Only 24 (34%) achieved tolerance at a mean age of 4.4 years. Vazquez-Ortiz et al. studied a large cohort of 44 children with fish FPIES and found a 25% resolution rate at 46 months, 50% at 54 months, and 75% at 60 months [15]. Another large cohort in Italy [22] described 70 children with fish or shellfish FPIES. Twenty-seven underwent OFC, and 63% (17/27) achieved tolerance at a mean age of 8.8 years.

Other smaller cohorts from Spain have described low tolerance rates varying from 18% (3/15) [23] to 33% (4/12) [20] at mean and median ages of 4.5 and 4 years, respectively.

Unlike other foods, abdominal pain with ingestion of fish may persist after resolution of FPIES up to 10 years [23]. In addition, some children with FPIES to one fish species are at risk of developing FPIES to other fish species, with two reports of loss of tolerance to other fish species that the child previously tolerated [24].

Fish FPIES may develop later than other solid foods. In Caubet et al.'s cohort [9], median age of diagnosis was 30 years, including five patients with fish/shellfish FPIES after 5 years of age. None tolerated fish by the age of 5 years. Tan et al. [25] described a series of adults with non-IgE-mediated gastrointestinal food hypersensitivity, and the major causes of symptoms were crustaceans, molluscs, and fish, with a median age of symptom onset at 29 years. Tolerance was not assessed due to the retrospective nature of the study, although symptoms were reproduced through accidental reactions in some patients over a period of up to 30 years.

Fruits

Although FPIES to fruits have been described in 7.8% (36/462) [10] to 10% (22/230) [16] of cohorts, little data is available in the literature concerning their natural history. Ludman et al. [18] reported a case of FPIES to blueberries with an initial presentation at the age of 10 months and a negative OFC at 34 months. Thus, more data is required to further clarify the natural history of FPIES to fruits.

Vegetables/Legumes

Vegetable FPIES varies from 8% (18/230) [16] to 11.6% (54/462) [10] of patients with FPIES in the Australia and USA, respectively, although no information is provided on resolution rates in these studies. In Ruffner et al.'s cohort [10], the most common vegetables were sweet potato (4.1%), followed by peas (3.2%). Nowak-Wegrzyn et al.'s [4] cohort included a few patients with vegetable FPIES, including peas ($n = 2$), string beans ($n = 2$), squash ($n = 1$), and sweet potato ($n = 1$), with resolution dates varying between 14 and 34 months. All of these were accidental exposures reported by parents and not OFCs.

Comparison of the Natural History of Solid and Liquid FPIES

Four major studies have provided specific data on the natural history of patients with solid FPIES as compared to liquid (CM and soy) FPIES:

- Nowak-Wegrzyn et al. [4] compared children with solid FPIES (n = 14) to CM and/or soy FPIES (n = 30). Solid FPIES included children with FPIES to grains, vegetables, and poultry. Median age of onset of solid FPIES was 5.5 months and significantly higher when compared to CM at 0.5 months and soy at 1.5 months. Median age of resolution of solid FPIES was 2 years compared to 2.33 years for CM and 2.37 years for soy.
- Ruffner et al. [10] performed the largest study to date in the USA in which 462 patients with FPIES were included. They found a mean age of onset of 7 months for CM FPIES compared to 12 months for solid FPIES. They did not find a statistically significant different age of resolution between solid and liquid FPIES (3.5 years compared to 2.7 years, respectively), although there was clearly a trend towards a higher age of resolution for solid foods.
- In Spain, Ruiz-Garcia et al. [14] performed a retrospective study involving 16 children with FPIES to solids and liquids. Mean age of resolution for solid foods (mainly fish but also rice, chicken, wheat, and legumes) was 5.5 years compared to 2.2 years for liquid FPIES. This difference was statistically significant ($p = 0.017$). Of note, this is the cohort with the highest mean age of resolution for solid FPIES, but data may be skewed upwards due to a higher proportion of fish FPIES (31%). Also, this study has a small number of patients (eight with solid FPIES compared to eight with liquid FPIES) which limits interpretation.
- In Italy, Miceli Sopo et al. [13] found a statistically significantly lower age at initial presentation for CM FPIES (3.5 months) compared to other foods (10.6 months), which were mostly solids (fish, egg, rice, egg) except for two patients with soy FPIES. In addition, age of tolerance for CM FPIES was significantly lower than other foods (2 years compared to 4.4 years, respectively), although interpretation is difficult due to the low number of patients with solid FPIES (n = 6).

Thus, some comparative studies support a younger age of resolution in patients with liquid FPIES compared to solid FPIES [13, 14], whereas others do not [4, 10]. While global resolution data for solids is not always higher than liquids, individual resolution rates of specific solids (i.e. fish) are clearly higher than CM and soy (Table 11.1). Further multicentric and prospective studies are needed to further assess the differences in between solid and liquid FPIES because of large methodological differences in studies.

Natural History of Multiple FPIES Compared to Single FPIES

Most children with FPIES react to only one food (65–80%) [26]. Nevertheless, in US cohorts, up to 35% of patients may react to multiple foods [9, 10] and may be at increased risk of poor growth and nutrient deficiencies [26]. Risk factors for multiple FPIES are not clear. Some studies support coallergy between soy and CM in around 10–30% of patients [9, 10], whereas others did not report this association [5, 11, 13]. Patients with FPIES to solid foods often have FPIES to more than one food [9], and FPIES to fruits and vegetables was associated with having multiple FPIES [16]. In the USA, 40% with grain FPIES reacted to two or more grains, and 20% reacted to soy or CM and a grain [10]. FPIES to both rice and oats are common in Australia [11].

The natural history of patients with multiple FPIES as compared to single FPIES is relatively unknown. Mehr et al. [16] found a statistically significant lower age of onset of multiple FPIES when compared to single FPIES (median 5.0 vs 5.5 months, respectively). They also found an association between a shorter length of exclusive breastfeeding (less than 4 months) and multiple FPIES. However, natural history of these patients was not mentioned. In Caubet et al.'s study [9], 35% of patients ($n = 56$) reacted to multiple foods, and more than 50% of patients with solid FPIES reacted to two or more foods. Children with multiple FPIES including CM did not have a significantly different age of resolution when compared to children with only CM FPIES.

Risk of Secondary IgE-Mediated Food Allergies in Patients with FPIES

FPIES is classified as a non-IgE-mediated allergy, and skin prick tests and specific IgE to the incriminated food are usually negative. However, a subgroup of FPIES patients test positive to the culprit food (i.e. atypical FPIES). These children may eventually develop IgE-mediated allergic reactions to the culprit food, although they initially presented typical clinical manifestations of FPIES. Most reported cases involve CM FPIES [5, 9, 13, 27, 28], although cases have been rarely described with fish and egg [3, 4, 10, 21, 22]. The opposite has also been reported, with a switch from an IgE-mediated allergy phenotype to a FPIES phenotype [29, 30].

The largest study evaluating the natural history of patients with atypical FPIES was performed by Caubet et al. [9], in which 39 children (24%) had detectable specific IgE to the food causing FPIES. Seven out of 17 (41%) children with CM FPIES and detectable CM-specific IgE developed symptoms of IgE-mediated food allergy at follow-up [9]. CM IgE-mediated allergy was confirmed by OFC in five patients, whereas two of these patients had reactions suggestive of anaphylaxis. The presence of specific IgE to CM was a risk factor for persistence of CM FPIES beyond 3 years of age. Indeed, subjects with persistent CM FPIES after age 3 years had a higher proportion of positive CM-specific IgE (46%) compared to the children with CM FPIES resolved by age 3 years (0%) [9]. Interestingly, none of the children with IgE sensitization to CM resolved their CM allergy while in the study. Of note, the majority of patients were atopic in this cohort, which could explain the high rate of positive specific IgE and switch to IgE-mediated reactions compared to other European cohorts. Similarly, Lee et al. in Australia noticed that children with a positive skin prick test at diagnosis ($n = 4$ including CM, egg, and soy) had a slower rate of tolerance compared to children with no evidence of sensitization (median age of tolerance being 4.5 years compared to 1.3 years, respectively) [12].

Little data is available concerning switch to IgE-mediated reactions in solid FPIES. Nowak-Wegrzyn et al. studied 14 patients with FPIES caused by solid and liquid foods and observed that only three of their patients subsequently developed detectable IgE to the causal food, one of which was a solid food (rice) [4]. In Ruffner et al.'s cohort of 462 patients with FPIES to liquids and solids, 19.6% of patients had positive skin prick tests, mainly due to CM, eggs, peanuts, and tree nuts, although specific evolution of these patients is not mentioned [10]. Katz et al. describe personal communications of three cases with fish and egg FPIES who developed secondary IgE-mediated reactions [3]. Miceli Sopo et al. [22] and Infante et al. [21] described a few cases of patients with detectable specific IgE to fish in children with fish FPIES.

Since children with FPIES and positive specific IgE may be at risk of more persistent FPIES and/or progression towards secondary IgE-mediated food allergies, skin prick tests and/or measurement of specific IgE levels should be considered both at the initial evaluation and at follow-up before repeat OFC, as the protocol will be adapted [9].

Eliciting Dose and Natural History

Eliciting doses to trigger symptoms of FPIES vary widely in studies. For CM, this may range from 30 to 150 mL [5]. Due to the delayed onset of symptoms, it is very difficult to estimate the true eliciting dose [31]. Nonetheless, the quantity of protein required to elicit symptoms may decrease on subsequent reactions. Bansal et al. [32] described four cases of FPIES caused by different solid foods, in which the eliciting doses decreased by more than tenfold between the first reaction and the most recent reaction. The delay between the first reaction and last reaction was not specified. Monti et al. [33] described a child with FPIES after ingestion of 50 mL of CM, who 2 weeks later presented with a similar reaction with only one spoonful of CM. Another report by Tan et al. [34] described an infant with soy FPIES after a bottle of soy formula, who subsequently reacted after to traces of soy in breast milk after the mother ate a soy ice cream. These findings were corroborated by Katz et al. [3] who made the same observations. However, interpretation of these reports requires caution, since they were not designed to calculate the threshold dose; the initial threshold dose may have been overestimated since the FPIES trigger was unknown at the time of introduction and a large quantity may have been ingested rapidly. Also, patients may subsequently refuse to eat larger quantities of foods that may cause them to have symptoms [31], which can bias the data. Future studies with threshold dose calculations during repeat OFCs are required to validate whether eliciting doses in FPIES vary with time.

Conclusion

The natural history of FPIES is heterogeneous and depends on multiple factors including country of origin, food triggers, atopic status, age of food introduction, referral patterns, and methodological differences in studies. Clear disparities exist in resolution rates reported by different centres. CM and soy FPIES have a good prognosis with most cases resolving by the ages of 3–5 years. On the other hand, prognosis of solid FPIES is much more variable with some foods resolving at a generally young age (i.e. grains) and others with more protracted courses, sometimes persisting or developing in adulthood (i.e. fish). Factors associated with a longer duration of symptoms include positive specific IgE and later onset of symptoms. As secondary IgE-mediated CM allergy may occur in patients with CM FPIES, SPTs and specific IgE should be monitored before repeat OFC. In addition, patients should be aware that threshold of reaction may vary with time, with some reports of patients reacting at lower thresholds after initial episodes (although subject to confounding factors). The current approach is to perform OFCs in children with FPIES every 12–18 months after beginning of symptoms. However, many children may outgrow FPIES earlier, and more frequent challenges may be indicated. Future prospective studies are urgently needed to better delineate the natural history of FPIES to different individual foods. To do so, the optimal duration between initial symptoms and rechallenge needs to be defined. Prospective studies with OFCs at regular close intervals will help to gather more precise data and ultimately provide more accurate recommendations for the follow-up of patients with FPIES.

Key Points/Clinical "Pearls"

- The natural history of FPIES is heterogeneous and depends on multiple factors including country of origin, food triggers, atopic status, age of food introduction, referral patterns, and methodological differences in studies.
- CM and soy FPIES have a good prognosis with most cases resolving by the ages of 3–5 years.
- Prognosis of solid FPIES is much more variable with some foods resolving at a generally young age (i.e. grains) and others with more protracted courses, sometimes persisting or developing in adulthood (i.e. fish).
- Factors associated with a longer duration of symptoms include positive specific IgE (atypical FPIES) and later onset of symptoms.
- The current approach is to perform OFCs in children with FPIES every 12–18 months after beginning of symptoms. However, many children may outgrow FPIES earlier, and more frequent challenges may be indicated.
- Prospective studies with OFCs at regular close intervals will help to gather more precise data and ultimately provide more accurate recommendations for the follow-up of patients with FPIES.

References

1. Savage J, Sicherer S, Wood R. The natural history of food allergy. J Allergy Clin Immunol Pract. 2016;4(2):196–203; quiz 4. https://doi.org/10.1016/j.jaip.2015.11.024.
2. Sampson HA, Aceves S, Bock SA, James J, Jones S, Lang D, et al. Food allergy: a practice parameter update-2014. J Allergy Clin Immunol. 2014;134(5):1016–25 e43. https://doi.org/10.1016/j.jaci.2014.05.013.

3. Katz Y, Goldberg MR. Natural history of food protein-induced enterocolitis syndrome. Curr Opin Allergy Clin Immunol. 2014;14(3):229–39. https://doi.org/10.1097/ACI.0000000000000053.
4. Nowak-Wegrzyn A, Sampson HA, Wood RA, Sicherer SH. Food protein-induced enterocolitis syndrome caused by solid food proteins. Pediatrics. 2003;111(4. Pt 1):829–35.
5. Katz Y, Goldberg MR, Rajuan N, Cohen A, Leshno M. The prevalence and natural course of food protein-induced enterocolitis syndrome to cow's milk: a large-scale, prospective population-based study. J Allergy Clin Immunol. 2011;127(3):647–53.e1-3. https://doi.org/10.1016/j.jaci.2010.12.1105.
6. Sicherer SH, Eigenmann PA, Sampson HA. Clinical features of food protein-induced enterocolitis syndrome. J Pediatr. 1998;133(2):214–9.
7. Li H, Nowak-Wegrzyn A, Charlop-Powers Z, Shreffler W, Chehade M, Thomas S, et al. Transcytosis of IgE-antigen complexes by CD23a in human intestinal epithelial cells and its role in food allergy. Gastroenterology. 2006;131(1):47–58. https://doi.org/10.1053/j.gastro.2006.03.044.
8. Hwang JB, Sohn SM, Kim AS. Prospective follow-up oral food challenge in food protein-induced enterocolitis syndrome. Arch Dis Child. 2009;94(6):425–8. https://doi.org/10.1136/adc.2008.143289.
9. Caubet JC, Ford LS, Sickles L, Jarvinen KM, Sicherer SH, Sampson HA, et al. Clinical features and resolution of food protein-induced enterocolitis syndrome: 10-year experience. J Allergy Clin Immunol. 2014;134(2):382–9. https://doi.org/10.1016/j.jaci.2014.04.008.
10. Ruffner MA, Ruymann K, Barni S, Cianferoni A, Brown-Whitehorn T, Spergel JM. Food protein-induced enterocolitis syndrome: insights from review of a large referral population. J Allergy Clin Immunol Pract. 2013;1(4):343–9. https://doi.org/10.1016/j.jaip.2013.05.011.
11. Mehr S, Kakakios A, Frith K, Kemp AS. Food protein-induced enterocolitis syndrome: 16-year experience. Pediatrics. 2009;123(3):e459–64. https://doi.org/10.1542/peds.2008-2029.
12. Lee E, Campbell DE, Barnes EH, Mehr SS. Resolution of acute food protein-induced enterocolitis syndrome in children. J Allergy Clin Immunol Pract. 2017;5(2):486–8 e1. https://doi.org/10.1016/j.jaip.2016.09.032.
13. Sopo SM, Giorgio V, Dello Iacono I, Novembre E, Mori F, Onesimo R. A multicentre retrospective study of 66 Italian children with food protein-induced enterocolitis syndrome: different management for different phenotypes. Clin Exp Allergy. 2012;42(8):1257–65. https://doi.org/10.1111/j.1365-2222.2012.04027.x.
14. Ruiz-Garcia M, Diez CE, Garcia SS, del Rio PR, Ibanez MD. Diagnosis and natural history of food protein-induced enterocolitis syndrome in children from a tertiary hospital in central Spain. J Investig Allergol Clin Immunol. 2014;24(5):354–6.
15. Vazquez-Ortiz M, Machinena A, Dominguez O, Alvaro M, Calvo-Campoverde K, Giner MT, et al. Food protein-induced enterocolitis syndrome to fish and egg usually resolves by age 5 years in Spanish children. J Allergy Clin Immunol Pract. 2017;5(2):512–5 e1. https://doi.org/10.1016/j.jaip.2016.12.029.
16. Mehr S, Frith K, Barnes EH, Campbell DE. Food protein-induced enterocolitis syndrome in Australia: a population-based study, 2012-2014. J Allergy Clin Immunol. 2017;140(5):1323–30. https://doi.org/10.1016/j.jaci.2017.03.027.
17. Sampson HA, Anderson JA. Summary and recommendations: classification of gastrointestinal manifestations due to immunologic reactions to foods in infants and young children. J Pediatr Gastroenterol Nutr. 2000;30. Suppl:S87–94.
18. Ludman S, Harmon M, Whiting D, du Toit G. Clinical presentation and referral characteristics of food protein-induced enterocolitis syndrome in the United Kingdom. Ann Allergy Asthma Immunol. 2014;113(3):290–4. https://doi.org/10.1016/j.anai.2014.06.020.
19. Holbrook T, Keet CA, Frischmeyer-Guerrerio PA, Wood RA. Use of ondansetron for food protein-induced enterocolitis syndrome. J Allergy Clin Immunol. 2013;132(5):1219–20. https://doi.org/10.1016/j.jaci.2013.06.021.
20. Vila L, Garcia V, Rial MJ, Novoa E, Cacharron T. Fish is a major trigger of solid food protein-induced enterocolitis syndrome in Spanish children. J Allergy Clin Immunol Pract. 2015;3(4):621–3. https://doi.org/10.1016/j.jaip.2015.03.006.

21. Infante S, Marco-Martin G, Sanchez-Dominguez M, Rodriguez-Fernandez A, Fuentes-Aparicio V, Alvarez-Perea A, et al. Food protein-induced enterocolitis syndrome by fish: not necessarily a restricted diet. Allergy. 2018;73(3):728–32. https://doi.org/10.1111/all.13336.
22. Miceli Sopo S, Monaco S, Badina L, Barni S, Longo G, Novembre E, et al. Food protein-induced enterocolitis syndrome caused by fish and/or shellfish in Italy. Pediatr Allergy Immunol. 2015;26(8):731–6. https://doi.org/10.1111/pai.12461.
23. Gonzalez-Delgado P, Caparros E, Moreno MV, Clemente F, Flores E, Velasquez L, et al. Clinical and immunological characteristics of a pediatric population with food protein-induced enterocolitis syndrome (FPIES) to fish. Pediatr Allergy Immunol. 2016;27(3):269–75. https://doi.org/10.1111/pai.12529.
24. Miceli Sopo S, Fantacci C, Bersani G, Romano A, Monaco S. Loss of tolerance for fishes previously tolerated in children with fish food protein induced enterocolitis syndrome. Allergol Immunopathol. 2018;46:394. https://doi.org/10.1016/j.aller.2017.09.029.
25. Tan JA, Smith WB. Non-IgE-mediated gastrointestinal food hypersensitivity syndrome in adults. J Allergy Clin Immunol Pract. 2014;2(3):355–7 e1. https://doi.org/10.1016/j.jaip.2014.02.002.
26. Nowak-Wegrzyn A, Chehade M, Groetch ME, Spergel JM, Wood RA, Allen K, et al. International consensus guidelines for the diagnosis and management of food protein-induced enterocolitis syndrome: Executive summary-Workgroup Report of the Adverse Reactions to Foods Committee, American Academy of Allergy, Asthma & Immunology. J Allergy Clin Immunol. 2017;139(4):1111–26 e4. https://doi.org/10.1016/j.jaci.2016.12.966.
27. Onesimo R, Dello Iacono I, Giorgio V, Limongelli MG, Miceli Sopo S. Can food protein induced enterocolitis syndrome shift to immediate gastrointestinal hypersensitivity? A report of two cases. Eur Ann Allergy Clin Immunol. 2011;43(2):61–3.
28. Kessel A, Dalal I. The pendulum between food protein-induced enterocolitis syndrome and IgE-mediated milk allergy. Acta Paediatr. 2011;100(10):e183–5. https://doi.org/10.1111/j.1651-2227.2011.02257.x.
29. Duffey H, Egan M. Development of Food Protein-Induced Enterocolitis Syndrome (FPIES) to egg following Immunoglobulin E (IgE)-mediated egg allergy. Ann Allergy Asthma Immunol. 2018;121:379–80. https://doi.org/10.1016/j.anai.2018.05.028.
30. Banzato C, Piacentini GL, Comberiati P, Mazzei F, Boner AL, Peroni DG. Unusual shift from IgE-mediated milk allergy to food protein-induced enterocolitis syndrome. Eur Ann Allergy Clin Immunol. 2013;45(6):209–11.
31. Leonard SA, Nowak-Wegrzyn A. Clinical diagnosis and management of food protein-induced enterocolitis syndrome. Curr Opin Pediatr. 2012;24(6):739–45. https://doi.org/10.1097/MOP.0b013e3283599ca1.
32. Bansal AS, Bhaskaran S, Bansal RA. Four infants presenting with severe vomiting in solid food protein-induced enterocolitis syndrome: a case series. J Med Case Rep. 2012;6:160. https://doi.org/10.1186/1752-1947-6-160.
33. Monti G, Castagno E, Liguori SA, Lupica MM, Tarasco V, Viola S, et al. Food protein-induced enterocolitis syndrome by cow's milk proteins passed through breast milk. J Allergy Clin Immunol. 2011;127(3):679–80. https://doi.org/10.1016/j.jaci.2010.10.017.
34. Tan J, Campbell D, Mehr S. Food protein-induced enterocolitis syndrome in an exclusively breast-fed infant-an uncommon entity. J Allergy Clin Immunol. 2012;129(3):873,. author reply -4. https://doi.org/10.1016/j.jaci.2011.12.1000.
35. Hsu P, Mehr S. Egg: a frequent trigger of food protein-induced enterocolitis syndrome. J Allergy Clin Immunol. 2013;131(1):241–2. https://doi.org/10.1016/j.jaci.2012.08.045.

Food Challenges 12

Kathleen Y. Wang and Antonella Cianferoni

Indications

An oral food challenge (OFC) is a procedure performed in food protein-induced enterocolitis syndrome (FPIES) for diagnosis or follow-up and can be performed for several reasons: to confirm that a FPIES reaction occurs after ingestion of a specific food, to assess for tolerance to cross-reactive foods, or, most commonly, to monitor for the resolution of FPIES.

FPIES is largely a clinical diagnosis. While some laboratory tests can help support the diagnosis, there is not a single laboratory or diagnostic procedure that is specific for FPIES [1]. Thus, in the majority of cases, careful history taking is key in making the diagnosis and identifying the trigger food. The ability to make a diagnosis based on clinical presentation is especially true if symptoms are reproducible upon subsequent exposure to the trigger food [2]. In these cases, confirmation with an OFC may be unnecessary, and the risk of an OFC may outweigh the benefits. However, in cases where the diagnosis is unclear and/or a food trigger is not identified, OFC is the gold standard to confirm a diagnosis of FPIES. This is especially helpful in confirming chronic FPIES, where symptoms can be non-specific and share overlapping features with other non-IgE-mediated food allergies such as food protein-induced allergic proctocolitis (FPIAP). While it can be used as a diagnostic procedure, more commonly, OFCs are performed to assess development of tolerance in FPIES, so that the trigger food may be reintroduced into the diet.

K. Y. Wang (✉)
Allergy and Immunology, Children's Hospital of Philadelphia, Philadelphia, PA, USA

A. Cianferoni
Division of Allergy and Immunology, University of Pennsylvania, Perelman School of Medicine, Children's Hospital of Philadelphia, Philadelphia, PA, USA

T. F. Brown-Whitehorn, A. Cianferoni (eds.), *Food Protein Induced Enterocolitis (FPIES)*,
https://doi.org/10.1007/978-3-030-21229-2_12

Risks and Benefits

Risks and benefits have to be considered and discussed with the patient and family when deciding to proceed with an OFC. Though no fatalities have been reported in the literature secondary to reactions during OFC, there are risks associated with a positive challenge including the possibility of a severe reaction leading to hypovolemic shock and/or requiring hospitalization. The risk of reaction is dependent on a number of factors, including the indication for OFC, time since index reaction, and the offending food. Table 12.1 highlights the outcomes of some published studies of FPIES OFC, including rates of reaction and hospitalization.

The benefits of a positive challenge include confirming that FPIES reaction exists to a food and knowledge about foods to avoid. The benefits of a negative challenge are even greater and allow for the introduction of the food into the diet, which may lead to improved nutrition, reduced anxiety, and improvement in quality of life.

Timing

The timing of OFC to monitor for the resolution of FPIES depends on many factors, including the food trigger in question, the country of origin of the patient, and patient and family preference. With regard to the type of food, the development of tolerance in cow's milk or soy FPIES has been reported to occur at an earlier age than grain and other solid FPIES [1]. Data from Korean, Israeli, and Australian cohorts suggest earlier ages of resolution for cow's milk and soy FPIES compared to the United States, as early as 1 year of age in Korean children [5, 8, 9]. Considerations such as the prevalence of the food in the patient and family's diet and patient anxiety can dictate the timing of OFC. A conservative approach and one that is commonly taken in the United States is to attempt OFC 12–18 months after the last reaction [13].

Choosing a Location

Deciding where to conduct an OFC in suspected or confirmed FPIES should take into consideration several factors, including the patient's risk assessment, parent's/caregiver's preference, the availability of support staff for prolonged observation, the availability of supportive treatments for reactions, and the availability of emergency services or distance to the hospital in case of severe reactions. While inpatient, day hospital, or office setting may be appropriate, it is of utmost importance that OFC should be conducted under medical supervision, in a setting where, at the minimum, access to intravenous fluids (IVF) is readily accessible. Access to a laboratory may also be a consideration to obtain supporting evidence of a positive reaction. Conducting OFC in the home setting or in other non-medically supervised settings can be risky due to the possibility of severe reactions and hypotension. In fact, up to 50% of positive OFCs might require treatment with IVF, and

Table 12.1 Published FPIES OFCs, protocols, and outcomes

Study	Year	Country	Type	No. of challenges	Triggers	Protocol	Positive challenges	Hypotension	IVF	Ondansetron	Steroids	Admission	ICU
							(%)	(% positive challenges)					
Wang et al. [3]	2019	USA	Assessment of tolerance, cross-reactivity	169	CM, soy, egg, grain, vegetable, fruit, meat, nut	1/3 serving size for age in a single dose with 4-hour observation; home titration to full serving size over 9–12 days	18	7	47	40	–	10	3
Vazquez-Ortiz et al. [4]	2017	Spain	Assessment of tolerance	81	CM, egg, grain, fish	0.3 g protein/kg body weight in three equal doses with 90-minute intervals with 24-hour observation	41	0	58	–	–	100 (protocol)	0
Lee et al. [5]	2016	Australia	Assessment of tolerance	81	CM, soy, grain, egg, meat, fruit, vegetable, fish, peanut	≥3 g protein or ≥1 g rice protein in a single dose with 4-hour observation	25	5	30	65	–	5	0
Caubet et al. [6]	2014	USA	Assessment of tolerance, cross-reactivity	180	CM, soy, egg, grain, vegetable, fruit, meat, fish/shellfish	0.06–0.6 g protein/kg body weight in three equal doses over 45 minutes with 4–8-hour observation	41	19	96	–	94	0	0

(continued)

Table 12.1 (continued)

Study	Year	Country	Type	No. of challenges	Triggers	Protocol	Positive challenges	Hypotension	IVF	Ondansetron	Steroids	Admission	ICU
							(%)	(% positive challenges)					
Sopo et al. [7]	2012	Italy	Diagnostic Assessment of tolerance	35 39	CM, soy, egg, grain, meat, fish, goat milk CM, soy, egg, grain, fish	Rome: 1/2 serving size for age with 2-hour observation and then full serving size for age with 4-hour observation Florence: 1/4, 1/2, and full serving size, for age each followed by 4-hour observation Benevento: 0.4 g protein/kg body weight in 3 equal doses over 3 hours with 4-hour observation, then full serving size followed by 2-hour observation	100 41	– –	43 (IVF or steroids; not differentiated in study) –	– –	43 (steroids or IVF; not differentiated in study) –	– –	– –
Katz et al. [8]	2011	Israel	Diagnostic	28	CM	150 mg, 600 mg, 900 mg, 1.8 g, 3.6 g, and 4.5 g of protein with 10–45 minutes of observation between doses and 3-hour of observation after the final dose	100	0	–	0	0	0	0
Hwang et al. [9]	2008	Korea	Assessment of tolerance, cross-reactivity	72	CM, soy	0.03–0.05 g protein/kg body weight	38	11	–	–	–	–	–

Fogg et al. [10]	2006	USA	Diagnostic, assessment of tolerance	33	CM, soy, egg, grains	0.05–0.15 g protein/kg body weight in two increasing doses over 30 minutes with 4-hour observation and titration over 9 days to goal (0.05–0.15 g/kg days 1–3, 0.1–0.3 g/kg days 4–6, 0.15–0.45 g/kg days 7–9)	48	–	9	–	–	–	–
Nowak-Wegrzyn et al. [11]	2003	USA	Diagnostic, assessment of tolerance	8	Oat, rice, chicken	≤0.6 g protein/kg body weight in increasing doses over 45–60 minutes with 6–8-hour observation	100	–	–	–	–	–	–
Sicherer et al. [12]	1998	USA	Diagnostic, assessment of tolerance, cross-reactivity	26	CM, soy, grain, vegetable, meat	0.6 g protein/kg body weight (0.15–0.3 g protein/g body weight in patients with history of severe reaction with small ingestion) in increasing doses over 45–60 minutes with 6–8-hour observation	42	–	27	–	12	–	–

–, not available, *CM* cow's milk

approximately 15% can develop hypotension [1, 2]. Success with oral rehydration has been described to be helpful in a small cohort, but the risk of a severe reaction still necessitates that FPIES OFCs be performed in a medical setting for all foods that have previously caused severe reaction and protracted vomiting and for high-risk foods [8]. Despite the risks, when there is a good working relationship between families and clinicians, some families will opt to administer challenged food at home for foods that have never been ingested before even if they are at high risk with the understanding that severe reactions require a visit to the nearest emergency room.

Preparing Patients for Challenge

As FPIES OFC is a procedure, verbal or written informed consent should be documented. Indication for the challenge, risks, benefits, implications, and limitations of positive and negative challenges should be discussed. The patient should be in good health to avoid confounding challenge outcome. Fasting prior to the procedure ensures that any reactions are a result of the challenged food. It is recommended that in challenges for delayed reactions, as is the case for FPIES, the fasting period should be as long as 12 hours. In infants and young children, this period of fasting may prove to be difficult, and a light meal of half the usual amount can be given 2 hours before the challenge [14]. Performing the challenge in the morning during breakfast time is helpful for fasting and allows the challenge to serve as a meal. The anticipated duration of the challenge should be discussed so that the patient and family can plan accordingly.

Challenge Protocol

Due to the risk of severe reactions necessitating IVF resuscitation, establishing secure intravenous access before starting an OFC is recommended in many cases. This is especially important if there is a prior history of severe reaction or anticipated difficulty obtaining IV access in case of a reaction. At the minimum, immediate access to IV fluids should be available [1]. Currently, risk factors for developing a reaction requiring IV fluids are not well characterized.

Prior to the start of OFC, it may be helpful to obtain a baseline complete blood count (CBC) with differential, though this is optional in non-research settings [1]. In positive OFCs, a post-challenge CBC demonstrating increased neutrophil count can aid with interpretation [6, 15].

FPIES OFCs are generally unmasked, and food is fed in its natural form since objective symptoms are expected and the potential for bias is low.

The total dose and dosing regimen for performing FPIES OFCs have not been systemically studied. Therefore, protocols and practices vary by provider and

Table 12.2 Dosing protocol for FPIES OFCs [1]

Dose	0.03–0.6 grams of food per kilogram of body weight
Administration	3 equal doses over 30 minutes
Maximum	3 grams protein, 10 grams food, or 100 mL liquid
Observation	4–6 hours
Modifications	For patients with history of severe reactions, start with low initial dose, and if there is no reaction after 2–3 hours, administer an age-appropriate serving size and observe for 4 hours

institution. The current international consensus guidelines recommend administering 0.06–0.6 g protein/kg of body weight, usually 0.3 g protein/kg of body weight, in three equal doses over 30 minutes. It is recommended to not exceed 3 g protein, 10 g total food, or 100 mL of liquid for dosing. Initial dosing is followed by a 4- to 6-hour observation period. For patients with a history of severe reactions, the challenge may begin with a low initial dose, followed by 2–3 hours of observation, then a full age-appropriate serving size, and 4 hours of observation [1]. Table 12.2 summarizes these recommendations.

Modifications of these recommendations are at the discretion of the supervising physician and are made with the individual patient's history in mind. Some protocols advocate for the administration of the food in a single dose [3, 5]. Due to the variance between protocols, time spent in OFC may greatly vary. Table 12.1 summarizes protocols of some published FPIES OFCs.

Practical Food Administration

The challenged food can be brought in by the family or provided by the physician. The food may be administered in different forms, depending on the patient's age, taste preferences, and form of the food encountered in the diet. Given the unmasked nature of these challenges, food may be administered in its natural form, such as for milk, soy, meats, fish, fruits, and vegetables. Consider lactose-free milk in patients with history of possible or confirmed lactose intolerance, as to prevent confounding challenge outcome.

In cases where the volume of food needed exceeds the amount likely to be eaten by the patient or there is desire to mask the taste, odor, or texture of the food, powder or flour forms may be available for mixing with different vehicles. Powder and flour forms are available for milk, soy, egg, and grain. Select the vehicles based on patient's age and taste preference. Examples of vehicles are listed in Table 12.3.

Special considerations should be given to those with enteral feeding tubes. While most formulas and powders can be given through enteral tubes, the administration of non-liquid foods may be difficult or not possible with some small-bore tubes and can lead to clogging. Consultation with a nutritionist or gastroenterologist may be helpful prior to OFC in these patients.

Table 12.3 Sample vehicles for the administration of challenge dose [14]

Infant formula	Oatmeal
Apple sauce	Tapioca fruit mixture cereal
Grape juice	Mashed potato
Milk smoothie	Chocolate pudding
Fruit smoothie	Lentil soup
Popsicle	Ice cream

Table 12.4 Diagnostic criteria for the interpretation of FPIES OFCs [1]

Major criterion	Vomiting in the 1- to 4-hour period after ingestion of the challenged food and the absence of classic IgE-mediated allergic skin or respiratory symptoms
Minor criteria	Diarrhea in the 5- to 10-hour period after food ingestion Lethargy Pallor Hypotension Hypothermia Increased neutrophil count ≥1500 neutrophils above baseline
Interpretation	One major criterion and two minor criteria are considered a diagnostic/positive challenge*

*Supervising physician may decide that a challenge is positive in the absence of minor criteria because (1) rapid use of ondansetron may prevent the development of minor criteria and (2) not all facilities are equipped to perform neutrophil counts in a timely manner

Interpretation of Challenge Outcomes

Unlike OFC for IgE-mediated food allergies which involves the interpretation of subjective symptoms, the interpretation of OFC for FPIES relies largely on objective symptoms. The original diagnostic criteria proposed by Powell included delayed vomiting and diarrhea, fecal eosinophils, fecal leukocytes, and increase in neutrophil count. Meeting ≥3 criteria constitutes a positive challenge, meeting 2 criteria is deemed equivocal, and meeting ≤1 criteria is considered a negative challenge [16]. Critiques of these diagnostic criteria include that it was established based on challenge outcomes in young infants with recent removal of the food from their diet. In clinical practice, infants are generally not challenged and challenges are delayed after a period of avoidance, when the inflammatory and clinical response could be diminished [17]. In addition, diarrhea is only seen in a minority (<50%) of patients, with vomiting being the consistent symptom during a reaction [6–8, 18–20]. Finally, complete blood counts (CBC) are rarely collected as a baseline or after a reaction, and the ability to perform labs in a timely manner is dependent on the institution. Based on these observations and critiques, the international consensus guidelines proposed revised criteria for the interpretation of OFCs in patients with possible or confirmed FPIES. These criteria require fulfillment of a major criterion of vomiting and two minor criteria of lethargy, pallor, diarrhea, hypotension, hypothermia, or increased neutrophil count from baseline (Table 12.4) [1]. In some cases, challenges can be considered diagnostic even if minor criteria are not met since early use of IVF and ondansetron may prevent the development of progressive symptoms, and not all facilities are able to perform labs.

Treatment for Positive Challenges

In all reactions, vital signs should be monitored and airway, breathing, and circulation (ABC) assessed. Patients with acute FPIES reactions are at risk of dehydration and hypovolemic shock. Therefore, the mainstay of treatment for acute FPIES reactions during OFC is aggressive fluid resuscitation with isotonic IVF, to be repeated as clinically indicated. Maintenance fluids with dextrose can also be helpful. Up to 50% of positive OFCs may require treatment with IVF, and approximately 15% of patients can develop hypotension [1, 2]. Oral rehydration may be attempted and successful in mild-moderate reactions, but caution should be taken in patients with a history of severe reaction [13]. The use of ondansetron in acute FPIES reactions during OFCs has not been well established. Two small case series suggest that intravenous and intramuscular ondansetron can lead to rapid resolution of symptoms, and a retrospective review suggests its efficacy over IVF and corticosteroids, though no difference was found between patients who received ondansetron and no therapy, and therapies were administered according to the severity of reaction [20–22]. Therefore, the available data on ondansetron use is limited and conflicting, but it has been anecdotally helpful, and the guidelines recommend its use to be considered as an adjunctive treatment for emesis [1]. Although no studies support the use of corticosteroids in FPIES reactions, a single dose of intravenous methylprednisolone may be helpful for the presumed inflammatory reaction that occurs in FPIES and can be considered for severe reactions [2]. Epinephrine is not routinely recommended for acute FPIES reactions, though it may be helpful in severe reactions leading to hypovolemic shock and should be used if there is concern for concomitant IgE-mediated anaphylaxis. In cases of severe hypotension, shock, and severe lethargy, the patient should be transferred to the intensive care unit for further care. Tables 12.5 and 12.6 summarize these treatment modalities, and Table 12.1 summarizes the medical interventions and outcomes of some published FPIES OFC studies.

Table 12.5 Treatment modalities for acute FPIES reactions during OFCs

First-line therapy	Normal saline (0.9% sodium chloride) 10–20 mL/kg IV
Adjunctive therapy	Ondansetron 0.15 mg/kg IV or IM (maximum 16 mg per dose)[a] Methylprednisolone 1 mg/kg IV (maximum 60–80 mg per dose) Epinephrine 0.01 mg/kg IM (maximum 0.5 mg per dose) in case of low blood pressure; if blood pressure continues to be low despite IM epinephrine, IV epinephrine may be indicated while transferring to PICU. IV infusion: Initial, 0.05–2 mcg/kg/minute (3.5–140 mcg/minute in a 70-kg patient); titrate to desired mean arterial pressure (MAP). May adjust dose every 10–15 minutes by 0.05–0.2 mcg/kg/minute to achieve desired blood pressure goal. After hemodynamic stabilization, may wean incrementally every 30 minutes over 12–24 hours

[a]Special caution in those with arrhythmia risk factors as ondansetron has the potential of prolonging QT interval [23]

Table 12.6 Management of acute FPIES reactions during OFCs [1]

Severity	Mild	Moderate	Severe
Symptoms	1–2 episodes of emesis No lethargy	≥ 3 episodes of emesis Mild lethargy	≥ 3 episodes of emesis Severe lethargy, hypotonia, cyanotic, or ashen appearance
Vital signs	Normal blood pressure Normal heart rate	Normal blood pressure Normal/high heart rate	Normal/low blood pressure High heart rate
Management ABC and vital sign assessment	1. Attempt oral rehydration (breastfeeding or clear fluids) 2. If age 6 months and older, consider ondansetron intramuscular, 0.15 mg/kg/dose; maximum, 16 mg/dose 3. Monitor for resolution about 4–6 h from the onset of a reaction	1. Attempt oral rehydration (breastfeeding or clear fluids) 2. Consider placing a peripheral intravenous line for normal saline bolus 20 mL/kg; repeat as needed 3. If age greater than 6 months, administer ondansetron intramuscular 0.15 mg/kg/dose; maximum, 16 mg/dose 3. Transfer the patient to the emergency department or intensive care unit in case of persistent or severe hypotension, shock, extreme lethargy, or respiratory distress 4. Monitor vital signs 5. Monitor for resolution at least 4–6 h from the onset of a reaction 6. Discharge home if patient is able to tolerate clear liquids	1. Place a peripheral intravenous line and administer normal saline bolus, 20 mL/kg rapidly; repeat as needed to correct hypotension 2. If age 6 months and older, administer intravenous ondansetron, 0.15 mg/kg/dose; maximum, 16 mg/dose 3. If placement of intravenous line is delayed because of difficult access and age is 6 months or older, administer ondansetron intramuscular, 0.15 mg/kg/dose; maximum, 16 mg/dose 4. Consider administering intravenous methylprednisolone, 1 mg/kg; maximum, 60–80 mg/dose 5. Monitor and correct acid base and electrolyte abnormalities 6. Correct methemoglobinemia, if present 7. Monitor vital signs 8. Discharge after 4–6 h from the onset of a reaction when the patient is back to baseline and is tolerating oral fluids 9. Transfer the patient to the emergency department or intensive care unit for further management in case of persistent or severe hypotension, shock, extreme lethargy, respiratory distress

Discharge Instructions

After a positive challenge, the patient should be instructed to continue food avoidance and follow-up plans should be discussed. After a negative challenge, the patient should be encouraged to introduce the food into the diet, though advised to avoid the challenged food for the remainder of the day for concerns of delayed reactions. In some protocols where challenges are performed with a cumulative dose less than serving size for age, patients are provided instructions to slowly increase the dose to a goal of full serving size over the subsequent days. In these cases, there is the possibility of reaction with home titration to full dose, though low (8% and 9% in studies by Wang et al. and Fogg et al.) [3, 5]. Patients should be instructed to contact the office with delayed reactions or reactions with home introduction; alternatively, telephone follow-up can be conducted. Patients should be provided with an updated emergency FPIES letter to be used in the event of reaction and need to seek medical care.

Clinical Pearls

- FPIES is largely a clinical diagnosis though OFC can help confirm the diagnosis in cases where the diagnosis is unclear and/or a food trigger is not identified. OFC can also help assess tolerance of cross-reactive foods and assess the resolution of FPIES.
- IVF is of utmost importance for patients developing an acute FPIES reaction during OFC; therefore, OFC should always be performed in a medical setting with access to IVF.
- Food challenge protocols vary, but all require prolonged observation to monitor for delayed GI manifestations that are the hallmark of FPIES reactions.

References

1. Nowak-Węgrzyn A, Chehade M, Groetch ME, Spergel JM, Wood RA, Allen K, et al. International consensus guidelines for the diagnosis and management of food protein-induced enterocolitis syndrome: Executive summary-Workgroup Report of the Adverse Reactions to Foods Committee, American Academy of Allergy, Asthma & Immunology. J Allergy Clin Immunol. 2017;139:1111–26.
2. Sicherer SH. Food protein-induced enterocolitis syndrome: case presentations and management lessons. J Allergy Clin Immunol. 2005;115:149–56.
3. Wang KY, Lee J, Cianferoni A, Ruffner MA, Dean A, Molleston JM, et al. Food protein-induced enterocolitis syndrome food challenges: experience from a large referral center. J Allergy Clin Immunol Pract. 2019;7(2):444–50.
4. Vazquez-Ortiz M, Machinena A, Dominguez O, Alvaro M, Calvo-Campoverde K, Giner MT, et al. Food protein-induced enterocolitis syndrome to fish and egg usually resolves by age 5 years in Spanish Children. J Allergy Clin Immunol Pract. 2017;5:512–5.
5. Lee E, Campbell DE, Barnes EH, Mehr SS. Resolution of acute food protein-induced enterocolitis syndrome in children. J Allergy Clin Immunol Pract. 2017;5:486–8.

6. Caubet JC, Ford LS, Sickles L, Järvinen KM, Sicherer SH, Sampson HA, et al. Clinical features and resolution of food protein-induced enterocolitis syndrome: 10-year experience. J Allergy Clin Immunol. 2014;134:382–9.
7. Sopo SM, Giorgio V, Dello Iacono I, Novembre E, Mori F, Onesimo R. A multicentre retrospective study of 66 Italian children with food protein-induced enterocolitis syndrome: different management for different phenotypes. Clin Exp Allergy. 2012;42:1257–65.
8. Katz Y, Goldberg MR, Rajuan N, Cohen A, Leshno M. The prevalence and natural course of food protein-induced enterocolitis syndrome to cow's milk: a large-scale, prospective population-based study. J Allergy Clin Immunol. 2011;127:647–53.
9. Hwang J-B, Sohn SM, Kim AS. Prospective follow-up oral food challenge in food protein-induced enterocolitis syndrome. Arch Dis Child. 2009;94:425–8.
10. Fogg MI, Brown-Whitehorn TA, Pawlowski NA, Spergel JM. Atopy patch test for the diagnosis of food protein-induced enterocolitis syndrome. Pediatr Allergy Immunol. 2006;17:251–5.
11. Nowak-Wegrzyn A, Sampson HA, Wood RA, Sicherer SH. Food protein-induced enterocolitis syndrome caused by solid food proteins. Pediatrics. 2003;111:829–35.
12. Sicherer SH, Eigenmann PA, Sampson HA. Clinical features of food-protein induced enterocolitis syndrome. J Pediatr. 1998;133:214–9.
13. Järvinen KM, Nowak-Węgrzyn A. Food protein-induced enterocolitis syndrome (FPIES): current management strategies and review of the literature. J Allergy Clin Immunol Pract. 2013;1:317–22.
14. Nowak-Wegrzyn A, Assa'ad AH, Bahna SL, Bock SA, Sicherer SH, Teuber SS. Work Group report: oral food challenge testing. J Allergy Clin Immunol. 2009;123(6Supp):S365–83.
15. Powell GK. Milk- and soy-induced enterocolitis of infancy. Clincal features and standardization of challenge. J Pediatr. 1978;93:553–60.
16. Powell GK. Food protein-induced enterocolitis of infancy: differential diagnosis and management. Compr Ther. 1986;12:28–37.
17. Feuille E, Nowak-Węgrzyn A. Definition, etiology, and diagnosis of food protein-induced enterocolitis syndrome. Curr Opin Allergy Clin Immunol. 2014;14:222–8.
18. Mehr S, Kakakios A, Frith K, Kemp AS. Food protein-induced enterocolitis syndrome: 16-year experience. Pediatrics. 2009;123:e459–64.
19. Ruffner MA, Ruymann K, Barni S, Cianferoni A, Brown-Whitehorn T, Spergel JM. Food protein-induced enterocolitis syndrome: insights from review of a large referral population. J Allergy Clin Immunol Pract. 2013;1:343–9.
20. Holbrook T, Keet CA, Frischmeyer-Guerrerio PA, Wood RA. Use of ondansetron for food protein-induced enterocolitis syndrome. J Allergy Clin Immunol. 2013;132:1219–20.
21. Miceli Sopo S, Battista A, Greco M, Monaco S. Ondansetron for food protein-induced enterocolitis syndrome. Int Arch Allergy Immunol. 2014;164:137–9.
22. Miceli Sopo S, Bersani G, Monaco S, Cerchiara G, Lee E, Campbell D, et al. Ondansetron in acute food protein-induced enterocolitis syndrome, a retrospective case-control study. Allergy. 2017;72:545–51.
23. Freedman SB, Uleryk E, Rumantir M, Finkelstein Y. Ondansetron an the risk of cardiac arrhythmias: a systematic review and postmarketing analysis. Ann Emerg Med. 2014;64:19–25.e6.

Food Protein-Induced Enterocolitis Syndrome and Quality of Life

13

Ashley A. Dyer, Ozge Nur Aktas, Jialing Jiang, Christopher M. Warren, and Ruchi S. Gupta

Introduction: Food Protein-Induced Enterocolitis Syndrome (FPIES)

Food protein-induced enterocolitis syndrome (FPIES) is a non-IgE-mediated food allergy that typically affects infants and young children [1]. FPIES is characterized by the following symptoms that occur 1–4 hours post-ingestion of an allergenic food: projectile, repetitive emesis; dehydration; lethargy; diarrhea; and even hypovolemic shock. Due to FPIES-related feeding issues, longer-term health outcomes often result in the infant's inability to meet milestones for weight gain and height [1, 2]. In the United States, the most common FPIES food triggers include cow's milk, soy, rice, and oat. As more foods are introduced into an infant's diet, FPIES triggers have been shown to also include beans, egg, poultry, seafood, and vegetables [3].

Delay in an FPIES diagnosis is a common experience for families as there are currently no diagnostic tests for FPIES food triggers and physician awareness of the condition remains low [4–6]. Gold standard diagnosis requires physicians to differentially diagnose FPIES based on clinical history alone, which is then confirmed

A. A. Dyer · J. Jiang · C. M. Warren
Northwestern University Feinberg School of Medicine, Chicago, IL, USA

O. N. Aktas
Pediatrics, University of Illinois at Chicago, Chicago, IL, USA

R. S. Gupta (✉)
Northwestern University Feinberg School of Medicine, Chicago, IL, USA

Ann & Robert H. Lurie Children's Hospital of Chicago, Chicago, IL, USA
e-mail: r-gupta@northwestern.edu

T. F. Brown-Whitehorn, A. Cianferoni (eds.), *Food Protein Induced Enterocolitis (FPIES)*,
https://doi.org/10.1007/978-3-030-21229-2_13

by a food challenge [7]. The mainstay for current management of FPIES is avoidance of the known food trigger. Unlike IgE-mediated food allergy, which responds to epinephrine if there is an accidental ingestion, the only effective treatment for FPIES is intravenous fluid resuscitation within an inpatient setting [1, 8–10]. The limited tools for FPIES diagnosis, compounded by the lack of physician ability to provide tailored guidance for individualized avoidance diets, contribute to impaired quality of life (QoL) among caregivers [11]. Moreover, additional drivers of QoL impairment include children undergoing unnecessary medical workups and surgical consultations as well as inappropriate treatment for sepsis [12].

Compared to IgE-mediated food allergy, very few rigorous studies have been conducted to systematically assess QoL among families caring for a child with FPIES. Nevertheless, existing exploratory studies and recent FPIES caregiver assessments of unmet needs provide a window into the current lived experiences of affected families [13]. These initial studies can serve as the bedrock of inquiry—shedding light on how researchers, clinicians, and advocates can better ask questions, develop management plans, and meaningfully advocate for affected FPIES families to ultimately enhance caregiver self-efficacy aimed at improving overall QoL.

Caregiver Assessment of Unmet Needs

In a survey conducted by an international FPIES advocacy group assessing the greatest personal and family challenges caregivers face, several unmet needs were identified (Table 13.1). The following unmet needs will be used to guide this chapter exploring the current literature regarding FPIES-related QoL, including (1) nutritional, social, and emotional burdens that accompany avoidance of FPIES triggers, (2) lack of FPIES awareness among providers, (3) lack of diagnosis and treatment guidelines, and (4) lack of collaborative care among providers and integrative care teams [13].

Unmet Need

Emotional, Social, and Nutritional Burdens

Social and Emotional Considerations

Parental Stress

Our current understanding of the natural history of FPIES may provide caregivers with some hope. Overall, among infants and young children with FPIES, there is an exceptionally high rate of recovery with more than 85–90% of patients resolving the condition between the ages of 3 and 5 [14]. Moreover, while FPIES reactions can be severe and affect the child for days or even weeks at a time, there are currently no documented fatalities due to an FPIES reaction [14].

Table 13.1 Comparing Caretaker Assessment of Unmet Needs with the 2017 Consensus Guidelines Assessment of Future Needs [7, 13]

Caretaker Assessment of Unmet Needs	Consensus Guidelines Assessment of Future Needs
Epidemiology	
Limited operational definition of disease	Characterize chronic FPIES
Poor definition and understanding of acute versus chronic FPIES	Establish FPIES prevalence
Poorly understood prevalence	Identify FPIES risk factors
	Perform longitudinal cohort studies to better determine outcomes and the natural history of FPIES in children and adults
Basic science	
	Determine pathophysiology of acute and chronic FPIES
	Understand relationship between atopy and FPIES
Clinical diagnosis and clinician management	
Lack of FPIES awareness among providers	Validate the proposed diagnostic criteria
Poor definition and understanding of acute versus chronic presentations	Standardize the OFC protocol and criteria for challenge positivity
Obstacles and delay in finding diagnosis	Develop non-invasive biomarkers for diagnosis and monitoring resolution
Lack of diagnostic and treatment guidelines	
Lack of collaborative care among providers	
Lack of collaboration with alternative providers many families turn to due to lack of support and available treatment	
Therapeutics	
	Develop therapeutic approaches to accelerate FPIES resolution
	Determine role of ondansetron in managing FPIES reactions
	Determine whether extensively heated (baked) cow's milk and egg white proteins can be tolerated by children with FPIES
Patient management	
Poor quality of life	Perform systematic evaluation of the prevalence of nutrient deficiencies, poor growth, and feeding difficulties in patients with FPIES and provide guidance for preventative intervention
Nutritional, social, and emotional burdens that come with avoidance	
Financial burden to pay for expensive and often uncovered elemental formula	
Other	
Limited representation in the literature	
Lack of active funding to support initiatives and studies	

Nevertheless, many questions remain unanswered, leaving families to confront their child's FPIES with little support from the larger medical community regarding how to effectively manage FPIES-related social, emotional, and nutritional burdens. Moreover, FPIES typically strikes during a particularly stressful transitional period. It is well known that parents of healthy young children often experience a myriad of factors that impair their QoL, including feeding difficulty and sleep issues [15–18]. Such typical parenting stressors are often compounded among parents managing their child's FPIES due to common symptoms like abdominal pain and further feeding issues, which have been shown to worsen sleep, namely, due to the inability to calm a crying baby [15, 17, 19, 20].

A recent article by Lozinsky et al. [21] reports factors affecting psychological health and stability of families in a population of caregivers and general practitioners managing children with either non-IgE-mediated and IgE-mediated cow's milk protein allergy (CMPA) [21]. Caregivers of children with CMPA often report feeling exhaustion due to lack of sleep as well as stress or anxiety related to their child's health. Families disclose that they are not able to enjoy their time together as a family and other children within the family without CMPA receive less time and attention. Strikingly, many families also report that they are perceived to be overacting, worrying too much, and they do not feel like they are taken seriously. Moreover, caregivers of children with CMPA identify that the amount of time taken to reach diagnosis impacts not only their stress level but also has implications within the caregiver–child relationship, which includes reports of frustration with the child and over 40% of caregivers seeking medical support for depression [21].

Caregiver Comparison

FPIES Versus IgE-Mediated Food Allergy

One exploratory study conducted by Greenhawt [22] suggests that the caregiver burden of disease is distinctly different for families managing FPIES versus families managing IgE-mediated food allergy (Fig. 13.1). Comparison of QoL measures between FPIES and IgE-mediated food allergy revealed that social (e.g., social activities), psychological (e.g., parents feeling unable to help), and dietary (e.g., meal preparation) domains contribute to greater QoL impairment among caregivers of children with FPIES. Particular demographic factors and disease characteristics were also shown to impact caregiver QoL. For example, the biological sex of the caregiver adversely affected QOL with female caregivers of children reporting worse QoL than male caregivers [22]. This finding parallels previous research by Warren et al. [23], which found greater impairments among maternal caregivers when compared to paternal caregivers of children with IgE-mediated food allergy [23]. Moreover, caregivers of children with both liquid and solid food FPIES were shown to impair QoL when compared to caregivers managing a child with a single FPIES food trigger. No differences in QoL comparing caregivers of children with FPIES and caregivers of children with IgE-mediated food allergies were found with regard to socioeconomic status, family income, and caregiver education [22].

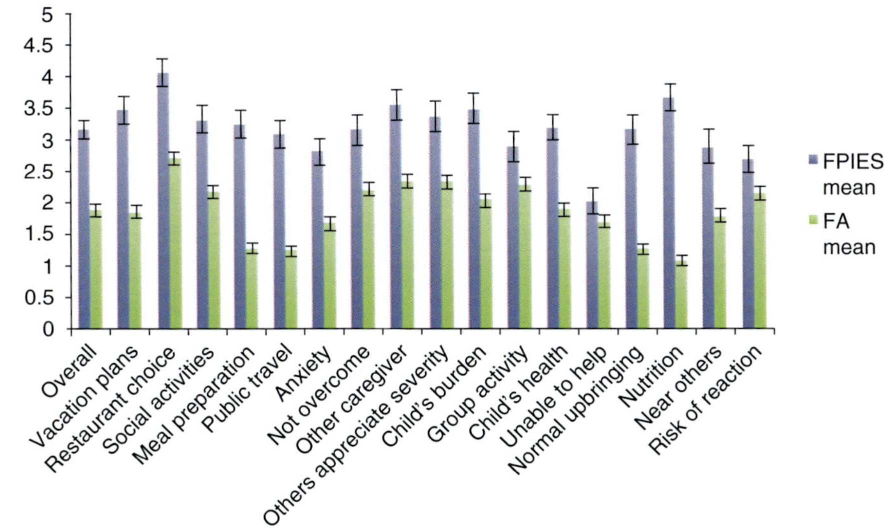

Fig. 13.1 Comparison of mean total FAQL-PB scores between CCF and CFAs. The difference was statistically significant ($P < 0.05$) in all QoL domains. *Error bars* represent SEs. (Reprinted from Greenhawt et al. [22], Copyright 2016, with permission from Elsevier)

Patient Comparison

Non-IgE-Mediated Food Allergy Versus IgE-Mediated Food Allergy

A recent study by Foong et al. [24] compared patients with non-IgE-mediated food allergy versus patients with IgE-mediated food allergies across physical, emotional, social, and psychosocial domains. Patients with non-IgE-mediated food allergy had worse QoL within the physical functioning domain, which included questions regarding sports participation and exercise, doing household chores, and reporting aches and low energy levels. Patients reported abdominal pain, persistence of flatus, and gastrointestinal symptom severity even after undergoing an elimination diet, which also contributed to QoL impairment. In addition, having to eliminate a greater number of foods from the diet was also associated with greater QoL impairment among patients with non-IgE-meditated food allergy. Differences in QoL between non-IgE-mediated food allergy and IgE-mediated food allergy were only observed within the physical domain; no differences were observed in QoL across the emotional, social, and psychosocial domains [24].

QoL Comparison

Non-IgE-Mediated Gastrointestinal Food Allergies, Intestinal Failure, and Sickle Cell

Previous research by Meyer et al. [15] measured QoL of caregivers of non-IgE-mediated food allergy before and after an elimination diet [15]. These data were then compared to two historical cohorts of patients with sickle cell disease and intestinal failure. Overall, factors that significantly impacted family QoL of families managing non-IgE-mediated food allergies included the child being younger in age, having to exclude more foods during the elimination diet, experiencing higher symptom severity, and reporting nasal congestion [15].

Compared to the sickle cell cohort, caregivers of children with non-IgE-mediated food allergy fared significantly worse across all family impact domains including physical functioning, emotional functioning, social functioning, cognitive functioning, communication, worry, daily activities, and family relationships. The greatest differences between the sickle cell cohort and non-IgE-mediated food allergy cohort included the following domains: emotional functioning, cognitive functioning, and daily activities. Compared to the intestinal failure cohort, caregivers of children with non-IgE-mediated food allergy fared worse across all domains; however, statistically significant differences between the two groups were only reported across the following domains: physical functioning, emotional functioning, and worry [15].

Nutritional Management Considerations

Key factors that greatly impact nutritional management of FPIES include (1) number of foods avoided, (2) role of breastfeeding and appropriate weaning advice, and (3) identifying a suitable formula choice [3]. For patients with FPIES, strict avoidance of an offending food is the current mainstay for daily management as even small amounts of food or oral mucosal contact can act as an FPIES trigger [25]. Avoidance can be difficult for families as they seek food alternatives or allergen-free food. Allergen labeling is often vague; labels do not often indicate potential cross-contact during production, and US law only requires labeling of the top 8 allergens of peanut, tree nut, milk, egg, wheat, finfish, shellfish, and soy. Not surprisingly, this leads to caregivers having difficulties in reliably identifying less common allergens in products [26].

FPIES is particularly challenging as it affects infants, young children, and parents experiencing the stress of caring for a young child with a chronic condition while trying to manage other aspects of the child's development (e.g., maintaining sleep schedules). Previous literature suggests that patients with FPIES to cow's milk may confront malnutrition and failure to thrive [27]. Moreover, one-third of infants with FPIES to cow's milk and/or soy may develop FPIES to rice and other grains that are commonly introduced to children as introductory solid foods throughout weaning. This can compound the stress of nutritional management for caregivers due to avoiding multiple foods while trying to maintain adequate nutrition.

Alternatives to cow's milk-based formula may include exclusive breastfeeding [28], hydrolyzed formula, or amino acid-based formula [29].While nutrition guidelines and best practices for breastfeeding and weaning approaches for children with FPIES will be explored in other chapters, one area for further exploration related to QoL is the added cost of elemental formulas [13]. Previous research assessing the economic burden of IgE-mediated food allergy in the United States estimated that over $24.8 billion is spent annually in the United States, with a significant proportion of those costs covering special diets and allergen-free food [30]. Further research assessing the economic and structural factors that support breastfeeding, as well as lessen the financial burden of alternative formulas when breastfeeding, remains critical to improving public health policies and programs to support families managing FPIES.

Unmet Need

Lack of FPIES Awareness Among Providers

The lack of FPIES awareness among clinicians leads to much confusion and can yield emotional and financial burdens for families trying to navigate the medical system to adequately address their child's health needs. As much time, money, and energy is spent on caregivers navigating the medical system to receive an appropriate FPIES diagnosis, one area that may help to reduce confusion and improve QOL would be to better equip providers with the skills to correctly identify and diagnose the FPIES more efficiently. To date, there have been three surveys assessing the current FPIES knowledge and management practices of general pediatricians and allergists. [4, 6, 31]

In a 2013 study assessing a small cohort of randomly selected pediatricians subscribed to a national US-based advocacy organization ($N = 86$), more than 80% of clinicians had limited understanding or never heard of FPIES [6]. Furthermore, in a 2017 study assessing FPIES knowledge among a larger cohort of general pediatricians, over 50% of the pediatricians indicated they had a poor understanding of the condition even though 73% of the practitioners indicated they had cared for a patient with FPIES. Pediatricians varied in their ability to recognize hallmark symptoms of FPIES with 83.5% identifying severe vomiting and 70.3% recognizing failure to thrive as FPIES manifestations. The more severe symptoms (e.g., hypotension, cyanosis) were recognized less frequently. Regarding management, 65% of pediatricians identified the need for prompt emergency care and rehydration; however, many pediatricians still incorrectly advised first-line treatment known to be ineffective at treating FPIES including epinephrine (16%) and antihistamines (5%) [4, 31].

While the aforementioned studies underscore the need to bolster training among general pediatricians, a 2017 study sought to further assess the level of familiarity with FPIES regarding diagnosis and management among practicing allergists. Among 470 allergy providers, almost one-third of respondents did not report "full understanding" of the condition. In addition, diagnostic and management practices from the types of diagnostic testing employed (e.g., skin testing, specific IgE) to the varying guidance around "safe" nutrition and alternate feeding options to FPIES triggers varied substantially among practitioners. While over 70% of surveyed allergists provided their patients with allergy action plans, over 20% incorrectly prescribed these patients an epinephrine auto-injector. In addition, the more years you were in practice, the less likely you were to indicate having a "full understanding" of FPIES. While enhancing allergists' knowledge, particularly those who have been in practice longer, remains integral to improving clinical diagnosis and management of FPIES, the wide variance of diagnosis and management practices signaled the need for more explicit practice parameters regarding FPIES diagnosis and management [4].

Unmet Need

Lack of Diagnosis and Treatment Guidelines

The first international consensus guidelines for the diagnosis and management of FPIES were published in 2017 by a working group comprised of over 40 physicians, dieticians, researchers, and advocates. The guidelines address many of the unmet needs outlined earlier in the chapter and are outlined in Table 13.2. While the

Table 13.2 Summary of 2017 International Consensus Guidelines for the Diagnosis and Management of Food Protein-Induced Enterocolitis Syndrome: Executive Summary–Workgroup Report of the Adverse Reactions to Foods Committee, American Academy of Allergy, Asthma, and Immunology [7]

Section overview	Subsection summary statements
Section 1: Definition and clinical manifestations	Recognize FPIES as a potential medical emergency, which presents as delayed onset of protracted emesis and/or watery/bloody diarrhea, culminating in hemodynamic instability and hypotension in 15% of patients
	Recognize the symptom phenotype in patients with FPIES is determined by the frequency of food ingestion
Section 2: Epidemiology	Recognize that onset of FPIES to cow's milk and soy can occur at younger ages compared with FPIES to solid foods. Patients can have a single trigger or multiple triggers.
	Consider specific IgE testing of children with FPIES to their trigger food because comorbid IgE-mediated sensitization to triggers, such as cow's milk, can infer a greater chance of persistent disease
	Do not recommend any specific prenatal or postnatal food introduction/avoidance or health behaviors or advise patients regarding any specific genetic factors known to moderate the risk of a patient with FPIES
	Consider FPIES a heterogeneous disorder associated with a number of geographic variations in the features of the disease, representing a spectrum of "syndromes" as opposed to a uniform "syndrome"
Section 3: Diagnosis of FPIES	Diagnose FPIES primarily based on a clinical history of typical characteristic signs and symptoms with improvement after withdrawal of the suspected trigger food. Exclude other potential causes and use of oral food challenge (OFC) to help confirm the diagnosis if the history is unclear and there is a favorable risk/benefit ratio
	Conduct OFC in patients with suspected FPIES in medically supervised settings in which access to rapid fluid resuscitation is available and prolonged observation can be provided, if necessary
	Do not routinely perform testing for food IgE-mediated process. However, because some patients with FPIES can exhibit coexisting IgE-mediated allergies, testing can be considered in patients with certain comorbid conditions. Assessment of chemistry of blood counts can help rule out other causes of symptoms if obtained in the acute setting
	Do not obtain radiographic testing in the routine diagnostic work-up of suspected FPIES
	Consider a broad differential for a patient presenting with acute vomiting in making a diagnosis of FPIES
	Use distinct criteria to diagnose FPIES in the outpatient/community setting compared with the monitored setting in which OFC are being used to rule in the diagnosis

Table 13.2 (continued)

Section overview	Subsection summary statements
Section 4: Pathophysiology of FPIES	Classify FPIES as a non-IgE-mediated food allergy but be aware that postulated T cell-mediated mechanism of FPIES requires further validation
Section 5: Gastrointestinal manifestations of FPIES	Do not routinely obtain endoscopic evaluation as part of the evaluation of FPIES
	Do not use stool tests to make the diagnosis of FPIES
	Consider a work-up to rule out other gastrointestinal diseases resulting in symptoms that overlap with FPIES
Section 6: Management of acute FPIES	Treat acute FPIES as a medical emergency and be prepared to provide aggressive fluid resuscitation because approximately 15% of patients can have hypovolemic shock
	Manage acute FPIES individually according to severity and review treatment strategies with the caregivers of each patient
	Consider ondansetron as an adjunctive management of emesis in patients with acute FPIES
	Use dietary elimination for trigger food or foods for the primary management of FPIES and educate caregivers and other care providers regarding avoidance strategies
	Do not recommend routine maternal dietary elimination of offending triggers while breastfeeding if the infant is thriving and remains asymptomatic
	Reintroduce the foods triggering FPIES under a physician's supervision
	Recognize that infants with cow's milk - or soy-induced FPIES might be at increased risk of having FPIES to other foods
Section 8: Nutritional management for FPIES	Provide guidance during the introduction of complementary foods to ensure nutritional adequacy during this time and beyond
	Do not routinely recommend avoidance of products with precautionary allergen labeling in patients with FPIES
	Use hypoallergenic formula in formula-fed infants or infants who can no longer breastfeed and are given a diagnosis of FPIES caused by cow's milk
	Monitor growth (weight and height/length) regularly in children with FPIES
	Recommend foods that enhance developmental skills in infants in the complementary feeding period to prevent aversive feeding behaviors and delay in the development of food acceptance and feeding skills
Section 9: Natural history of FPIES	Recognize that the age of development of tolerance in patients with FPIES varies by type of food trigger and country of origin
	Evaluate patients with FPIES at regular intervals according to the patient's age and food allergen to determine whether she or he is still allergic

guidelines will evolve and be updated as researchers and practitioners further hone best practices, the establishment of guidelines remains a promising first step in communicating current knowledge and best practices. Publication of these guidelines may provide an opportunity for caregivers and practitioners to better communicate and work together toward improving every step of the FPIES diagnosis and management journey by encouraging adoption of current best practices among caregivers and practitioners alike (Guidelines 2017) [7]. When comparing the guideline working group's *Assessment of Future Needs* with the FPIES advocates *Assessment of Unmet Needs* (Table 13.1), there is considerable overlap regarding how best to move forward. These overlaps include (1) improving epidemiological understanding (e.g., FPIES prevalence, risk factors, natural history), (2) establishing and promoting adherence to guidelines-based diagnosis and management practices (e.g., validating proposed diagnostic criteria, standardizing OFC protocols), and (3) developing therapeutic treatment options to potentially accelerate FPIES resolution [7, 13]. The development of further effective strategies for improving QoL among families caring for children with FPIES would further strengthen the consensus guidelines and help to facilitate comprehensive care.

While the development and dissemination of consensus guidelines remain a promising first step in improving FPIES care, further work remains necessary regarding how to best educate clinicians and disseminate clinical guidelines within both the primary care and specialist settings. Additionally, delineating the most appropriate and effective roles for general practitioners and medical subspecialists remains critical to better manage expectations and clearly communicate a care plan to caregivers of children with FPIES.

One model to consider within the FPIES community would be to extend the NIH-funded Food Allergy Support Tool, which was developed to improve clinical diagnosis and management of IgE-mediated food allergy. This clinical decision support tool could be extended to incorporate the 2017 FPIES consensus guidelines to encourage clinicians to (1) better document clinical history, (2) adhere to diagnostic guidelines as to not over treat, (3) provide comprehensive counseling, (4) provide an FPIES emergency action plan, and (5) refer to an allergist for confirmatory OFC and management. This systems-level intervention has the potential to streamline and facilitate provision of consistent, guidelines-based care, as well as encourage clear communication to caregivers throughout the FPIES diagnosis and management process [5].

Unmet Need

Lack of Collaborative Care Among Providers and Integrative Care Teams

The lack of collaborative care among healthcare providers is one of the main concerns families managing FPIES report regarding barriers to receiving a timely diagnosis [13]. Consulting a physician and nutritional expert can be crucial in identifying appropriate feeding alternatives. The burden of management and potential health effects posed may also further prompt and exacerbate feelings of stress, anxiety, worry, and substantially impact QoL of patients and families as they navigate the nutritional terrain while living with FPIES, which may also call for targeted family-level psychological support. In addition to collaboration between physicians and nutritionists, families have also indicated that they are interested in more targeted collaboration with integrative practitioners (e.g., Western herbalists, Chinese medicine practitioners) that families readily consult, largely due to reported lack of support and current lack of treatment options [13].

Conclusion

To date, few peer-reviewed studies assessing QoL among FPIES affected families have been published. Future research should consider incorporating the QoL tool validated by Greenhawt et al. [22] to better understand how to guide families through the process of FPIES diagnosis and management as well as to provide support on how to navigate the social, emotional, and nutritional challenges associated with daily living. Incorporating management supports aimed at improving patient and caregiver QoL into the 2017 international consensus guidelines will only strengthen the ability of families to communicate with informed practitioners to reduce caregiver stress and anxiety and to support families living with FPIES in their overall well-being.

Clinical Pearls: FPIES Quality of Life (QoL)

- *Improve FPIES Awareness Among Providers*: FPIES remains a challenging diagnosis for clinicians, which can lead to much confusion and yield emotional and financial burdens for families trying to navigate the medical system. The limited tools available to help guide an FPIES diagnosis, particularly the lack of tailored guidance for individualized avoidance diets, contribute to impaired QoL among caregivers. Additional drivers of QoL impairment include children undergoing unnecessary medical work-ups, surgical consultations, and inappropriate treatment.
- *Accelerate Systematic Implementation of Diagnosis and Treatment Guidelines*: A working group comprised of over 40 physicians, dieticians, researchers, and advocates published the first international consensus guidelines for the diagnosis and management of FPIES in 2017. Better tools and systems level interventions are needed to systematically implement the evidence-informed guidelines into wide scale practice.
- *Enhance FPIES Research*: Compared to IgE-mediated food allergy, a limited number of studies have been conducted to systematically assess QoL among families caring for a child with FPIES. In addition to research focused on the epidemiology and pathophysiology of FPIES, studies focused on FPIES-related QoL are needed.

References

1. Feuille E, Nowak-Wegrzyn A. Definition, etiology, and diagnosis of food protein-induced enterocolitis syndrome. Curr Opin Allergy Clin Immunol. 2014;14(3):222–8.
2. Fiocchi A, Claps A, Dahdah L, Brindisi G, Dionisi-Vici C, Martelli A. Differential diagnosis of food protein-induced enterocolitis syndrome. Curr Opin Allergy Clin Immunol. 2014;14(3):246–54.
3. Venter C, Groetch M. Nutritional management of food protein-induced enterocolitis syndrome. Curr Opin Allergy Clin Immunol. 2014;14(3):255–62.

4. Greenhawt M, Bird JA, Nowak-Wegrzyn AH. Trends in provider management of patients with food protein-induced enterocolitis syndrome. J Allergy Clin Immunol Pract. 2017;5(5):1319–1324 e1312.
5. Otto AK, Dyer AA, Warren CM, Walkner M, Smith BM, Gupta RS. The development of a clinical decision support system for the management of pediatric food allergy. Clin Pediatr (Phila). 2017;56(6):571–8.
6. Menon N, Feuille E, Huang F, Nowak-Wegrzyn AH. Knowledge of Food Protein-Induced Enterocolitis (FPIES) among general pediatricians. J Allergy Clin Immunol. 2013;131(2):AB177.
7. Nowak-Wegrzyn A, Chehade M, Groetch ME, et al. International consensus guidelines for the diagnosis and management of food protein-induced enterocolitis syndrome: Executive summary-Workgroup Report of the Adverse Reactions to Foods Committee, American Academy of Allergy, Asthma & Immunology. J Allergy Clin Immunol. 2017;139(4):1111–1126 e1114.
8. Miceli Sopo S, Battista A, Greco M, Monaco S. Ondansetron for Food Protein-Induced Enterocolitis Syndrome. Int Arch Allergy Immunol. 2014;164(2):137–9.
9. Holbrook T, Keet CA, Frischmeyer-Guerrerio PA, Wood RA. Use of ondansetron for food protein–induced enterocolitis syndrome. J Allergy Clin Immunol. 2013;132(5):1219–20.
10. Jarvinen KM, Nowak-Wegrzyn A. Food protein-induced enterocolitis syndrome (FPIES): current management strategies and review of the literature. J Allergy Clin Immunol Pract. 2013;1(4):317–22.
11. Wang J, Fiocchi A. Unmet needs in Food Protein Induced Enterocolitis Syndrome (FPIES). Curr Opin Allergy Clin Immunol. 2014;14(3):206–7.
12. Andrews T, Tsarouhas N, Spergel J. Food allergy presenting as a "septic"-appearing infant. Pediatr Emerg Care. 2004;20(10):677–9.
13. Schultz F, Westcott-Chavez A. Food protein-induced enterocolitis syndrome from the parent perspective. Curr Opin Allergy Clin Immunol. 2014;14(3):263–7.
14. Katz Y, Goldberg MR. Natural history of food protein-induced enterocolitis syndrome. Curr Opin Allergy Clin Immunol. 2014;14(3):229–39.
15. Meyer R, Godwin H, Dziubak R, et al. The impact on quality of life on families of children on an elimination diet for Non-immunoglobulin E mediated gastrointestinal food allergies. World Allergy Organ J. 2017;10(1):8.
16. Eronen R, Pincombe J, Calabretto H. Support for stressed parents of young infants. Neonatal Paediatric Child Health Nurs. 2007;10
17. Hildingsson I, Thomas J. Parental stress in mothers and fathers one year after birth. J Reprod Infant Psychol. 2014;32:41–56.
18. Skreden M, Skari H, Malt UF, et al. Parenting stress and emotional wellbeing in mothers and fathers of preschool children. Scand J Public Health. 2012;40:596–604.
19. Meyer R, Rommel N, Van OL, Fleming C, Dziubak R, Shah N. Feeding difficulties in children with food protein-induced gastrointestinal allergies. J Gastroenterol Hepatol. 2014;29:1764–9.
20. Rouf K, White L, Evans K. A qualitative investigation into the maternal experience of having a young child with severe food allergy. Clin Child Psychol Psychiatry. 2012;17:49–64.
21. Lozinsky AC, Meyer R, Anagnostou K, et al. Cow's milk protein allergy from diagnosis to management: a very different journey for general practitioners and parents. Children. 2015;2(3):317–29.
22. Greenhawt M, Schultz F, DunnGalvin A. A validated index to measure health-related quality of life in patients with food protein-induced enterocolitis syndrome. J Allergy Clin Immunol. 2016;137(4):1251–1253.e1255.
23. Warren CM, Gupta RS, Sohn MW, et al. Differences in empowerment and quality of life among parents of children with food allergy. Ann Allergy Asthma Immunol. 2015;114(2):117–25.
24. Foong RX, Meyer R, Godwin H, et al. Parental perception of their child's quality of life in children with non-immunoglobulin-E-mediated gastrointestinal allergies. Pediatr Allergy Immunol. 2017;28(3):251–6.

25. Mane SK, Bahna SL. Clinical manifestations of food protein-induced enterocolitis syndrome. Curr Opin Allergy Clin Immunol. 2014;14(3):217–21.
26. Joshi P, Mofidi S, Sicherer SH. Interpretation of commercial food ingredient labels by parents of food-allergic children. J Allergy Clin Immunol. 2002;109(6):1019–21.
27. Yang M, Geng L, Xu Z, et al. Severe food protein-induced Enterocolitis syndrome to Cow's Milk in infants. Nutrients. 2016;8(1):1.
28. Leonard SA, Nowak-Węgrzyn A. Food protein–induced enterocolitis syndrome: an update on natural history and review of management. Ann Allergy Asthma Immunol. 2011;107(2):95–101.
29. Caubet JC, Ford LS, Sickles L, et al. Clinical features and resolution of food protein-induced enterocolitis syndrome: 10-year experience. J Allergy Clin Immunol. 2014;134(2):382–389. e384.
30. Gupta R, Holdford D, Bilaver L, Dyer A, Holl JL, Meltzer D. The economic impact of childhood food allergy in the United States. JAMA Pediatr. 2013;167(11):1026–31.
31. Feuille E, Menon NR, Huang F, Greenhawt M, Nowak-Wegrzyn A. Knowledge of food protein-induced enterocolitis syndrome among general pediatricians. Ann Allergy Asthma Immunol. 2017;119(3):291–292 e293.

14 Creation of IFPIES

Fallon Schultz Matney

Dark Ages: Our Story Begins

My son Landon was born the pinkest, fullest baby on the unit. I always say that he was born different. He had this seriousness about him, his eyes always give away exactly how he is feeling; in time, they would become my compass for navigating his FPIES. As a first-time parent, we have big dreams for motherhood and for our babies. We imagine the joy we will feel watching our child's first steps, hearing their first words, and taking their first bites. When these milestones don't come as planned or at all, our core is rocked.

I never imagined feeding my child would become the greatest challenge I have faced in my life, and I have been through some serious challenges. I never imagined that food could make a child so sick. I never guessed my child would become a "patient" and spend nearly 10 years battling food.

Landon was born in the dark ages of FPIES, when a Google search yielded zero results. Maybe 20 physicians in the USA knew about FPIES then. FPIES was believed to be an ultra-rare food allergy. My son was called "a rare case of a rare disease," and he suffered for nearly 2 years before he received his diagnosis. In that time, he reacted to over 30 foods, many of which lead him to shock. I was a frantic mother, trying to help my baby with no support, guidance, or experience. This wasn't the vision I had for him or for my experience as a mother.

I was determined to figure this out and make it better. I never imagined that our struggles would lead to answers, support, and guidance for others in the form of the International FPIES Association (IFPIES).

My son's experience with FPIES started at 2 weeks old. He was an exclusively breastfed baby. He would nurse every 2–3 hours and always seemed hungry. He would cry during all his feeds and hours later would vomit profusely and have

F. Schultz Matney (✉)
International FPIES Association (IFPIES), Point Pleasant Beach, NJ, USA

T. F. Brown-Whitehorn, A. Cianferoni (eds.), *Food Protein Induced Enterocolitis (FPIES)*,
https://doi.org/10.1007/978-3-030-21229-2_14

numerous diapers filled with blood. His bottom was raw and blistered, he never seemed content, and no matter how many visits we made to the lactation consultant or pediatrician, nothing seemed to help.

At 3 months, when Landon began to fall off the growth chart, I heard the words "food allergy." I grew up in an Italian family where every problem is cured by food. Italians live to eat, and feeding your baby is a rite of passage. What was this talk about "food allergy?" I had no experience in this so learning what it meant took time.

His pediatrician suspected he was suffering from milk protein allergy and suggested he switch from breastmilk to formula. This was my first experience with "FPIES robbery", as I like to call it. I was going to breastfeed until he was at least 1 year old. I was going to be that mom who did everything by the book.

I did what every stubborn woman would do to challenge this idea of food allergy. I tortured myself and refused to give up. But the more I did, the worse he got. It took my ob-gyn's plea to stop and reassurance that my son would still be everything he is meant to be before I finally gave up breastfeeding.

Liquid Gold

Trialing formulas was a nightmare. We started with the traditional "go-to" formulas, then transitioned to hydrolyzed formulas. He did not get any better. I would cry in the shower so no one could see me breakdown or witness the fear and self-doubt I felt inside. I felt like I didn't know how to be a mother and maybe I would never be good at it.

It wasn't until elemental formula (aka "liquid gold") was introduced that every single symptom disappeared. No more bloody diapers, no more vomiting. No more comfort feeding, sleepless nights. It took 6 months. Six months!

However, this liquid gold came with a price…and a battle. Our insurance company would not cover the cost, and to feed my son I would need to pay $2000 a month. I refinanced my home. I begged for samples from our pediatrician. I warred with our insurance company.

Over the course of 2 months, I logged 482 phone calls to our insurance company, providing adequate medical documentation, attending all the appeals and required meetings, only to be denied. This was the only thing my child could consume safely and no one could help.

One day, I received an anonymous letter accusing me of Munchausen by proxy, a psychiatric disorder in which a parent lies or fabricates a child's symptoms for their personal attention. When a parent is suspected of Munchausen's, Child Protective Services steps in and may remove the child from the home. I lived in fear that someone would take my son from me.

Years later, our assigned case manager shared it was the insurance company that sent the letter. She was the reason my son's formula was finally covered. I had spent months on the phone with her, and she heard Landon screaming on a daily basis. She heard the desperation in my voice. She advocated for us, and we were "awarded" a 1-month supply of formula at a time. Every month, I would go through this same stressful appeal process. This went on for 2 years. Even now, nearly 10 years later, even with my connections and advocacy skills, formula coverage is still a battle.

The Road to CHOP

When Landon was 6 months old, it was time to start trialing solid foods. We started with rice cereal, which he seemed to tolerate at first, but over time, blood re-appeared to his diapers and the screaming cry returned. I was told to trial foods one by one and document what happened. When I tried a new food, he would look incoherent and sleepy, followed by vomiting and many, many diapers. His doctors would either tell me it was a virus, to trial the food again, or discontinue food all together. This went on with over 30 foods.

A wheat and a sweet potato trial are what ultimately led us to CHOP, where I finally met the team of doctors that ultimately would diagnose and care for Landon: Dr. Brown, Dr. Maqbool and Sarah Weston RD, CSP, LDN. Over the years they have become our "dream team", always consulting one another and working with so much dedication on Landon's behalf.

I was struggling to get my family to understand what was happening to Landon (remember, we are Italian and food fixes everything!). The team offered to meet with them to explain FPIES and provide them with realistic expectations.

During this meeting, the missing pieces and real gaps in FPIES became blaringly obvious. There was no treatment except avoidance. There was no diagnostic test to determine if a food would cause a reaction. It was all trial and error. There was no diagnosis code. There was no research or publications. They had no idea how many cases there were worldwide, but it was ultra-rare and Landon may be the rarest of them all. Even at CHOP, the number one children's hospital in the country, the only answer for FPIES was a resounding "we don't know."

Everything seemed bleak. But I am a known rebel and relentless fighter. I could not accept what I was hearing, and I wanted to know how to fix it.

Finally, I spoke up. I had to ask if anyone was "doing anything" about FPIES? Was there a nonprofit or research fund out there? Was anyone moving the needle forward on this disease? The next day, the Development Team at CHOP came to visit Landon's room and the next phase of our journey began.

A Light in the Dark Ages of FPIES

It started as a research fund, The FPIES United Family Fund, and I had no clue what I was doing. All I knew was that I wanted to make a difference, and there were other children and parents like us who were struggling daily without support. The Development Team helped me to craft a research page through CHOP and I turned to the FPIES groups on Facebook to share this initiative.

During the dark ages of FPIES, there were groups of parents banding together out of desperation and fear. We lived on Facebook in the wee hours of the night, in between feedings and vomiting sessions. We'd stay up chatting, comparing stories, sharing recipes and meal plans, and laughing and crying together. Up until this point, we didn't understand what FPIES meant; all we knew was that our children all had it and that there weren't any answers. I shared the FPIES United Family Fund in these groups and on my social media pages. My goal was to not only raise awareness, but to raise funds to advance FPIES.

When donations began pouring in to the FPIES United Family Fund, I met with the Chief of the Allergy Department at CHOP, Dr. Jonathan Spergel. I knew I wanted to create something big, something meaningful and something immediate. Dr. Spergel shared this vision and pledged his support to me. He became my biggest cheerleader and confidante in this journey. We worked cohesively and concisely to ensure that every patient and family had the support they deserved and to him I am forever grateful.

Dr. Spergel connected me with Beth Allen, the Founder of the American Partnership for Eosinophilic Disorders (APFED). APFED has a similar story to IFPIES. Beth is a mom who worked to champion eosinophilic esophagitis, the same disease I thought Landon had that led us to CHOP. Beth became my mentor, leading me through the logistics of starting a nonprofit. For a year, I listened and learned, researched and asked questions, and jumped in and backed out.

She and Dr. Spergel helped me to craft the structure of the organization with my wish list and needs assessment in mind. We identified the major societies and organizations to forge partnerships with selected the potential members of our Medical Advisory Board.

Spergel would become the first Medical Advisory Chair, and Beth became Chair of our Board of Trustees. With their help, influence, and support, the framework was in place to create what is now the International FPIES Association (IFPIES).

Our First Steps

Our first task was to create basic materials that could be disseminated to families and providers. We drafted a brochure and some handouts and utilized funding from the FPIES United Family Fund for some basic research. I relied on social media to keep families informed. As a result, many families began scheduling appointments to be seen at CHOP. There was a growing energy in the community, and families wanted to get involved. An executive board was formed with a group of FPIES mothers I had met along the way, and we each volunteered our time to launch the organization as the International Association for Food Protein Enterocolitis (IAFFPE) in September 2011. When Amity Westcott-Chavez, our current Vice President, joined the organization, she single-handedly catapulted us into new growth and development. Amity has two sons who were both diagnosed with FPIES. She had the same intense passion to create change but she was far more poised, succinct and deliberate in her execution. When we started to work together, we immediately recognized we were a dynamic team, I had a vision and she had the skill set and brilliance to bring it to fruition. We often jokingly refer to one another as "work wives" as we have had to build trust and reliance in once another to take on these tasks while caring for our families and working full-time. Amity has been a gift to IFPIES and is the reason it has succeeded in the way it has.

Seven years ago, I attended my first Annual Meeting of the American Academy of Allergy, Asthma and Immunology (AAAAI). This was the first time I met in person with many of the medical advisors who had agreed to pursue this mission. I was a nervous wreck. When we gathered, I shared my vision for the organization. I asked for their feedback and invited them to teach me all that they knew. I didn't hide my passions or my fears.

In the end, I have never felt more supported in my life, and I was blown away by their insights and perspectives. In the FPIES world, there is a great deal of frustration with doctors. Families are often turned away by the medical community, making this a parent-managed disease. To sit with a group of expert physicians who not only believed in this vision, but also shared in the frustrations, was magical. It was as if everything had aligned in these moments.

The rest of my first AAAAI Annual Meeting was another story. I sat at our booth trying to give out materials on FPIES to allergists, gastroenterologists and other conference attendees. I received a lot of backlash and negative feedback. "FPIES isn't real." "Do you know how rare that is?" "You're wasting your time." I knew then we had our work cut out for us, and it was going to take patience to convey our message, educate patients and the medical community, and make an impact. We needed an aggressive, methodical plan to voice the concerns and needs of the FPIES community and get the medical professionals' attention and commitment.

Bridging the Gaps

It was my son's own battle with FPIES that in many ways, crafted the agenda for IFPIES. He and I had experienced so much in those first 2 years without a diagnosis. I often jokingly say that we lived through every challenge FPIES could throw at us and we are still winning. But these challenges came with a great deal of suffering and a fight. Everything was a battle. From finding a diagnosis, to learning there was no treatment, to navigating elemental formula and food challenges, insurance coverage, passes and fails, expanding a very limited diet, and most of all, accepting that my son could not eat normally.

To make change happen, I needed the best of the best. I walked into the allergy world not knowing anyone. I had to draw on the sincerity of my mission to build the best team I could for our community. I needed to speak the language to properly advocate for these families, to gain the respect of the medical community, and to convince them to come on this journey with us.

First on my list was to unite patients and families with the medical community. This would become our organizations tagline: "Bridging the Gap between patient, family and provider." And for the first 2 years, that was our primary mission.

Without the medical community's support, families would never be heard or accomplish change. We had to work in unison. We had to look at FPIES realistically, together, and accept that while the current state of treatment was unacceptable, it could be changed.

This was often difficult for the FPIES patients and families to understand. Initially IFPIES was viewed as an organization that was provider-focused. I will admit, this was somewhat intentional. Without the medical community's support, we wouldn't have any success in moving the needle for FPIES. We had to build a strong foundation with the partnership of both providers and the food allergy community. This had to be done strategically and in stages to be effective. I was methodical about how I envisioned progress for our community.

I also needed to understand why providers could not offer solid guidance to their patients. The medical world is evidence based. When there is a lack of publications or research in any disorder, providers are simply not able to "guess" at treatment recommendations. A huge gap existed between the research and what was happening in the providers' offices. This was reflected in the many patients and families living without a diagnosis, treatment or guidance. I took the time to listen not only to the patients and families, but to the providers as well. I needed to understand both perspectives so we could marry the two and make real, impactful change.

Armed with knowledge, I started to meet individually with the published thought leaders and appealed to them to join our medical advisory board. I attended all of the allergy/immunology academy meetings, pleaded to attend any and all talks on FPIES, and snuck in meetings between presentations to connect with these providers one by one.

At one point, I was denied access to the only talk on FPIES being held during that meeting. I asked the speaker for admission; when denied, I stood outside listening through a crack in the door taking notes for the FPIES community until the speaker invited me in.

This presentation was an opportunity for our community to be heard, so I spoke up. A lot. I answered questions. I asked questions. I shared what it was really like for these families and these children. I challenged the accepted beliefs on FPIES and referenced the papers I had learned to quote inside and out. The speaker would later become one of our medical advisors. I became less afraid of being vocal and more interested in finding answers. I would no longer accept "we don't know" as an answer for FPIES.

Making FPIES Official

Having a separate, distinct ICD-10 code was crucial. The disease needed its own name and number. The code was also the only way to track prevalence—or how common the disorder is. The code would make FPIES official. I learned the process from APFED Founder Beth Allen, who had worked to get ICD-9 codes passed for eosinophilic disorders. Volunteers from the IFPIES Medical Advisory Board helped draft the medical information. I lead this initiative and submitted all the necessary paperwork, anxiously waiting for months for the CDC (Centers for Disease Control) to respond.

The CDC responded with an invitation to come speak at their annual meeting regarding a specific code for FPIES. I couldn't believe it. We advanced to the second round and were being offered the opportunity to present. Dr. Anna Nowak-Wegrzyn, our current Medical Chair, attended the meeting and spoke on the topic. She is responsible for most of the publications currently available on FPIES and has spearheaded nearly every major initiative on the disorder. During the CDC meeting, she spoke on the medical and research perspective of FPIES. I also spoke on the patient perspective.

Dr. Nowak delivered a brilliant presentation that led us to a public comment period. This meant, we had to wait while the public chimed in to support or decline our petition. Thousands of families wrote to the CDC in support and after a few weeks, I received a phone call from the CDC Director politely asking us to not send anymore letters of support, they had been flooded with letters and it was evident that this community would stop at nothing for their children.

Three months later, we received the final verdict. The ICD-10 code for FPIES is official; we passed unanimously. The FPIES community was now visible. I was so thrilled to share this news with our medical advisors who shared in this excitement. We had made a giant leap for FPIES.

This was our first lesson that a group of determined people could work hard toward a common goal and create real, impactful change. This experienced fueled my passion. From here we could start, from here we could grow.

Putting It in Print

The lack of literature on FPIES posed a significant issue for the patients and families living with the disorder. Time after time, families would return to the online boards after leaving their appointments with treatment plans that were not applicable. Some families could not even locate a provider in their area who had heard of FPIES, so they were forced to travel great distances to see a knowledgeable provider or rely on the Facebook groups for information and guidance. As a result, children were suffering. Our organization decided to shift focus and champion the motto, "Lack of awareness is 100% curable."

We knew we had to intervene in areas that were not being reached. But how could a small organization with no real funding engage the medical community? How could we generate answers or a plan for these families without the support of the medical community?

As it happens, providers were also looking for support. They were also frustrated with the lack of guidance to navigate FPIES and often had to rely solely on their own clinical experiences with patients. Providers wanted answers just as much as parents did, and they were open and honest about this with me during our meetings. All these questions created a confusing time in FPIES. It became apparent that to address these issues, we would need to increase publications on FPIES.

With this in mind, our organization set out to examine the needs of the FPIES community. First, we looked at quality of life for FPIES patients. The findings were compelling. Compared to traditional food allergy, FPIES patients reported a significantly worsened quality of life. This made sense given the fact that there were no established diagnostic or treatment guidelines, leaving families to manage this disorder largely on their own.

Next, we needed to define acute versus chronic FPIES. At the time, there was great controversy in the medical community about whether chronic FPIES even existed, which often led to dismissal of patient reports. This was creating a real panic in the community, with many families being turned away for help, and in some cases, even being accused of Munchausen by proxy, a psychiatric disorder in which parents fabricate their children's symptoms for attention. These were not isolated incidents. These claims were happening more and more within the community and there were even reports of children being taken from their parents due to physician disbelief. I would share these stories at the academy meetings and with the IFPIES Medical Advisory Board. We all came to a consensus that the literature did not adequately reflect or address the needs of the community and there was an urgent need to remedy this.

During conference calls, I discussed these gaps with our dedicated medical advisors. Through our insightful conversations, we outlined the needs and from these needs, we crafted ways to increase publications. What sets IFPIES apart from other organizations is that our team members are not only experts, published researchers, and world-renowned clinicians, but they have deep passion and sincerity for this cause, which is evident in all they have done for our organization.

IFPIES has a true partnership with our medical community and a commitment to work tirelessly on behalf of these patients and families. There is a real commitment to find answers and improve lives. Every initiative we have completed together has been accomplished on donated time, after work hours, and in the spirit of the IFPIES mission, vision, and values.

Since our organization was founded, publications on FPIES have expanded dramatically. From 2010 to this writing, 123 articles were published on FPIES. Compare this to just 19 articles on FPIES published between 2000 and 2009. That is expansive growth for a rare disorder that was not even official on paper until passage of the ICD-10 code in 2013.

These accomplishments have a direct impact on FPIES patients and families and also work to support and inform providers. Further, they have demonstrated the value of evidence-based practice and have called attention to the gaps that exist in the literature. We have built this organization for growth and will continue to expand research and support publications that reflect the true needs of the FPIES community.

The FPIES Guidelines: A Clinical Compass

To mark our third anniversary in September 2014, the organization launched an exciting new chapter with a more streamlined name as the International FPIES Association (I-FPIES). During this time, we had also taken on our largest initiative to date: the publication of the "International Consensus for the Diagnosis and Treatment of Food Protein-Induced Enterocolitis Syndrome."

This was a 3-year project for our organization, led by Drs. Anna Nowak-Wegrzyn and Matthew Greenhawt. We invited over 40 FPIES experts across the globe to help define FPIES and to provide a framework for providers and families. Each provider was hand-selected by IFPIES for their expertise and ability to see large cohorts of FPIES patients.

Our aim was to examine FPIES as a whole and remove any preconceived ideas we had so FPIES could be openly and objectively evaluated in its present form. We all lived in different time zones and the initial work that needed to be accomplished was daunting. Over 900 citations had to be combed through for their relevance to FPIES. This was no easy feat. It took 1 year of work just evaluating the literature. We held only two face-to-face meetings at two consecutive Annual Meetings of the American Academy of Allergy, Asthma and Immunology annual meeting. During that first meeting in 2014, we shaped our master outline and delegated assignments. At our next meeting in 2015, we planned how we would compile, edit, and publish what would become the largest publication ever on FPIES.

As the IFPIES representative and sole layperson, I fought for the inclusion of acute and chronic FPIES. It was an incredible experience to be heard among the experts and have the parent perspective valued and incorporated into these guidelines. Sometimes, I was very vocal and relentless. Other times, I sat back to learn and understand the medical perspective, which yielded amazing findings.

Together, we learned that the first foods of introduction in each country were the most common triggers in that country. That gave us clues into the pathophysiology of FPIES, which would give us a productive and fruitful outline for research needs. Uncovering one of the basic principles of FPIES was one of the most exciting experiences not only in my FPIES journey, but in my lifetime.

In the end, we created a 99-page document that serves as a go-to reference for the diagnosis and management of FPIES. I knew we had accomplished something big and life-changing for patients living with this once invisible food allergy. As a group, we were writing the history of this disorder, and the guidelines would serve as a jumping off point for the organization's future initiatives.

The next hurdle was to make the guidelines accessible to everyone, not just medical providers. I asked for a quote to have them published open access. When the quote came back $60,000, I felt deflated. As a volunteer-run organization, funding is extremely limited. We rely on donor funding for many of our initiatives, and many of our potential donors are financially challenged by the costs of caring for their children.

I couldn't accept this. We had an answer within reach that would directly and positively impact the patients living with this disorder. I called on our medical advisors to rally with me to request a reduction in the quote. Together and separately, we held meetings with the decision makers. We were relentless. In a few weeks, we learned that the guidelines would be published, open access, free of charge. All 99 pages. Three years of hard work, determination, and answers for the FPIES community are now available to everyone who needs them through *The Journal of Allergy and Clinical Immunology* [1].

May the Fourth be with you

Many of our initiatives have been the direct result of parent advocacy and involvement. National FPIES Awareness Day is a wonderful example. Our organization has been blessed with some of the most amazing volunteers over the years. One thing every volunteer has shared is a determination for change based on their child's own journey with FPIES. This is certainly true for Christine Quigley.

Christine is mother to Connor, a beautiful little boy who suffered greatly with FPIES for many years. He went months without food, and Christine fought as his advocate through many food reactions and little progress. She, too, turned to the internet looking for answers and evaluating ways to manage FPIES.

I got to know Christine and Connor well, and she was deeply frustrated with the lack of support and guidance in FPIES. "What foods do I trial? Why can't anyone tell me what will be safe for my son to eat? Who is addressing nutritional needs and ways to promote a healthy gut?" On our phone calls, I heard a desperation in her voice that was oh-so-familiar. I knew we needed this amazing woman on board with IFPIES.

Christine made it her mission to raise awareness of FPIES. As an IFPIES volunteer, she petitioned the US Congress in 2015 for a national awareness day. She partnered with a lobbyist to find bipartisan support for this bill. After meeting with FPIES families and hearing their stories, Senators Cory Booker (D-NJ) and Patrick Toomey (R-PA) agreed to cosponsor this bill and advocate for its passage in Congress. More than 1000 supporters joined IFPIES' national campaign by signing and sharing the I-FPIES petition to make this day official, and countless others sent letters of support that detailed their own struggles with FPIES.

Within 6 months, we had a day to call our own. This is one of many shining examples of the power and unity of the FPIES community. Four years prior, a diagnosis code did not even exist for FPIES. A mother on a mission, determined to make her son's disease known, moved the US Congress to officially recognize May fourth as National FPIES Awareness Day.

In May of 2018, we celebrated the fourth annual National FPIES Awareness Day as a community. Celebrated? Yes! Every year we celebrate that we have created change. We celebrate those who have outgrown FPIES and those still bravely in the thick of the fight. We celebrate the caregivers who weather the storms of FPIES and let the sun shine on its victories.

With FPIES like so many other conditions, the answers only begin to emerge with increased awareness. National FPIES Awareness day is also a time to call attention to the needs of the community. What better time is there to teach others who may be indirectly impacted by FPIES in the hopes they can keep our children safe? The day also honors the medical professionals who fight tirelessly on our behalf, and recognizes that we are no longer invisible, crazy parents with children suffering from a mysterious food virus. As a community, we have arrived, but we won't stop until all FPIES patients worldwide have what they need to have the best possible quality of life.

A Community, a Conference

Hosting the FPIES Education Conferences are truly the best days we have had at IFPIES. There is something so incredible and poignant about seeing so many FPIES families together in one space. As volunteer conference organizers who pull together these events on a shoestring budget, there is nothing more gratifying than to witness the "a ha" moments, see the bonds of shared experience, and send families home with a feeling of empowerment and hope.

At our first conference held at the Children's Hospital of Philadelphia in 2013, FPIES was still in its embryotic phase, and there wasn't much data or evidence to provide to our attendees about how to navigate this disorder. That did not affect the power of the day. It was the first time a large group of FPIES families were all in one room.

It was the first time our medical advisors had a chance to directly educate and interact with an audience of families—and they came away learning just as much as the attendees. We set out to provide the families with access to the experts, and we ended up igniting a passion in the providers to do more.

At the close of that first conference, I spoke with parents who had come to the conference completed deflated by FPIES. They left with new sense of purpose, a charge to keep going, and a feeling that they could do this. Our conferences are crafted to educate, but more importantly, to empower these parents.

Something happens every time we host a conference that is simply inspiring. You can see the shackles lifted. You can see the sadness being replaced by a fuel to fight. Over the last 7 years, we have hosted three national conferences. Attendees come from all over the country and even outside of the USA. Our speakers donate their time and develop presentations to meet the needs of the families. Attendees can interact with the leading experts in a supportive environment and learn to advocate for their children in a way that produces positive outcomes.

Ultimately, our wish list is to have 2-day conferences in multiple areas across the USA and internationally because the need is so great. The conference agenda is created by surveying families directly. With the increase in publications, resources, and understanding of FPIES over the years, the needs and topics have shifted. We can see the difference in the newcomers each conference. They are more educated, they are diagnosed, they are inquisitive, and they ask in-depth questions. As an organization, we are witnessing the impact of the progress on FPIES, and this motivates us to continue pushing forward.

The First FPIES Center

While online resources were becoming more plentiful and online support communities flourished, FPIES still needed a place to call home. It needed a hub that patients could come to for a plan and providers could reference or connect with for questions and expertise.

During our early days as the FPIES United Family Fund, our community raised money for the Children's Hospital of Philadelphia (CHOP), which is where our organization first started. The funds the FPIES community had raised were used in part to create the first and only FPIES Center in the world at CHOP in 2014 with allergy and nutrition, and 2016 with allergy, gastroenterology and nutrition.

My son had been diagnosed at CHOP at 2 years old after suffering over 20 acute and chronic reactions. It was honestly the worst time of my life. After 2 years and 8–10 specialists, it took CHOP only 10 minutes to diagnose my son.

With a diagnosis had come hope, as the broken pieces of what he had been experiencing were finally coming together. Prior to diagnosis, I had been dismissed at every turn, even accused of making up my son's symptoms, and I was desperate to find a physician who could help. Help came in the form of Dr. Terri Brown-Whitehorn, who is now the Director of the FPIES Center at CHOP.

Currently, the FPIES Center has an allergist, gastroenterologist and registered dietitian on staff who work together in best interests of FPIES patients. The International FPIES Association has always advocated for collaborative care as we saw the positive impact this had on the patients and families. Those who were fortunate enough to gain access to collaborative care seemed to be the patients and families who had the most success.

Because FPIES can be so tricky, our experts often learned that what we thought was FPIES was another condition entirely or another condition layered on top of FPIES. Initially, this was very difficult for our community to process because FPIES alone seemed too much. This is where the FPIES Center comes in. It is a hub for all patients and families and a support for all providers. It is a vision we shared as an organization, born from a group of parents who all experienced the confusion and complexity of FPIES. It's been a dream that Dr. Brown, Dr. Spergel, and I have shared and a service we urgently wanted to provide the community.

In upcoming years, it is our hope to expand the FPIES Center model into multiple centers across the globe and to utilize the CHOP FPIES Center as a pilot for these centers. We want every family to have access to collaborative care and the experts specializing in FPIES. We want providers, new and seasoned, to have a connection to FPIES patients that will yield answers and guidance that will lead to the empowerment of our patients and families. Ultimately, it is our hope that these centers will someday champion a cure.

Forming Partnerships

I-FPIES partners with national and international health organizations and the major medical societies and academies to get the word out about FPIES and share resources.

Since 2012, IFPIES has been a recognized lay organization with the American Academy and College of Allergy, Asthma, and Immunology (AAAAI). We have also worked in partnership with the American Academy of Pediatrics and are referenced as a go-to resource for credible information on FPIES. While many of the initiatives have been driven by IFPIES, our participation with these organizations is crucial to the advancement of FPIES.

Each year, we exhibit at AAAAI Annual Meeting and provide resources and educational materials to thousands of providers from across the globe. I have also had the privilege of becoming a member and faculty speaker at these conferences. In 2017, I was asked to give a talk on "The Burden of FPIES." This talk was special to me because it was the first opportunity for many providers to truly understand what it is like to live with FPIES. I spent a few months preparing my presentation because I wanted to deliver a compelling message: "All families need support and validation of their struggles."

While giving my talk, I remember looking out into the audience and seeing providers who were moved. Some were in tears; others nodded their heads in agreement, while others fervently took notes. It was the first time that the gaps in the FPIES treatment plan and the difficulty of implementing treatment recommendations were highlighted. I firmly believe that to be successful clinically, we must also address the practical needs of the patient. This led me to call for action within AAAAI's Adverse Reactions to Food Committee to included practical management consideration in all FPIES treatment plans.

I have been honored to travel abroad to give similar talks and to conduct educational webinars for providers who have seen FPIES patients but who may not have a thorough understanding of the challenges they face. It is something that I am deeply passionate about. I feel that it has been a blessing to many burdens.

As an organization, we deliver a message of empowerment and teach both families and providers effective ways to navigate the pitfalls of living with FPIES. Based on practical experience, we have created unique ways to manage this disorder and have made it our mission to share this knowledge and create a sense of empowerment within our community.

I have made it my life's work to advocate on behalf of the estimated 1000,000 individuals living with FPIES and to deliver their message to providers so that we can find solutions. By working in the trenches with families and connecting directly with providers at these conferences, I've become keenly aware of the gaps and needs that exist on both ends. Having the ability to speak at medical conferences, with no medical degree, has been a responsibility I take very seriously. I have learned that all it takes is a few minutes to initiate change, awareness, and growth.

As the "new kid on the block," I've been so appreciative of the support and generosity our organization has received from the food allergy community. It truly is a community of inclusion. More so than ever before, non-IgE allergies like FPIES are being included in the broader dialogue on food allergy. The "unknown" food allergy is quickly becoming known with the continued expansion of educational resources, research studies, and global outreach and awareness.

Going Global

Our reach has expanded since we became an international organization in 2012. From the beginning, our goal has been to create global consistency in FPIES. After all, we represent EVERY patient and EVERY provider.

FPIES has its unique challenges in that it behaves differently in different countries. As we learned when we worked on the guidelines, there were clues to be found when working with our international partners. I slowly began to explore the international FPIES pages online and evaluated the needs in these different countries. Some of the challenges were similar to the USA, but many countries had different structures in place for access to care, emergency care, and treatment recommendations.

In recent years, I began to connect online with international advocates who were trying to spearhead change in their respective countries. As an organization, we developed a plan for international chapters that would link into our main organization and our medical advisors and would channel back the needs within the country represented. A prime example is our interaction with the FPIES Brazil Chapter, led by Renato Aschar. As a father to a daughter with FPIES, Renato had great frustration with the lack of knowledgeable providers and access to care and guidance for FPIES patients in Brazil. He and I began to discuss the needs of the Brazilian FPIES patients and families.

When Renato traveled to meet me at the Annual Meeting of the American Academy of Allergy, Asthma and Immunology, I was inspired by his dedication, his eagerness to learn and his ability to make connections with others. We discussed how IFPIES has tackled some of the US-based issues, which he then replicated and adapted for his country. He formed a medical advisory board and he translated materials and disseminated them throughout the Brazil. He met with many providers and educated them about FPIES. He continues to make a difference in his country.

Our relationship with Renato and FPIES Brazil embodies the spirit of partnership and collaboration that runs throughout our organization. Families across the globe have access to support thanks to people like Renato and our other volunteers who work selflessly and with compassion to make FPIES known. We have created several chapters of IFPIES in multiple countries around the world. In addition, our medical advisory board is comprised of national and international experts who connect globally to support their peers.

The International FPIES Association's mission is to create and implement FPIES awareness campaigns and support channels in all countries where access to information about FPIES is critically lacking. After all, awareness is an integral part of diagnosing this condition, and an early diagnosis can make a huge difference in the battle against FPIES.

Funding Research to Unlock the Answers

- It is the dream of IFPIES to fund research that will ultimately lead to a cure. However, getting research funded is a global difficulty. Across the board, there is limited funding and high demand. In FPIES, the opportunities for funding are even more difficult. We do not have a treatment. We do not have prevalence data to establish how common the disease is. We do not have funding sources like the

National Institute of Health because most of our children will outgrow FPIES. That means we have to be creative in how we tackle and expand research into FPIES.

Much of the research that has been conducted or funded by IFPIES has been administered through surveys. Through this means, we have called attention to key topics that significantly impact our patient and families, including quality of life, acute vs. chronic FPIES and the psychosocial aspects of living with FPIES. Several of these surveys were conducted at our three FPIES Education Conferences, as well as through online participated by the FPIES community. We are fortunate to have providers and researchers who are willing to conduct these surveys with the goal to increase publications and awareness. These studies are also performed to gain a greater insight into how FPIES behaves and impacts patients and families. But to truly advance FPIES, we need to advance research in a much bigger way.

As an organization, we have created a needs assessment and have methodically structured our research initiatives to yield results with limited funding. Our first initiative was to encourage our providers to publish case studies to demonstrate the presentation of FPIES and to highlight that any food could cause a reaction. It was awareness-based research in the formative years that was necessary to interest the providers and represent the community. Since our founding, publications on FPIES have increased dramatically. Between 2010 and 2015, 99 articles were published on FPIES, with 66 of those publications featuring an IFPIES medical advisor.

Once we laid the groundwork, we were able to start looking more deeply into FPIES and pair our research goals with our other initiatives. For example, to study how common FPIES is, we first had to create an ICD-10 code. Over time, the utilization of this code will yield free data to use for prevalence information. We have had to think outside the box to study this disorder so that while we have sparse funding, we are still moving the needle to be able to obtain larger scale funding in the future.

The first few studies challenged the idea that FPIES was ultra-rare. We did this by encouraging our providers to assess their patient data and publish the data they found. When CHOP evaluated data from its FPIES patient database, they were astonished at the findings. They were seeing far more FPIES patients than expected. Most patients reported one or two triggers, but the next most common report was 6+ triggers. These types of findings began to generate a buzz around FPIES at the medical conferences and put the disorder on the map in the world of food allergy. The studies began to reflect the real-life experiences that patients and families faced. The parent was no longer seen as crazy or anxious, and the child was no longer misrepresented in the literature. It was no longer accepted that there were only two types of food allergic conditions: IgE and eosinophilic. There was this other food allergic condition called FPIES that was delayed, understudied, and in great need of awareness. We had finally begun to bring FPIES on par with other food allergic disorders.

As our most recent effort, IFPIES is funding our first major study looking into the pathophysiology and genetics of FPIES. In true IFPIES spirit, this study is multicultural and is being conducted internationally with two centers in two different countries participating. It is our hope that this study may identify a genetic marker that could be further studied and lead to a diagnostic tool for FPIES. It is also important that we finally uncover the true pathophysiology of FPIES so that biomarkers—or measurable indicators of the disorder—can be identified.

This is the promise of FPIES research. It is not a shot in the dark. We are extremely selective and purposeful with our funding. We are intentional with our initiatives and spend every dollar to have the greatest impact for the FPIES community.

Food trials can be a traumatizing experience filled with multiple obstacles and residual aftermath. The more we are learning about FPIES, the more we are recognizing that it can be a chronic condition that snowballs into other challenges: feeding therapy, emotional support, financial burden, poor quality of life. These are only a few of the lingering post-reaction issues that impact patients and families.

Imagine a world where a patient does not have to trial a food and risk having a reaction to determine if it is safe or not. The answers lie in the research, which is why it is a cornerstone of our organization. As we move toward our first decade of supporting families and providers, IFPIES will dive deeper into research needs and apply what we learn to practical care. We know in research we will find the answers.

The Invisible Made Visible

I am often asked if I plan to run this organization forever. I usually laugh because I didn't think I would be running an organization at all. I also never imagined I would have a child born with a puzzling disorder and the assorted hurdles it has presented. I know in my heart that I would be forever restless if I didn't try and fight as hard as I could to prevent another family from the experiences we have had. Leading this organization has been one of the greatest pleasures of my life.

FPIES has been a struggle, but it has also been a blessing. I have learned so much, and it has created a bond between my son and I that words cannot explain. The trust and security we have in one another, born from the experiences he has endured, are unlike any other.

The relationships we have built and the unbelievably strong and brilliant people we have met along the way have changed us as individuals and reshaped our FPIES experience. My hope is that IFPIES can be that for someone else. My hope is that our organization can not only empower and educate, but also heal and inspire. To know that FPIES is now recognized and credible information is widely available that makes all the sadness, confusion, anxiety, and fighting worth it. No one will ever have to live in the "dark ages" of FPIES again.

The dedicated team that has volunteered their time and talents to grow this organization won't ever allow it to give up. IFPIES started as a band of warrior mothers who refused to give up. Today, we are a group of moms and dads who know what it is like to hold our children in shock, to have many sleepless nights in fear and worry, and who believe that a better future is possible. Some have children who outgrew

FPIES years ago, yet their commitment to helping families still in the thick of FPIES is unwavering. We all have seen that with hard work and determination, we CAN make change.

We can move the needle forward. We can get to a place where this is manageable, and we can live meaningful and engaging lives with FPIES. The International FPIES Association will keep working until there is a diagnostic tool, until there is a treatment. We will continue to educate, empower, and support our families through their hardships and their successes. We will continue to represent the patient, family, and provider. We will continue to educate ourselves so that we can be productive advocates on behalf of our community and be a safe place for them to lean on. We will be fierce when called for and gentle when needed. We will never turn away anyone who needs support. We won't stop fighting until there is a cure.

FPIES has been set on fire. In many ways, it is a torch. It is the food allergy that is increasing in prevalence, is growing in awareness, and is being acknowledged across the globe. There is still so much to do, but we have solid groundwork to build upon. I hope that our children's children will not know of FPIES. I hope that 10 years from now, we will all look back and say, "Remember when?"

Key Points

The International FPIES Association (I-FPIES) is a non-profit patient organization dedicated to advancing the awareness and understanding of food protein-induced enterocolitis syndrome (FPIES) while promoting and addressing the needs of patients with FPIES and their families.

Like many other families living with FPIES, I-FPIES Founder Fallon Schultz Matney went through a long, confusing struggle to diagnose her son Landon. The organization was founded in 2011 to establish a formal channel of support and information for families, as well as increase education and awareness in the global medical community.

The organization's accomplishments include the approval of an ICD-10 code specific to FPIES, the publication of the first international consensus guidelines for FPIES, passage of a resolution by the US Congress declaring a National FPIES Awareness Day, and support of groundbreaking research on quality of life, pathophysiology, and genetics.

Acknowledgment/Thanks Writing a chapter is harder than I thought and more rewarding than I could have ever imagined. None of this would have been possible without the support of my work wife and Vice President of IFPIES, Amity Chavez. She has been the brain behind this organization and has stood by me during every struggle and success. Amity is the real backbone to IFPIES and so much more to me than she will ever know.

Dedication

- To the believers (and the doubters): Thank you for shaping this beautiful organization into what it is today. May you always know your worth, your importance, and your impact on the lives you touch; and the eternal gratitude I have for you.
- To my fellow mothers...Always know you are not alone, you have a hand in me. You WILL make it through.
- To my son, Landon, my fearless rebel who has united and inspired a community out of your personal struggle and boundless resilience...Being your mother has been my life's greatest honor. You were born to change the world, and I promise I will never stop fighting for you.

Reference

1. Nowak-Wegrzyn A, Chehade M, Groetch ME, Spergel JM, Wood RA, Allen K, Atkins D, Bahna S, Barad A, Berin C, Burks AW, Caubet JC, Chavez A, Cianferoni A, Conte M, Davis C, Fiocchi A, Grimshaw K, Gupta R, Hofmeister B, Hwang JB, Katz Y, Konstantinou G, Lightdale J, McGhee S, Mehr S, Micelli Sopo S, Monti G, Muraro A, Noel S, Nomura I, Noone S, Sampson HA, Schultz F, Sicherer SH, Thompson C, Turner P, Venter C, Whitehorn-Brown T, Greenhawt M. International consensus guidelines for the diagnosis and management of food protein-induced enterocolitis syndrome: executive summary—workgroup report of the adverse reactions to foods committee, American Academy of Allergy, Asthma & Immunology. J Allergy Clin Immunol. 2017;139:1111–26.

Food Protein-Induced Enterocolitis Syndrome: A Healthcare Professional Parent Perspective

15

Maria S. White

Chow, fare, nosh, edibles, grub, nutriment, snack, or eats, the word *food* can go by many names. Merriam-Webster [1] defines *food* as "a material consisting essentially of protein, carbohydrate, and fat used in the body of an organism to sustain growth, repair, and vital processes and to furnish energy." When consuming food, do we reflect on "the necessity to sustain growth, repair, and vital processes" with each meal consumption? Possibly, we do reflect on this when we are trying "to eat healthy." Do we consider the details of protein involvement and breakdown on the molecular level in what we consume to satisfy our nutritional needs? We probably do not.

The nomenclature and idea of food in everyday life can be strongly shaped by culture. Some cultures are food-centric. Others may not be. My culture is food-centric. Food and it's timing, also known as our meals, strongly shape my Italian and Polish ethnicity-based notion of food. My family is finishing one meal and already discussing the next. My Polish aunt or *ciocia* is already prepping the place setting for lunch shortly after breakfast is cleaned up. Food is a way of life. We "live to eat." However, over the past 18 months, "eating to live" brought a whole new perspective into my family's life. Food started making one of us sick, and we could not figure out why. The following will discuss my family's journey leading to and through a diagnosis of food protein-induced enterocolitis syndrome (FPIES). Perspectives below not only come from a mother of a child with FPIES but also a seasoned adult critical care nurse and an academic nurse educator.

M. S. White (✉)
Wilmington, DE, USA

T. F. Brown-Whitehorn, A. Cianferoni (eds.), *Food Protein Induced Enterocolitis (FPIES)*,
https://doi.org/10.1007/978-3-030-21229-2_15

Life Before FPIES

I was determined to make all of my children flexible eaters and not to be picky. I was aggressive in solid food trials with my oldest child, mindful of what I gave him, read books on what food to trial first based on color and taste, and made food fun. Feeding and eating were fun. My oldest was fed breast milk without formula supplementation until his first birthday when it was time to transition to whole milk. He did great with solid food trials, and 3.5 years later, he is one hearty eater.

Baby number two came 22 months later after the firstborn. I was determined to breastfeed baby number two the same length of time and initiate food introduction like I did with my oldest child. Here is where the challenges came, solid food introduction. Meet DJ. He is a blue-eyed, bubbly, mellow-mannered yet persistent, resilient 2-year-old little warrior. He is my secondborn who is growing on the 50th percentile of the growth curve, has adorable plump cheeks, and is extremely active. DJ loves to eat, play with trucks and his older brother, read books, and cook on his red Little Tikes kitchen set. I could see his future enrolling in culinary school because of his love for play cooking and food at an early age. However, DJ did not always have a great relationship with food.

Pre-diagnosis of FPIES

DJ, like my oldest child, was exclusively breastfed without formula supplementation. Around month 4.5, it was time to start teaching him how to eat solid pureed food. I was so excited about making my next child a flexible foodie and enjoy the beauty and flavors of food. It started with a popular brand of infant rice cereal. First serving went great. He tongued a majority of it out, but he was learning a new texture. I was excited for him. I put DJ down for his nap an hour or so later. Our aunt said he spit up in bed and slept a bit longer than his normal nap time frame. We thought nothing of this as my oldest often spit up without concern. Day 2 trial was quite a different experience. DJ started violently vomiting 2.5 hours after he consumed the rice cereal. He wretched to the point of vomiting bile, a yellow-green-tinged clear fluid of digestive enzymes. He looked pale. He was sluggish and cool to touch. I was terrified and so was my husband. With my clinical nurse background, I knew I had to be calm, so I did not send anyone else in my house into a panic. My husband cuddled him. My nurse mode turned on, and in my mind, I am thinking: identify the underlying cause. What were the causative factors with the process of elimination? Was this a bad container of infant cereal since he vomited 2 days in a row after eating? Later that day, he had a strange mucus-like diarrhea that resolved within 24 hours. Once our little guy was settled and symptoms resolved, I ran to the local store to pick up another container of the same brand of rice cereal. Day 3 trialing rice cereal with the same brand but different container resulted in the same result or "reaction." My husband, mother, and I did not know what to do. He, again, vomited so frequently to the point of bile and was sluggish, pale, and cool to the touch. I immediately called our pediatrician's office for guidance and was told to monitor him. The nurse said it could be a GI bug, he is probably tired from the vomiting, and must be given Pedialyte; if the vomiting persists over the next day or two, call back for an appointment. We held off rice cereal for 2 days. Fourth attempt of rice cereal with a different brand and he had the same symptoms. We saw a pediatrician the next day with a possible diagnosis of reflux. I was specifically told not to use the word "lethargic" because in the pediatric population, it had neurologic implications. Well, yes, of course it has neurologic implications. I am an adult trauma critical care nurse. Talk to me about lethargy all day. The provider prescribed ranitidine and told us to give DJ's belly a rest from rice cereal for 2 days, stop rice cereal if reaction occurred again, and see a GI specialist. No way did I think this was reflux. Nursing school 101 or even life 101 trigger-reaction pattern was happening. I could not understand the mechanism of action here. The same thing happened with the fifth exposure to rice cereal. We cuddled DJ and called the nurse on-call, and the nurse told us the same thing. If a fever emerged or symptoms persisted or he had a decrease in wet diapers, we will schedule an appointment. I advocated for an appointment with GI. We did not give rice cereal again and held off on solids for 2 weeks until the GI appointment.

This GI specialist or pediatrician who specialized in GI cases was the answer to my prayers. He sat down and took the time to hear me, let me discuss my concerns, and focused on minute details that could have potentially been causal factors. He illustrated a plan of continued food introduction with a possible allergy consult if symptoms continued.

My husband, aunt, and I were primary caregivers of DJ, who next began an oat trial. After the sixth time the food was given to him, it became more and more difficult to feed him. He would clamp his mouth shut and turn his head. In retrospect, it was almost a Pavlovian conditioning with DJ having this innate sense that if he ate, food was going to make him sick. We carried on trialing foods for 4 days and calling them clear until DJ had blood-streaked mucus stool and vomited 2 hours after eating apples and oats mixed. We saw a pediatrician the next day, and an abdominal X-ray was done. The sick visit doctor stated he palpated a possible mass and just wanted to be sure it was nothing. Abdominal X-ray was negative. We gave apples without issues and were advised to have an allergy consult. We continued with more food trials. We gave DJ sweet potatoes on the fifth attempt with other pureed food trials in the interim. DJ had an identical reaction to sweet potatoes to that he had to the rice cereal. I called the GI specialist for a follow-up visit discussing DJ's reactions to other foods.

Diagnosis of FPIES

I sat on my iPhone and laptop for hours those few weeks trying to put the puzzle pieces together. I researched for "infant vomiting 2.5 hours after eating." Then, FPIES came up, food protein-induced enterocolitis syndrome. What on earth is this? I read more and more formulating differential diagnoses: infection, contaminated container, malrotation of the bowel, food allergy, grain intolerance, etc.

Nothing fit like FPIES did. I was sick to my stomach and could not wait to meet with the GI specialist again.

The GI specialist was the same GI provider we met with when symptoms first commenced. Again, he interviewed me, took the time to listen, and asked about every detail of the food behavior patterns, ingestions, and sequelae thereof. He suggested doing a barium swallow to rule out a volvulus due to bowel malrotation. I sat back in my seat the entire visit waiting for the appropriate time to interject about my suspicions. In healthcare, it is walking a fine line when challenging a provider. It is really important when inquiring to do so in a respectful manner where you are not questioning their judgment, but also advocating your thoughts and concerns from your own research. I have professionally challenged many providers in my years of nursing to advocate for my patients. This is my son. Why was this so difficult for me to do that day? At the end of the visit, I respectfully worked through my summary and differential diagnoses. "I just want to make sure I am understanding why we are crossing things off the list. Can I run a few things by you? It was not condition X because Y, correct? It was not condition A because of symptom B, correct?" Finally, I brought up FPIES. "What are your feelings about FPIES—food protein-induced enterocolitis syndrome?" He paused. I paused and then proceeded to discuss how I did a literature review that yielded exclusively breastfed infants are inclined to have a later-in-life diagnosis. This is because the syndrome is identified when solid food introduction occurs, which is not until 5–6 months of age or later. He paused again. DJ fit the criteria. You can see the in-depth contemplation and analysis of the situation on the GI specialist's face. He turned to me and said, "You may be right." I exhaled. He stated, "I think you are on to something here. I would like to proceed with the barium swallow to rule out a volvulus because that can be an emergent situation. If all is clear, the FPIES route is our next course of action."

We walked right over to the radiology department because the GI specialist ordered the barium swallow. I was on edge the entire time; I had to feed my little guy the dosed barium as they imaged his belly. As a bedside nurse, whenever I needed to control my emotions and be strong, I said Hail Marys, a type of Catholic prayer, in my head repeatedly. I repeatedly said these prayers the entire time in the X-ray room. At the end of the diagnostic test, the radiologist came to speak with me. I will never forget how the radiologist made me feel that day. He asked me why we were there. I described DJ's symptoms including lethargy and vomiting bile. The radiologist looked at me and said, "Your child cannot be vomiting bile. That is not physiologically possible. We need to be very careful when we say lethargic when describing your son's condition." I wanted to scream and tell him the challenges over the past few weeks, my level of education, healthcare experience, and training. Yes, my kid was lethargic and indeed vomiting bile. The barium swallow was negative. The next day, a diagnosis of FPIES was made.

The GI specialist who diagnosed DJ deserves immense accolades for how he handled our situation. The finesse, respect, "bedside manner," and intelligence of this man cannot be commended enough. He was in tune with how to speak with families, phenomenal with children, and one of the most important things was he was humble enough to listen and adjust his professional judgment based on my concerns. We as healthcare professionals can be so wrapped up in the day-to-day tasks that it is easy to forget the foundation of our professional training, which is to *listen to our patients*. They provide us with pertinent information that may be inadvertently omitted or not examined.

I experienced two very crucial things that day. If I could provide any feedback to any healthcare professional colleagues regardless of the discipline, it would be this: listen and do not dismiss your patients' and their families' concerns. The GI specialist knew I was a critical care nurse, yet he still gave me the same respect that he did prior to finding out my healthcare background. The radiologist talked down to me as though I was an uneducated incompetent family member who had no idea what I was talking about. Listen, explain simply in nonmedical jargon, and address the concerns of patients and families.

Post-diagnosis of FPIES

My husband and I received the phone call the next day from the GI specialist explaining the next steps and to seek an allergy consult. We continued with food trials, had an emergency letter to take to the local emergency department in the event DJ had another reaction, and awaited the allergy appointment. I felt relief in a very strange way. I cried because of the diagnosis, but also because the fear of the unknown was uplifted.

We continued with fruit and vegetable trials per the GI specialist and then saw the allergist a week or so later. She asked me if I was in healthcare because of the way I articulated DJ's story. I did tell her my background but reiterated how I have no experience in pediatrics and am just trying to be an educated mom here. She appeared nervous and disheveled, maybe she was new? She was also kind, empathetic, and listened to the whole story. However, I had a list of questions on where to go next, and she waffled back and forth with her responses. She printed out the entire excerpt of FPIES, Up-To-Date, a medical reference resource and handed it to me. I clearly read this cover-to-cover prior to coming to the visit, and this woman told me nothing new or illustrated a definitive plan moving forward. Maybe try this or maybe try that was not good enough for me.

After the appointment, I researched the leading FPIES clinicians on the East Coast and came across the FPIES clinic at a leading children's hospital in my area and in the country. Until, I had a confirmed appointment, I transitioned DJ's allergy care to this metropolitan institution. This metropolitan healthcare system was incredible. I will never forget that first appointment we had with this interdisciplinary team. DJ had an appointment at an FPIES clinic. If warranted, there was the opportunity to meet with an allergist, dietician, and gastroenterologist all in the same visit. I could not believe it. This was an amazing integration of an interdisciplinary team that truly conformed to the convenience of the patient while producing a seamless continuity of care. My son did not need a visit with the gastroenterologist. We saw the allergist and dietician. We left that appointment with a food trial plan of action, recipes and ideas on how to trial food, another emergency letter, and an immense sense of relief. DJ has/had four triggers—rice, oat, sweet potato, and beef—all with the "classic" acute FPIES reaction: vomiting, lethargy, pallor, cool to touch, and mucus diarrhea within 24 hours of the reaction. Many struggles can surface if a patient, especially a child with a chronic condition, is not well managed. The struggles that surfaced for us impacted family dynamics, food trialing, and parental anxiety which will be discussed below.

Management of a Chronic Condition

Many challenges arise from the management of a child with a chronic condition. I would cry often to my mother about what I was going through. Why did this happen to me? She would be empathetic yet always put the situation into perspective. She would gently say to me, "When you go to that FPIES clinic, look around and take a minute to reflect about your journey with DJ. There are children and parents in that world-renowned institution in much more challenging situations than DJ." She was right. She did not minimize what my husband and I were going through but really made me reflect, adapt, and overcome. Three of the main challenges experienced in DJ's FPIES journey included food trialing, my anxiety, and the strain on my family dynamics when managing our child with a chronic condition.

Food Trials

Food trialing was a great challenge amidst the management of this syndrome. My little guy would clamp his mouth shut and nestle his head into his high chair during meal time. I mentioned that it was almost like a Pavlovian effect or operant conditioning. DJ had this innate sense that when food was coming, he would get sick. So, he began to refuse food. How did this little 8-month-old know this? Stimuli plus stimulus-induced reaction yielded aversion behaviors. I was so anxious to make sure he was getting nutrients that there was a point among food trials where my husband and I were practically force-feeding DJ. We would hold his little arms down and gently spoon-feed him his trials. I was so distraught about this situation. I wrote to the allergist and dietician via the web-based healthcare portal. In the most professional and compassionate manner, the dietician strongly advised against this. She suggested letting him experience and trust the food again from a tactile and flavor perspective. It was quite a messy week after that conversation with the dietician. We allowed DJ to play with the safe pureed food, smear it on his tray, and play with his own spoon. It was back to the basics which was something I overlooked during the chaos of this syndrome management. Literally, a week later, DJ willingly ate food again. I was amazed. Were we making this possible food aversion worse? I believe we were. He began to trust food again. Was he feeling my stress and anxiety too? Once I relaxed, so did he.

Anxiety

DJ had a few breathing issues at birth which most likely initiated my anxiety. However, once this feeding issue came forth, I could have done well if I had an anxiolytic prescribed twice a day as needed. However, I was too stubborn and was focused on these food trials that I put my own emotional well-being on the side. This experience with DJ created an immense amount of anxiety for me. I am extremely grateful for the support system that my family has provided to me as well as in the management of DJ. My husband allowed me to take the reins of DJ's management. I managed all food trials and appointments and illustrated and implemented all the feeding preparations and schedules. I read every label, prepared everything from scratch, and logged everything DJ ate from day 1 of food trials at 6 months of age all the way through him passing the high-risk foods at 15 months of age. As I illustrated my story in this forum, I was able to refer back to the spreadsheet of food trial and provider consult documentation. Wow, I was pretty organized. My husband would call me crazy. I was anxious and determined to get my kid to eat more foods than just five foods. I am a member of a parent support group and would observe parents discussing that their children only have ten safe foods. I vowed, if it was in my control, to put my own feelings aside and brave through the food trials. I girded my loins and pushed forward. We trialed foods knowing that we have an emergency plan in place. I was on edge. I was tightly wounded. I dreaded each and every day around days 4–7 of food trials. However, I got DJ and myself through it with great support from our family unit. We persevered on.

Family Dynamics

The family dynamic patterns obviously change and adapt to the management of a chronic condition. Day-to-day life changes. Ours changed with the preparation of, shopping for, and oversight of food ingestion, incidence of reaction, stress of the aforementioned, and anxiety of the unknown with each ingestion.

My husband and I work full-time. We thankfully have our aunt to watch our children and was always on board with all of the direction for feeding while we were at work. The day-to-day life changes were substantial. However, we needed to adapt and continue on. Some members of our family thought we were overreacting with the strict routine or food introduction we maintained. This was a source of an argument between my husband and me depending on which side of the family it came from. The older generations of the family did not always understand the management of this disease and often had the mind-set to feed DJ anything. There was a level of frustration that developed with some of our family and friends because people felt we were exaggerating and did not truly understand the disease process. It was not until an accidental exposure to beef recently that had family members really observe the severity and alarm of a reaction with this syndrome. Family dynamics are greatly impacted with this syndrome. Thankfully, our family has adjusted and overcame the challenges. There are still great challenges to having a child with food allergies. The most important mindset I learned to adopt is to keep calm and continue on.

Conclusion

It has been a long 18 months since the first trigger ingestion. DJ now eats everything we eat with the exception of his triggers. We have re-trialed three of the four triggers in an in-office oral food challenge. DJ has outgrown rice, oat, and sweet potato with strict abstinence of each. We have recently had an accidental exposure to beef. We are not completely out of the woods yet. However, there is great light at the end of the tunnel. I no longer prepare special foods for DJ. He eats what we eat. I just do not cook the trigger. At the first FPIES clinic appointment, the dietician told me her goal was to have DJ eat everything we eat. We have met this goal and sustained it for the past 8 months. My husband and I are forever grateful for the amazing care the team has provided.

Back to my food-centric ethnicity-based heritage, my grandfather would say, "When life gives you lemons, make limoncello." I hope to one day make limoncello with some of the great FPIES clinicians and researchers. My goal is to help FPIES families and shape the world of FPIES management through my healthcare knowledge, FPIES child management experience, and future educational preparation.

Key Points/Clinical "Pearls"

- Food allergies present an array of challenges for both parents and children in daily functioning. Management of a chronic condition from a day-to-day perspective is equally as important as long-term goals.
- Continuity of care is critical for a child with a chronic condition who requires management by multiple specialties.
- *To healthcare providers, regardless of the discipline*: Always go back to the basics of your respective training. Take the time to listen to patients and family members, explain medical terminology in simple terms, and address the concerns of patients and families.
- *To families:* It can be challenging to discuss with a provider concerns or questions. Be organized, do your research, write down your questions, and when inquiring do so in a respectful manner. Your healthcare providers are present to help you and want the best for you and your family members.

Reference

1. Merriam-Webster. Merriam-Webster dictionary: definition of food. 2018. Retrieved from: https://www.merriam-webster.com/dictionary/food.

Development of the FPIES Center

16

Terri Faye Brown-Whitehorn, Gayle Diamond, and Amy Dean

In the Beginning

In the mid-1990s, we occasionally saw babies with streaks of blood or mucus in their stools in allergy. Most of the time, these babies were seen by their pediatricians, did well, and thrived. These babies were diagnosed with food protein colitis or food protein allergic proctocolitis [1]. If breastfed, their moms restricted their diets from milk and/or soy; and if babies were formula fed, they did better on extensively hydrolyzed milk formula. If there was an accidental ingestion, streaks of blood or mucus would return. Either way, by a year of age, the majority of these babies outgrew their reaction to milk, and very few developed worsening/persistent symptoms or iron deficiency anemia [2]. If babies were going to be referred to a specialist, they were seen in gastroenterology. If a baby was otherwise thriving, how concerned should one be? Was there anything else that needed to be done? As a parent, seeing blood in your baby's stool is upsetting, and over the course of time, we started seeing babies in allergy. After all, the reactions had to do with "food allergy," and we took care of babies with food allergy. However, these babies' histories were far different from babies with IgE-mediated food allergy who presented immediately to an emergency room following exposure to milk—with hives, swelling, vomiting, and/or respiratory distress. These reactions were not immediate and not IgE mediated. These babies were well even with accidental milk exposure. Allergy

T. F. Brown-Whitehorn (✉)
Division of Allergy and Immunology, University of Pennsylvania, Perelman School of Medicine, Children's Hospital of Philadelphia, Philadelphia, PA, USA
e-mail: brownte@email.chop.edu

G. Diamond
Gastroenterology, Hepatology, and Nutrition, Children's Hospital of Philadelphia, Philadelphia, PA, USA

A. Dean
Department of Clinical Nutrition, Children's Hospital of Philadelphia, Philadelphia, PA, USA

T. F. Brown-Whitehorn, A. Cianferoni (eds.), *Food Protein Induced Enterocolitis (FPIES)*, https://doi.org/10.1007/978-3-030-21229-2_16

testing looking for IgE-mediated sensitivity (either skin testing or lab work) was often performed, but the result was not indicative of what was happening to the patients. The majority of these tests were negative; however, when positive, another layer of complexity was added to these otherwise healthy babies in terms of possibility of immediate reaction and need for epinephrine auto-injectors.

Baby Alice

We then started seeing babies who actually ingested soy or milk and developed delayed-onset severe vomiting with/without diarrhea. Their presentations were different from the babies with IgE-mediated reactions as there was often a 2-hour delay in the onset of vomiting and hives or breathing difficulties were absent. I met Baby Alice, who was a 10.5-month-old healthy breastfed baby girl, with her parents. She had already been regularly ingesting all cereals, fruits, vegetables, and meats. A month earlier, she developed severe vomiting 2 hours after ingestion of cow's milk yogurt. Once she seemed better, she was able to be nursed without sequelae. She had two other episodes of severe vomiting, lethargy, and loose stools following dairy exposure. By the third exposure, her family knew that this was no coincidence; she was having a reaction to dairy. She presented to me with concerns of acute food protein-induced enterocolitis [3, 4]. She was otherwise a very happy and healthy baby. She had not required emergency department (ED) visit so lab work during episodes was not obtained. At times, we have seen elevated white blood cell count with left shift in babies with acute FPIES reactions [3, 4]. There was no reason to perform a food challenge as she had three reactions with the same symptoms. Allergy testing was negative to milk and soy, and her parents were told this was expected as she did not have an immediate IgE-mediated reaction. She had no reactions or symptoms noted when the mom ingested dairy and breastfed, so the mom's diet continued with dairy. As a high percentage of children with acute FPIES to milk have reactions to soy, we recommend to wait to introduce soy until ~15 to 18 months of age [5, 6]. We reviewed the diagnosis of FPIES with her family, gave them an emergency FPIES management plan, and recommended follow-up in 6–12 months (depending on whether she developed reactions to other foods). We also reviewed that she could outgrow these types of reactions, and she returned and tolerated an in-hospital milk challenge at 3 years of age. Although stressful initially, we managed Baby Alice with her pediatrician, and since she was doing so well, she did not need referral to our colleagues in nutrition or gastroenterology.

More and more patients similar to Baby Alice were being referred to the allergy division in the early 2000s. In fact, we noticed that a majority of babies similar to Alice had negative skin prick testing, and we wondered if atopy patch testing to foods would uncover non-IgE-mediated food reactions. We had been using similar testing for eosinophilic esophagitis patients and had some success but did not know about its utility in FPIES [7, 8]. In our initial paper by Fogg et al., we found that atopy patch testing predicted oral food challenge results in 28 of 33 instances:

including 12 negative patch testing yielding negative food challenge results, 16 positive patch testing yielding positive food challenge, and 5 patients with positive patch testing having negative food challenge (tolerated food). In that paper, the majority of children had reactions to milk (13), soy (12), rice (3), oat (3), eggs (1), and wheat (1). There was one child who reacted to three foods (milk, soy, and rice) and another who reacted to two (rice and oat). Unfortunately, the use of atopy patch testing in patients with food protein-induced enterocolitis did not pan out, as we soon had patients with negative atopy patch testing develop severe symptoms to the ingested food(s). Around this time, we noticed more children reacting to foods other than milk and soy and some children having reactions to more than one food.

Baby Jacob

In our institution, the majority of babies had FPIES reactions to milk or soy; however, like our colleagues in other institutions, we began seeing babies presenting following ingestion of solid foods [9, 10]. These babies were made known to us following emergency department visits or hospitalizations. I remember meeting the parents of a baby flown to our institution and hospitalized in our pediatric intensive care unit in hypovolemic shock at 20 weeks of age. Baby Jacob did not seem interested in rice cereal when his parents first tried to introduce it at 16 weeks. His parents then tried giving him applesauce a week later, but he seemed to play with the spoon rather than ingest the food. At 19 weeks of age, he was given a small amount of rice cereal mixed with applesauce. Two hours later, he had profuse, bilious vomiting. He was brought to an outside emergency room and underwent evaluation looking for pyloric stenosis, infection, or brain tumor. He was initially given intravenous fluids (IVF) and antibiotics. He was breastfed exclusively, and after a few days when all cultures and studies were normal/negative, he was discharged home. He was diagnosed with "apple allergy," with recommendation to avoid apples, and was discharged home with an epinephrine auto-injector. At the time, there was no mention of rice avoidance, so at 20 weeks of age, he was given rice cereal again. Two hours later, he had severe vomiting. He was limp, ill-appearing, and hypotensive, at the time of presentation to the outside ED. He was given epinephrine without improvement and IVF. He was flown to our institution and stabilized in our pediatric intensive care unit (PICU). Again, he had a negative infectious evaluation, despite having an elevated white blood cell count and left shift. As he improved and his workup was unrevealing, clinicians and parents wondered about the etiology of his symptoms. Could he have an allergy to rice? His clinical team consulted allergy, and I met him prior to discharge. "Yes, one could be allergic to rice." This confirmed everyone's suspicions. He had acute food protein-induced enterocolitis to rice. Diagnosis then and now relies on history. There would be no additional confirmatory food challenge necessary. Parents were given strict instructions to avoid cereals (rice, oat, and wheat), and the mom would continue breastfeeding. We discussed holding off on direct introduction of milk and soy as well. He was to return to see me in the outpatient allergy clinic, given an emergency letter on food protein-induced enterocolitis management, and we would begin the journey together with his pediatrician. His brave parents slowly introduced several foods at home (fruits, vegetables, and meats/poultry) overtime. As he got older, he underwent food challenges to higher-risk foods and was able to add dairy, soy, and wheat into his diet. As a toddler, he was seen by a registered dietician to ensure adequate nutrition. He did have some feeding difficulties which were managed with the help of our feeding team. He did not have concomitant gastroesophageal reflux, growth concerns, or abnormal stools and did not require consultation in gastroenterology.

Baby Jacob taught us two things about acute FPIES in babies. First, rice is definitely a cause of acute FPIES. Second, the differential diagnosis of acute FPIES is broad. Over the years, we have seen similar babies. Thankfully, the majority do not require hospitalization in an intensive care unit; however, some do present in shock (15%) [4, 11]. The diagnosis, especially after first ingestion of a food, is difficult. Babies do not present to their pediatric or emergency room clinicians with a sign that says "I am having an allergic reaction to a food." As a result, he/she undergoes testing that rules in or out diagnoses that are most severe and life threatening. Evaluations need to be performed, antibiotics given, and tests run. We would never want an emergency room clinician or surgeon to think that a baby had a reaction to rice when in fact the baby had a malrotation and needed surgery. We would not want clinicians to miss meningitis or a brain tumor in a 6-month-old blaming lethargy on sweet potatoes. So, unfortunately, even in 2019, the majority of babies need to have an exposure to a food more than once for the treating clinician to think that reaction is from food (except if there is either a family history of FPIES or a prior reaction to FPIES). We are hopeful that a biomarker or test specific to FPIES will be found to identify acute and chronic FPIES reactions as well as a special "test" to determine causative food(s) in each child. In the meantime, as clinicians, we must listen to their parents/families.

As Dr. William Osler once said, "Listen to your patient, he [she] is telling you the diagnosis" [12].

I also think that Baby Jacob would have benefitted from a multispecialty FPIES clinic. He was referred to, and saw, different subspecialists as deemed necessary. He did well overtime and received the care that he needed. There were no other options at the time. I worked with his family and his pediatrician and, when needed, referred him to a nutritionist and a feeding team specialist. I am and have been comfortable diagnosing FPIES, recommending avoidance, giving an emergency management letter, and recommending food trials. However, once a baby starts/started to have reactions to many foods, nutrition questions, growth concerns, stool changes, gastroesophageal reflux, constipation, or texture/feeding issues, I would have no issue calling a colleague and asking for help. Now, I refer the child to our joint FPIES clinic. I do think that if Baby Jacob was born in 2018, his parents would have been given the opportunity to be seen in the joint FPIES clinic in allergy/nutrition or allergy/gastroenterology and nutrition.

Development of a Center for Pediatric Eosinophilic Disorders

In the mid-2000s, the leaders at our institution recognized the importance of trialing a joint multisubspecialty clinic for eosinophilic esophagitis, a condition in which babies, children, and adolescents develop a variety of symptoms (gastroesophageal reflux, growth concerns, abdominal pain, difficulty swallowing, and/or food impaction) and are managed in allergy, gastroenterology, and nutrition. At the time, no one knew how this would work. Clinicians have different styles. What about the logistics? Would appointments take too long? Would patients and their families like this type of visit? Would there be a benefit? In January 2006, I was privileged to be one of two allergists working in the newly formed Center for Pediatric Eosinophilic Disorders at the Children's Hospital of Philadelphia. Each clinician group needed to figure out how to blend their respective styles. Would they see the child and obtain the history at the same time, or would they see the patient separately and convene at the end? Either way, the child and their parents/caregivers were/are able to see all clinicians at the same visit with one unified plan going forward. Questions could be answered then and there. As a clinician, I saw firsthand the benefit for both the families and the clinicians. We learned the logistics along the way and continue to strive to improve. Over the last 12 years, we have seen that clinic grow from two allergists, two gastroenterologists, and one dietitian to four allergists and four gastroenterologists—from four joint clinics a month to ten joint clinics a month including a transition clinic for adolescents in which an adult gastroenterologist is present to meet the patient and his/her family. This multispecialty program has helped children clinically with eosinophilic esophagitis and eosinophilic gastroenteritis. In addition, basic and translational research has benefitted. Our center is now one of the biggest center in the United States, and our colleagues are some of the world's experts. Questions that were previously asked and needed to be referred to nutritionists or gastroenterologists in the past are now answered immediately.

In the meantime, we continued to see more and more babies/patients with FPIES, and I continued to wonder about developing a joint FPIES clinic. We also met Landon Schultz and his family (see Chap. 14) where we were met with encouragement to start a center and ideas to make it work.

Baby Sarah

I met 6-month-old Baby Sarah and her parents, with concerns of acute FPIES to oat. The mom had removed milk early on from her diet (Sarah seemed a bit fussy with maternal ingestion). Otherwise, she had been thriving on breast milk and growing along the 75th percentile for height and weight. Similar to Baby Jacob, she developed severe vomiting after ingesting oat cereal, necessitating emergency room visit/overnight hospitalization at 5 months of age. Surprisingly, she had tolerated oat cereal in the past, but had not had it for a week prior to the day of reaction. Since no one suspected oat cereal as a culprit, she was given oat again and developed a similar severe reaction (confirming, although not knowingly, a diagnosis of acute

FPIES). I saw her in the allergy clinic, reviewed what we did and did not know about FPIES, gave an emergency management letter, and developed plans of additional food trials. I also recommended holding off on all grains, milk, and soy for Baby Sarah. Since the mom and Sarah were fine with maternal ingestion of grains, these could have been continued. The family was tearful and rightfully concerned, but I promised that overtime we would work together. I also referred the family to a nutritionist. I knew that she was growing well now, but I envisioned we would need guidance overtime. Food trials were slow initially, and by 12 months of age, she had tolerated a few safe foods. At the time, she was still breastfed. Her parents had good questions: Would she be able to transition to a non-dairy milk alternative? Would she need an elemental formula? Should she have a food challenge to milk or wheat? Based on her current limited diet, what nutrients was she missing? I was able to answer some questions and referred her back to our nutritionist. Sarah was seen again at 19 months of age; food trials were a bit slow. Her parents remembered her reaction in the past and were a bit hesitant to rush introduction of additional foods. Trials needed to be held when she was sick with viral illness, and it was winter time. However, she was able to add lamb, coconut, berries, and elemental formula as a supplement to breast milk. She had not had any acute reactions. She was to have in-home challenges to salmon, dark leafy vegetables, and quinoa. Parents were also to schedule in-hospital food challenge to milk and wheat. She developed hives with introduction to eggs at 2 years of age, necessitating carrying an epinephrine auto-injector. Allergy testing at that point was positive to eggs and almond (never ingested but thoughts were to trial it as a milk alternative). She also had GI symptoms with spinach (mild in comparison to oat and was managed at home). By 3 years of age, she had a number of safe foods (mushrooms, salmon, chick peas, chicken, broccoli, cauliflower, sweet potato, potato, avocado, banana, blueberries, raspberries, peaches, grapes, coconut, cucumber, green pepper, corn, tomato, quinoa, and sunflower seeds) along with her elemental formula. She had not yet been scheduled for in-hospital food challenges, but the family was now ready. She lived hours away by car from our institution and would need to arrange hotel stays for the day prior and the day of food challenges. By age 4 years, she had been able to add many foods into her diet (including wheat!), and by 6, she tolerated in-hospital food challenge to oats—and was only avoiding eggs and almonds. She did have viral gastroenteritis at one point in which the family was concerned she was losing a "safe" food, but then her sister developed the same symptoms. All along, Sarah did not have issues with feeding, textures, or food aversions. As long as she was on her "safe" foods, she did not have issues with gastroesophageal reflux, constipation, or abnormal stools. Sarah was co-managed with a nutritionist, but I knew we would have all benefited from a joint FPIES clinic with nutrition.

We learn from patients. Baby Sarah taught me that one could have an acute FPIES reaction early on if there is a break or delay in getting the food. We would have expected Baby Sarah to be fine with oat cereal, but she was not. We also do not know if she would have ultimately developed a more chronic FPIES version if she continued with oat in her diet affecting her growth or GI symptoms or if she would have been fine. What we do know is that a break by a week for her led to symptoms.

I do not think that what happened to Sarah is very common, but I am no longer surprised by similar stories. Sarah also developed an IgE-mediated reaction to a food (egg). Although I do not think that she or other babies with FPIES are at increased risk to develop IgE-mediated reactions to food (time will tell), awareness is key. We know that 8% of children in the United States have IgE-mediated food reactions, so it is not surprising that someone with FPIES would have one too [12].

I enjoy my relationship with Baby Sarah and her parents. They once invited me to go on an all-expense-paid vacation at an exotic location with them as I would be able to keep their daughter safe and treat her if there was a reaction. I remember smiling and laughing at the prospect, but I think deep inside, her parents were a bit serious. Although some of her food trials could have probably been a little earlier, I respected and supported their decisions. In medicine, it has been said (perhaps by Hippocrates): "Cure sometimes, treat often, comfort always" [13].

CHOP FPIES Center: Allergy and Nutrition

Based on patients like Baby Jacob and Baby Sarah and my experience with our EoE clinic, I knew that patients with FPIES would benefit from a joint clinic and that starting first with allergy/nutrition was an appropriate approach. With the knowledge that we would be starting a multispecialty FPIES clinic, we asked a group of parents/caregivers what they would want (Chap. 14). We found that their goals were not unique to FPIES: they wanted an accurate diagnosis, the ability to diagnose and treat other conditions, and improved care coordination/communication between specialists. If the specialists are in the same room at the same time, improved communication was bound to happen. I also believe that these parents/caregivers want to feel heard. Too many times, families tell me that we are the first to listen to their babies' histories. We may not be able to cure the disease and determine future food triggers; but we can listen, examine, and make suggestions based on the most up-to-date knowledge.

I knew that an educated, experienced, and caring dietitian was necessary to make this work. Our goals were as follows:

Ensure nutritionally complete diets for patients and breastfeeding moms.
Decide food trials.
Review the importance of meal time as a social time.
Address feeding questions.
Assess growth and address concerns.
Recommend laboratory assessments.
Refer for feeding therapy.
Review the need for elemental formulas.
Strategize publications based on our experiences.

We would continue referral to gastroenterology, if needed. Amy Dean MPH RD and I started this monthly clinic in May 2014. We saw patients referred to us by other colleagues within our institution (allergy, gastroenterology, nutrition, or feeding team) with the thoughts to expand to outside our institution. Our goal was to see four patients a session with thoughts to expand as deemed necessary. We expected phone calls (and now electronic medical record communication).

Baby Connor

Around the same time I met Baby Sarah, I also met 7-month-old Baby Connor and his parents. He was a former full-term infant whose delivery was quite complicated (the mom had a severe postpartum hemorrhage), and Connor started his life in the neonatal intensive care unit (for a week) receiving respiratory support (CPAP) and antibiotics for presumed sepsis. He developed blood streaks in his stool at 6 weeks of age. He went through a variety of formulas and ultimately tolerated breast milk (the mom avoiding milk and soy). At a few months of age, he had blood in his stool, described as "currant jelly" in appearance, and there were concerns of intussusception. He underwent extensive evaluations and ultimately did not have intussusception. However, he seemed to do best clinically on gut rest. Small food trials led to significant irritability, abdominal pain, and bloody stools. By a year of age, he was on elemental formula and elemental cereal. He was growing well, and unless you knew his medical history, you would not think that there was any issue. There was a team approach to the care of Baby Connor, but his parents would need to see all of us separately (different locations at the time), and we would correspond via email/phone calls. At times, his parents were messengers. At 16 months of age, he was hospitalized with persistent GI symptoms and, ultimately, was diagnosed with *C. difficile*, necessitating infectious disease consultation and ultimately treatment. Throughout, he joined his family in his high chair during meal time eating whatever food was safe at the time. He was learning the social aspects of eating. At 22 months of age, he tolerated broth. By 2.5 years of age, he had a dozen of "safe" foods. Some of his food trials were unsuccessful (he did develop diarrhea and abdominal pain), but he and his family did not give up. He continued to add foods into his diet, and by the time he was in kindergarten, he had an open diet (minus a few foods). During this time period, the mom took a leave from her job to take care of Connor as caring for him was a fulltime job. What would they do if he had a reaction and parents were at work? The family had developed food charts and spreadsheets, and during visits, we would review trying to figure out what food(s) to trial next. Although I am sure that they had times of wanting to give up, they did not. He and his family have taught me a lot about resilience. To this day, I am not sure if we were missing something beyond acute and chronic FPIES, but whatever he had, food seemed to trigger reactions, and overtime he improved. Connor received the care that he needed. His parents made it work. But having worked in the EoE center, I felt like we should be able to offer the same options to families with children with FPIES, the ability for a family to see allergy, nutrition, and gastroenterology specialists at the same time.

CHOP FPIES Center: Allergy, Gastroenterology, and Nutrition

We began to see more and more babies who, like Baby Connor, would benefit from a pediatric gastroenterologist in the room at the same time with allergy and nutrition specialists. We were also receiving referrals from out of state, necessitating coordinating visits with a gastroenterologist. Wouldn't it be best if we had a joint clinic that involved all three subspecialties for those who require it? I met with a lead physician in gastroenterology and was introduced to Dr. Gayle Diamond, a pediatric gastroenterologist, who was relatively new to our institution but had an interest in FPIES and being involved in our joint clinic. Outside of her knowledge in pediatric gastroenterology, she was/is compassionate and willing to learn/work alongside us. Having her opinion from a different lens and being in the visit at the same time would provide patients and caregivers our joint thoughts/recommendations. Dr. Diamond became an integral part of our team: "Inherent in the diagnosis of both acute and chronic FPIES, are gastrointestinal symptoms of vomiting and/or diarrhea. Patients often have multiple GI signs and symptoms, some of which can be attributed to FPIES, but perhaps not all… I see myself as a partner in helping to consider the alternate diagnoses from FPIES for symptoms including: vomiting, reflux, diarrhea, bloody stool, poor growth, and poor eating. These symptoms can occur acutely or persist chronically as patients move through food trials." She also works closely with the team to help order tests which can assess patients' overall nutritional status and evaluate for specific nutritional deficits. In January 2016, this second monthly FPIES clinic was begun with allergy, gastroenterology, and nutrition availability for patients diagnosed with FPIES on a separate day from the FPIES allergy and nutrition clinic.

Referral to the FPIES Clinic

We have a coordinator who works with us to help schedule patients. Over the years, we have expanded: there are two gastroenterologists, three allergists, and two dieticians working together. Patients are referred from within our institution or as a second opinion from an outside institution (either per parent request or clinician request). Records will be sent and reviewed prior to seeing the patient. Based on history and parental request, the child is scheduled in the appropriate clinic. Most patients from outside our tristate region will be seen in the FPIES allergy, gastroenterology, and nutrition clinic.

What Happens in the FPIES Clinic

When a family comes to see us in the FPIES clinic, we have already reviewed records that were available. We still want to hear the history from the parents/child. We are listening for "keywords" or concerns. Although one may have said something to another clinician and it may be redundant, we want to know. We observe the baby/toddler during the visit and then perform our examination. At times, we have had babies with poor growth or severe failure to thrive who underwent additional testing to assess for alternative or concomitant diagnosis. At the extreme, there have been a few times when admission to the hospital has been recommended for further evaluation, although the majority of patients have outpatient evaluations. We assess for very early-onset inflammatory bowel disease/concomitant immunodeficiency, vitamin deficiency, and eosinophilic gastrointestinal disease and, if there are concerns, refer for possible mitochondrial or metabolic disorders. We have recommended lab work (blood and urine), stool studies, radiographic studies, and endoscopies/sigmoidoscopies.

However, the majority of time, we confirm the original diagnosis of FPIES. We address constipation, gastroesophageal reflux, vitamin deficiency, diarrhea, atopic dermatitis, IgE-mediated food allergy, asthma, and allergic rhinitis. We address the nutritional status of the patient (and breastfeeding moms if they are on restricted diets—and, when necessary, we refer to their clinicians). We can screen the child's immune system if needed. Future food trials are recommended, and the locations of those trials are discussed (home or in hospital). We work with families acknowledging that all GI symptoms are not food related (Baby Sarah had gastroenteritis). We review when to push through food trials and when to stop (if there is gray area).

After the child is seen, we then decide an appropriate follow-up. We work with each family to decide what is best for their particular situation. We know that overtime, many of the babies and children outgrow either FPIES or their need for joint clinic. However, we are here if they need us. As Sir William Osler once said: "The good physician treats the disease; the great physician treats the patient who has the disease" [14].

While I personally do not think that every patient with FPIES needs to be seen in a multispecialty clinic, I strongly believe that having one available is important for those who do.

Clinical Pearls

- Our awareness and understanding of FPIES have evolved overtime. We have learned from individual patients and from the combined perspectives of different specialties.
- Including allergy, nutrition, and GI specialists in a team setting can allow coordinated care of the complex needs of children with FPIES and their caregivers.

References

1. Maloney J, Nowak-Wegrzyn A. Educational clinical case series for pediatric allergy and immunology: allergic proctocolitis, food protein-induced enterocolitis syndrome and allergic eosinophilic gastroenteritis with protein losing gastroenteropathy as manifestations of non-IgE mediated cow's milk allergy. Pediatr Allergy Immunol. 2007;18:360–7.

2. Lake AM, Whitington PF, Hamilton SR. Dietary protein-induced colitis in breast fed infants. J Pediatr. 1982;101:906–10.
3. Sicherer SH, Eigenmann PA, Sampson HA. Clinical features of food-protein induced enterocolitis syndrome. J Pediatr. 1998;133:214–9.
4. Nowak-Wegrzyn A, Chehade M, Groetch M, et al. International consensus guidelines for the diagnosis and management of food protein-induced enterocolitis syndrome: executive summary-Workgroup Report of the Adverse Reactions to Foods Committee, American Academy of Allergy, Asthma & Immunology. J Allergy Clin Immunol. 2017;139(4):1111–26.
5. Caubet JC, Ford LS, Sickles L, et al. Clinical features and resolution of food protein induced enterocolitis syndrome: 10 year experience. J Allergy Clin Immunol. 2014;134:183–9.
6. Ruffner MA, Ruymann K, Barni S, et al. Food protein-induced enterocolitis syndrome: insights from review of a large referral population. J Allergy Clin Immunol Pract. 2013;1(4):343–9.
7. Spergel JM, Brown-Whitehorn T, Beausoleil JL, et al. Predictive values for skin prick test and atopy patch test for eosinophilic esophagitis. J Allergy Clin Immunol. 2007;119(2):509–11.
8. Fogg MI, Brown-Whitehorn T, Pawlowski NA, et al. Atopy patch test for the diagnosis of food protein induced enterocolitis syndrome. Pediatr Allergy Immunol. 2006;17(5):351–5.
9. Nowak-Wegrzyn A, Sampson HA, Wood RA, Sicherer SH. Food protein induced enterocolitis syndrome caused by solid food protein. Pediatrics. 2003;111:829–33.
10. Mehr S, Kakakios A, Frith K, Kemp AS. Food protein-induced enterocolitis syndrome: 16-year experience. Pediatrics. 2009;123:e459–64.
11. Tim Andrews T, Tsarouhas N, Spergel J. Food allergy presenting as a "septic"-appearing infant. Pediatr Emerg Care. 2004;20(10):677–9.
12. Gupta RS, Springston EE, Warrier MR, et al. The prevalence, severity, and distribution of childhood food allergy in the United States. Pediatrics. 2011;128(1):e9–17.
13. Shaw Q. On aprhorisms. Br J Gen Pract. 2009:954–5.
14. Centor RM. To be a great physician you must understand the whole story. Med Gen Med. 2007;9(1):59.

Future Needs

17

Antonella Cianferoni and Terri Faye Brown-Whitehorn

When asked to edit a book on food protein-induced enterocolitis syndrome (FPIES), we were excited. There would be a book, focused on FPIES, for clinicians, researchers, students, and families. The book would provide opinions and knowledge of some of the world's experts taking care of patients with FPIES and those taking care of patients without FPIES but similar presentations (metabolic or other GI disorders). This book would also review current knowledge on pathophysiology and future needs. And finally, this book would provide insight from a parent's perspective on life and family, a parent's perspective leading to the development of an international organization, and a clinician's perspective on the development of a tertiary multispecialty center.

In doing so, we have learned a lot. We know much more than we did 20 years ago, even 10 years ago. International guidelines have been written, ICD-10 code developed, and parent groups formed, and clinicians and non-clinicians are working together [1]. There are more and more publications on FPIES. Instead of individual case reports or small series of patients, information is being written about cohorts of >100 patients. We will learn more about these patients over time.

- How many patients truly outgrow FPIES without sequelae or other gastrointestinal conditions? How many continue to have FPIES reactions?
- How many develop eosinophilic esophagitis (EoE) or inflammatory bowel disease?
- Why are adults developing FPIES reactions and who is at risk?

A. Cianferoni · T. F. Brown-Whitehorn (✉)
Division of Allergy and Immunology, University of Pennsylvania, Perelman School of Medicine, Children's Hospital of Philadelphia, Philadelphia, PA, USA
e-mail: brownte@email.chop.edu

T. F. Brown-Whitehorn, A. Cianferoni (eds.), *Food Protein Induced Enterocolitis (FPIES)*, https://doi.org/10.1007/978-3-030-21229-2_17

Many questions still exist and we are excited to learn the answers.

We have divided future needs into five categories: the individual child and family needs, cohort of patient needs, research, education, and development of referral centers.

For an individual with this condition, we need to accurately diagnose and treat the condition with the knowledge that we now have Many clinicians still may not have heard of FPIES, and patients often undergo many reactions before diagnosis and symptoms/relationship with food(s) are recognized. In addition, these patients and families must be referred to nutritionists, feeding therapists, and psychologists (very stressful on caregivers) as the need arises. Keeping in mind differential diagnosis of symptoms is key, and referral to other specialists may be warranted.

One of the major obstacles is that the diagnosis of FPIES is based solely on clinical criteria. As we learn more, we are seeing a variation in both the presentation and the duration of symptoms. It is clear that validation of these clinical criteria is needed. The international community came together to standardize and define FPIES. These guidelines were and remain a huge accomplishment [1]. Now, prospective studies on patients who present with a variety of symptoms can be studied together or separately. Patients may present with acute symptoms, chronic symptoms, atypical symptoms, or a combination. Patients may have symptoms with one food or multiple foods. Reactions may be mild or severe. Treatment will either be oral rehydration and treatment at home (possibly in the hospital) or intravenous fluid boluses and treatment in the hospital. Milder cohorts need to be defined to avoid unnecessary dietary restrictions and locations for safe food introduction compared to more severe cohorts, who may or may not require dietary restrictions, slower food trials, or in-hospital food trials/challenges. Each of these groups must be studied to further understand the long-term clinical implications of FPIES spectrum diagnosis.

At the present time, there are no specific biomarkers that can objectively help with disease diagnosis or identification of food allergy triggers. This is a major obstacle not only for symptom validation but also for in vitro diagnosis of food trigger(s) and individualization of management (personalized medicine). Therefore, development of a specific, ideally noninvasive biomarker(s) that confirms FPIES diagnosis and reaction is urgently needed. This biomarker would be used to correctly diagnose the first episode as well as future episodes and would be used to differentiate symptoms from other causes (i.e., gastroenteritis). We also do not have a test/biomarker that identifies specific trigger food(s) and determines when one has outgrown the reaction. So, as of 2019, patients must ingest the food and have a reaction to confirm diagnosis. In the absence of testing that correctly predicts food sensitivities, frequency, location, and protocols for oral food challenges (OFC) need to be determined, to establish natural history and severity of symptoms in larger population groups, as well as to avoid unnecessary prolonged dietary restrictions. Standardized OFC schedules may also be implemented to systematically address tolerance. Food challenges of less allergenic forms of food allergy triggers such as baked milk or egg (in those with FPIES reactions to milk and egg) are needed to determine if avoidance is necessary and if tolerance accelerates or induces immunotolerance as has been seen in IgE-mediated food allergy [2].

Additional information on patient cohorts is needed As a group of patients, we need more information on who and why one infant/child or adult is more susceptible than another. We also need to know why some children react to multiple foods and others one. Why does one develop chronic FPIES? Acute FPIES? Who is more likely to outgrow FPIES and why? What about family history? Concomitant disorders? We need a way to "block a reaction." In the event there is accidental exposure, most patients will start to react in a few hours. What can be given? In the event of a reaction, the mainstay of treatment is intravenous fluids and supportive care. Ondansetron can be helpful in some [1]. How can we make patients reacting feel better faster? Having validated symptoms and standardized OFC will greatly help to establish homogenous cohorts across centers to gather all the much needed information.

Basic science research on pathophysiology of acute and chronic FPIES reactions are needed Further studies addressing the pathophysiology of this syndrome are desperately needed. As long as the key cell type(s) responsible for antigen recognition, initiation, and progression of the inflammatory cascade is unknown, it will be impossible to move away from the largely empiric management that currently characterizes the global approach to the disease. The role of the innate immune system and the lack of understanding about which cells of the adaptive immune system are responsible for the specific recognition of small antigenic quantities continue to puzzle the scientific community at large.

Results from genetic studies, RNA arrays, metabolomics, microbiome analysis, and transcriptome analysis have improved the understanding and pathophysiology of other non-IgE-mediated food allergy diseases such as eosinophilic esophagitis (EoE) [3]. A similar approach could be used in studying FPIES. Given that FPIES is empirically diagnosed and less clean than the EoE population (where the diagnosis is made based on pathology criteria), larger populations and therefore collaboration between different centers may be needed.

Future needs must also include education of the medical community (from those in training to the most experienced clinicians), daycare providers and schools, and the lay public Not all in the medical community are aware of FPIES as a diagnosis. Special emphasis on students, pediatricians, primary care clinicians, and emergency room clinicians is important. Keeping disorder within the differential is key. Allergists, gastroenterologists, and nutritionists also should have updated information regarding care of patients with FPIES. Daycare providers, schools, and other caregivers who interact with infants and toddlers must be educated on different types of food allergy including FPIES. These children must also avoid food of concern. Accidental exposures lead to delayed severe reactions, and caregivers must recognize and contact families to obtain appropriate care. Outside of those families affected by FPIES, most people have never heard of FPIES. IFPIES is an example of a parent-led organization that has made and will continue to make a difference. Balance of FPIES information and support groups are needed. Many newly diagnosed families seek information on the internet; however, they often encounter information from parents of the most severely affected infants. Our hope is that there is a balance of information on these sites reviewing that most children have one or two affected foods and most will outgrow over time.

Development of referral centers knowledgeable in diagnosis and treatment will help current patients and help promote knowledge by publishing information they learn from patients Many infants and children with FPIES can be cared for by primary care clinician and an allergist knowledgeable in the condition. Tertiary referral centers with multispecialty clinics (gastroenterology, allergy, nutrition +/− psychology) are options for those newly diagnosed with many questions/concerns, those with more severe disease, or those with concomitant disorders. In addition, we anticipate collaboration with other centers for research, biomarker development, and future guidelines.

Clinical Pearls

- Future needs include improved recognition and treatment of FPIES.
- More research is needed to understand the underlying pathophysiology of both acute and chronic FPIES.
- Education needs involve the medical community as well as daycare centers, schools, and the lay public.

References

1. Nowak-Wegrzyn A, Chehade M, Groetch ME, Spergel JM, Wood RA, Allen K, et al. International consensus guidelines for the diagnosis and management of food protein-induced enterocolitis syndrome: executive summary—workgroup report of the Adverse Reactions to Foods Committee, American Academy of Allergy, Asthma & Immunology. J Allergy Clin Immunol. 2017;139:1111–26. PMID 28167094.
2. Upton J, Nowak-Wegrzyn A. The impact of baked egg and baked milk diets on IgE and non-IgE mediated allergy. Clin Rev Allergy Immunol. 2018;55(2):118–38. PMID: 29516263.
3. Ruffner MA, Kennedy K, Cianferoni A. Pathophysiology of eosinophilic esophagitis: recent advances and their clinical implications. Expert Rev Clin Immunol. 2019;15:83–95. PMID: 30394139.

Index

T. F. Brown-Whitehorn, A. Cianferoni (eds.), *Food Protein Induced Enterocolitis (FPIES)*,
https://doi.org/10.1007/978-3-030-21229-2